Medical Statistics from Scratch

Second Edition

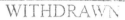

Medical Statistics from Scratch

An Introduction for Health Professionals

Second Edition

David Bowers
Honorary Lecturer, School of Medicine, University of Leeds, UK

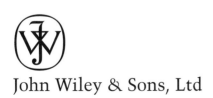

John Wiley & Sons, Ltd

Copyright © 2008   John Wiley & Sons Ltd, The Atrium, Southern Gate, Chichester,
West Sussex PO19 8SQ, England

Telephone   (+44) 1243 779777

Email (for orders and customer service enquiries): cs-books@wiley.co.uk
Visit our Home Page on www.wileyeurope.com or www.wiley.com

Reprinted October 2008, February 2009, October 2010
Reprinted with corrections December 2009

Other Wiley Editorial Offices

John Wiley & Sons Inc., 111 River Street, Hoboken, NJ 07030, USA

Jossey-Bass, 989 Market Street, San Francisco, CA 94103-1741, USA

Wiley-VCH Verlag GmbH, Boschstr. 12, D-69469 Weinheim, Germany

John Wiley & Sons Australia Ltd, 33 Park Road, Milton, Queensland 4064, Australia

John Wiley & Sons (Asia) Pte Ltd, 2 Clementi Loop #02-01, Jin Xing Distripark, Singapore 129809

John Wiley & Sons Canada Ltd, 6045 Freemont Blvd, Mississauga, Ontario, L5R 4J3

Wiley also publishes its books in a variety of electronic formats. Some content that appears in print may not be
available in electronic books.

Library of Congress Cataloging-in-Publication Data

Bowers, David, 1938–
    Medical statistics from scratch : an introduction for health professionals / David Bowers. — 2nd ed.
        p. ; cm.
    Includes bibliographical references and index.
    ISBN 978-0-470-51301-9 (cloth : alk, paper)
1. Medical statistics.   2. Medicine—Research—Statistical methods.   I. Title.
    [DNLM: 1. Biometry.   2. Statistics—methods. WA 950 B786m 2007]
    RA409.B669 2007
    610.72'7—dc22
                                        2007041619

British Library Cataloguing in Publication Data

A catalogue record for this book is available from the British Library

ISBN 978-0-470-51301-9 (P/B)

Typeset in 10/12pt Minion by Aptara Inc., New Delhi, India
Printed and bound in Great Britain by CPI Antony Rowe, Chippenham, Wilts

This book is for Susanne

Contents

Preface to the 2nd Edition

This book is a 'not-too-mathematical' introduction to medical statistics. It should appeal to anyone training or working in the health care arena – whatever their particular discipline – who wants either a simple introduction to the subject, or a gentle reminder of stuff they might have forgotten. I have aimed the book at:

- Students doing a first degree or diploma in clinical and health care courses.

- Students doing post-graduate clinical and health care studies.

- Health care professionals doing professional and membership examinations.

- Health care professionals who want to brush up on some medical statistics generally, or who want a simple reminder of a particular topic.

- Anybody else who wants to know a bit of what medical statistics is about.

The most significant change in this second edition is the addition of two new chapters, one on measuring survival, and one on systematic review and meta-analysis. The ability to understand the principles of survival analysis is important, not least because of its popularity in clinical research, and consequently in the clinical literature. Similarly, the increasing importance of evidence-based clinical practice means that systematic review and meta-analysis also demand a place. In addition, I have taken the opportunity to correct and freshen the text in a few places, as well as adding a small number of new examples. My thanks to Lucy Sayer, my editor at John Wiley, for her enthusiastic support, to Liz Renwick and Robert Hambrook, and all the other wiley people, for their invaluable help and special thanks to my copy-editor Barbara Noble, for her truly excellent work and enthusiasm (of course, any remaining errors are mine).

I am happy to get any comments and criticisms from you. You can e-mail me at: slothist@hotmail.com.

Preface to the 1st Edition

This book is intended to be an introduction to medical statistics but one which is not too mathematical—in fact has the absolute minimum of maths. The exceptions however are Chapters 17 and 18, on linear and logistic regression. It's really impossible to provide material on these procedures without some maths, and I hesitated about including them at all. However they are such useful and widely used techniques, particularly logistic regression and its production of odds ratios, that I felt they must go in. Of course you don't *have* to read them. It should appeal to anyone training or working in the health care arena—whatever their particular discipline—who wants a simple, not-too-technical introduction to the subject. I have aimed the book at:

- students doing either a first degree or diploma in health care-related courses

- students doing postgraduate health care studies

- health care professionals doing professional and membership examinations

- health care professionals who want to brush up on some medical statistics generally, or who want a simple reminder of one particular topic

- anybody else who wants to know a bit of what medical statistics is about.

I intended originally to make this book an amalgam of two previous books of mine, *Statistics from Scratch for Health Care Professionals* and *Statistics Further from Scratch*. However, although it covers a lot of the same material as in those two books, this is in reality a completely new book, with a lot of extra stuff, particularly on linear and logistic regression. I am happy to get any comments and criticisms from you. You can e-mail me at: slothist@hotmail.com.

Introduction

Before the spread of personal computers, researchers had to do most things by hand (by which I mean with a calculator), and so most statistics books were full of equations and their derivations, with many pages of the necessary statistical tables. Analysing anything other than small samples could be time-consuming and error prone. You also needed to be reasonably good at maths. Of course, for the statistics specialist there is still a need for books that deal with statistical theory, and the often complex mathematics which underlies the subject.

However, now that there are computers in most offices and homes, and many professionals have some access to a computer statistics programme, there is room for books which focus more on an understanding of the principal ideas which underlie the statistical procedures, on knowing which approach is the most appropriate, and under what circumstances, and on the interpretation of the outputs from a statistics program.

I have thus tried to keep the technical stuff to a minimum. There are a few equations here and there (most in the last few chapters), but those I have provided are mainly for the purposes of doing some of the exercises. I have also assumed that readers will have a nodding acquaintance of either SPSS or Minitab. Short courses in these programs are now widely available to most clinical staff. I also provide a few examples of outputs from SPSS and Minitab, for the commonest applications, which I hope will help you make sense of any results you get. Both SPSS and Minitab have excellent *Help* facilities, which should answer most of the difficulties you may have.

Remember this is an introductory book. If you want to explore any of the methods I describe in more detail, you can always turn to one of the more comprehensive medical statistics books, such as Altman (1991), or Bland (1995).

I

Some Fundamental Stuff

1

First things first – the nature of data

Learning objectives

When you have finished this chapter, you should be able to:

- Explain the difference between nominal, ordinal, and metric discrete and metric continuous variables.

- Identify the type of a variable.

- Explain the non-numeric nature of ordinal data.

Variables and data

A *variable* is something whose value can *vary*. For example, *age, sex* and *blood type* are variables. *Data* are the values you get when you measure[1] a variable. For example, *32 years* (for the variable *age*), or *female* (for the variable *sex*). I have illustrated the idea in Table 1.1.

---

[1] I am using 'measure' in the broadest sense here. We wouldn't measure the sex or the ethnicity of someone, for example. We would instead usually observe it or ask the person or get the value from a questionnaire. But we would measure their height or their blood pressure. More on this shortly.

Medical Statistics from Scratch, Second Edition   David Bowers
© 2008 John Wiley & Sons, Ltd

Table 1.1   Variables and data

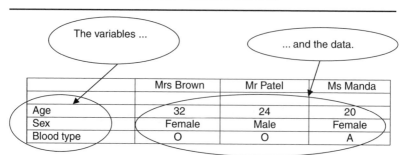

The good, the bad, and the ugly – types of variable

There are two major types of variable – *categorical* variables and *metric*[2] variables. Each of these can be further divided into two sub-types, as shown in Figure 1.1, which also summarises their main characteristics.

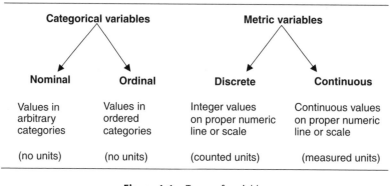

Figure 1.1   Types of variable

Categorical variables

Nominal categorical variables

Consider the variable *blood type*. Let's assume for simplicity that there are only four different blood types: O, A, B, and A/B. Suppose we have a group of 100 patients. We can first determine the blood type of each and then allocate the result to one of the four blood type categories. We might end up with a table like Table 1.2.

---

[2] You will also see metric data referred to as *interval/ratio* data. The computer package SPSS uses the term 'scale' data.

Table 1.2 Blood types of 100 patients (fictitious data)

Blood type	Number of patients (or frequency)
O	65
A	15
B	12
A/B	8

By the way, a table like Table 1.2 is called a *frequency table*, or a *contingency table*. It shows how the number, or frequency, of the different blood types is *distributed* across the four categories. So 65 patients have a blood type O, 15 blood type A, and so on. We'll look at frequency tables in more detail in the next chapter.

The variable 'blood type' is a *nominal categorical* variable. Notice two things about this variable, which is typical of all nominal variables:

- The data do not have any units of measurement.[3]

- The ordering of the categories is completely *arbitrary*. In other words, the categories cannot be ordered in any meaningful way.[4]

In other words we could just as easily write the blood type categories as A/B, B, O, A or B, O, A, A/B, or B, A, A/B, O, or whatever. We can't say that being in any particular category is better, or shorter, or quicker, or longer, than being in any other category.

Exercise 1.1   Suggest a few other nominal variables.

Ordinal categorical variables

Let's now consider another variable some of you may be familiar with – the Glasgow Coma Scale, or GCS for short. As the name suggests, this scale measures the degree of brain injury following head trauma. A patient's Glasgow Coma Scale score is judged by their responsiveness, *as observed* by a clinician, in three areas: eye opening response, verbal response and motor response. The GCS score can vary from 3 (death or severe injury) to 15 (mild or no injury). In other words, there are 13 possible values or categories of brain injury.

Imagine that we determine the Glasgow Coma Scale scores of the last 90 patients admitted to an Emergency Department with head trauma, and we allocate the score of each patient to one of the 13 categories. The results might look like the frequency table shown in Table 1.3.

---

[3] For example, cm, or seconds, or ccs, or kg, etc.
[4] We are excluding trivial arrangements such as alphabetic.

Table 1.3 A frequency table showing the (hypothetical) distribution of 90 Glasgow Coma Scale scores

Glasgow Coma Scale score	Number of patients
3	8
4	1
5	6
6	5
7	5
8	7
9	6
10	8
11	8
12	10
13	12
14	9
15	5

The Glasgow Coma Scale is an *ordinal categorical* variable. Notice two things about this variable, which is typical of all ordinal variables:

• The data do not have any units of measurement (so the same as for nominal variables).

• The ordering of the categories is *not* arbitrary as it was with nominal variables. It *is* now possible to order the categories in a meaningful way.

In other words, we can say that a patient in the category '15' has less brain injury than a patient in category '14'. Similarly, a patient in the category '14' has less brain injury than a patient in category '13', and so on.

However, there is one additional and very important feature of these scores, (or any other set of ordinal scores). Namely, the difference between any pair of adjacent scores is *not necessarily the same* as the difference between any other pair of adjacent scores.

For example, the difference in the degree of brain injury between Glasgow Coma Scale scores of 5 and 6, and scores of 6 and 7, is not necessarily the same. Nor can we say that a patient with a score of say 6 has *exactly* twice the degree of brain injury as a patient with a score of 12. The direct consequence of this is that ordinal data therefore *are not real numbers*. They cannot be placed on the number line.[5] The reason is, of course, that the Glasgow Coma Scale data, and

---

[5] The number line can be visualised as a horizontal line stretching from minus infinity on the left to plus infinity on the right. Any real number, whether negative or positive, decimal or integer (whole number), can be placed somewhere on this line.

the data of most other clinical scales, are *not properly measured* but *assessed* in some way, by the clinician working with the patient.[6] This is a characteristic of all ordinal data.

Because ordinal data are not real numbers, it is not appropriate to apply any of the rules of basic arithmetic to this sort of data. You should not add, subtract, multiply or divide ordinal values. This limitation has marked implications for the sorts of analyses we can do with such data – as you will see later in this book.

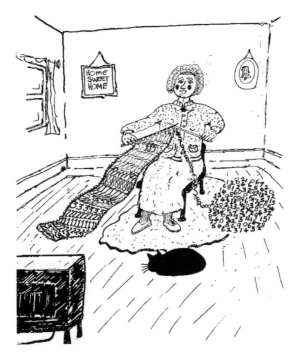

Exercise 1.2 Suggest a few more scales with which you may be familiar from your clinical work.

Exercise 1.3 Explain why it wouldn't really make sense to calculate an average Glasgow Coma Scale for a group of head injury patients.

Metric variables

Continuous metric variables

Look at Table 1.4, which shows the weight in kg (rounded to two decimal places) of six individuals.

---

[6] There are some scales that may involve *some* degree of proper measurement, but these will still produce ordinal values if even one part of the score is determined by a non-measured element.

Table 1.4 The weight of six patients

Patient	Weight (kg)
Ms V. Wood	68.25
Mr P. Green	80.63
Ms S. Lakin	75.00
Mrs B. Noble	71.21
Ms G. Taylor	73.44
Ms J. Taylor	76.98

The variable 'weight' is a *metric continuous* variable. With metric variables, proper measurement *is* possible. For example, if we want to know someone's weight, we can use a weighing machine, we don't have to look at the patient and make a guess (which would be approximate), or ask them how heavy they are (very unreliable). Similarly, if we want to know their diastolic blood pressure we can use a sphygmometer.[7] Guessing, or asking, is not necessary.

Because they can be properly measured, these variables produce data that *are* real numbers, and so can be placed on the number line. Some common examples of metric continuous variables include: birthweight (g), blood pressure (mmHg), blood cholesterol (μg/ml), waiting time (minutes), body mass index (kg/m^2), peak expiry flow (l per min), and so on. Notice that all of these variables have units of measurement attached to them. This is a characteristic of all metric continuous variables.

In contrast to ordinal values, the difference between any pair of adjacent values is exactly the same. The difference between birthweights of 4000 g and 4001 g is the same as the difference between 4001 g and 4002 g, and so on. This property of real numbers is known as the *interval property* (and as we have seen, it's not a property possessed by ordinal values). Moreover, a blood cholesterol score, for example, of 8.4 μg/ml is exactly twice a blood cholesterol of 4.2 μg/ml. This property is known as the *ratio property* (again not shared by ordinal values).[8] In summary:

- Metric continuous variables can be properly *measured* and have units of measurement.

- They produce data that are real numbers (located on the number line).

These properties are in marked contrast to the characteristics of nominal and ordinal variables.

Because metric data values are real numbers, you can apply all of the usual mathematical operations to them. This opens up a much wider range of analytical possibilities than is possible with either nominal or ordinal data – as you will see.

> **Exercise 1.4**   Suggest a few continuous metric variables with which you are familiar. What is the difference between, and consequences of, assessing the value of something and measuring it?

---

[7] We call the device we use to obtain the measured value, e.g. a weighing scale, or a sphygmometer, or tape measure, etc., a *measuring instrument*.

[8] It is for these two reasons that metric data is also known as 'interval/ratio' data – but 'metric' data is shorter!

Table 1.5 The number of times that a group of children with asthma used their inhalers in the past 24 hours

Patient	Number of times inhaler used in past 24 hours
Tim	1
Jane	2
Susie	6
Barbara	6
Peter	7
Gill	8

Discrete metric variables

Consider the data in Table 1.5. This shows the number of times in the past 24 hours that each of six children with asthma used their inhalers.

Continuous metric data usually comes from *measuring*. Discrete metric data, such as that in Table 1.5, usually comes from *counting*. For example, number of deaths, number of pressure sores, number of angina attacks, and so on, are all discrete metric variables. The data produced are real numbers, and are invariably integer (i.e. whole number). They can be placed on the number line, and have the same interval and ratio properties as continuous metric data:

- Metric discrete variables can be properly *counted* and have units of measurement – 'numbers of things'.

- They produce data which are real numbers located on the number line.

Exercise 1.5 Suggest a few discrete metric variables with which you are familiar.

Exercise 1.6 What is the difference between a continuous and a discrete metric variable? Somebody shows you a six-pack egg carton. List (a) the possible number of eggs that the carton could contain; (b) the number of possible values for the weight of the empty carton. What do you conclude?

How can I tell what type of variable I am dealing with?

The easiest way to tell whether data is metric is to check whether it has *units* attached to it, such as: g, mm, °C, $\mu g/cm^3$, *number of* pressure sores, *number of* deaths, and so on. If not, it may be ordinal or nominal – the former if the values can be put in any meaningful order. Figure 1.2 is an aid to variable type recognition.

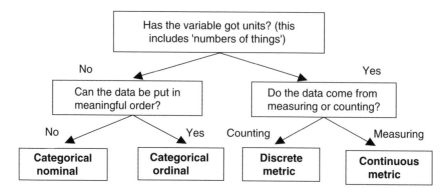

Figure 1.2 An algorithm to help identify variable type

Exercise 1.7 Four migraine patients are asked to assess the severity of their migraine pain one hour after the first symptoms of an attack, by marking a point on a horizontal line, 100 mm long. The line is marked 'No pain', at the left-hand end, and 'Worst possible pain' at the right-hand end. The distance of each patient's mark from the left-hand end is subsequently measured with a mm rule, and their scores are 25 mm, 44 mm, 68 mm and 85 mm. What sort of data is this? Can you calculate the average pain of these four patients? Note that this form of measurement (using a line and getting subjects to mark it) is known as a visual analogue scale (VAS).

Exercise 1.8 Table 1.6 contains the characteristics of cases and controls from a case-control study[9] into stressful life events and breast cancer in women (Protheroe *et al.*1999). Identify the type of each variable in the table.

Exercise 1.9 Table 1.7 is from a cross-section study to determine the incidence of pregnancy-related venous thromboembolic events and their relationship to selected risk factors, such as maternal age, parity, smoking, and so on (Lindqvist *et al.* 1999). Identify the type of each variable in the table.

Exercise 1.10 Table 1.8 is from a study to compare two lotions, Malathion and *d*-phenothrin, in the treatment of head lice (Chosidow *et al.* 1994). In 193 schoolchildren, 95 children were given Malathion and 98 *d*-phenothrin. Identify the type of each variable in the table.

At the end of each chapter you should look again at the learning objectives and satisfy yourself that you have achieved them.

---

[9]Don't worry about the different types of study, I will discuss them in detail in Chapter 6.

Table 1.6 Characteristics of cases and controls from a case-control study into stressful life events and breast cancer in women. Values are mean (SD) unless stated otherwise. Reproduced from *BMJ*, **319**, 1027–30, courtesy of BMJ Publishing Group

Variable	Breast cancer group ($n = 106$)	Control group ($n = 226$)	P value
Age	61.6 (10.9)	51.0 (8.5)	0.000*
Social class[†] (%):			
I	10 (10)	20 (9)	
II	38 (36)	82 (36)	
III non-manual	28 (26)	72 (32)	0.094[‡]
III manual	13 (12)	24 (11)	
IV	11 (10)	21 (9)	
V	3 (3)	2 (1)	
VI	3 (3)	4 (2)	
No of children (%):			
0	15 (14)	31 (14)	
1	16 (15)	31 (13.7)	0.97
2	42 (40)	84 (37)	
≥3	32 (31)[†]	80 (35)	
Age at birth of first child	21.3 (5.6)	20.5 (4.3)	0.500*
Age at menarche	12.8 (1.4)	13.0 (1.6)	0.200*
Menopausal state (%):			
Premenopausal	14 (13)	66 (29)	
Perimenopausal	9 (9)	43 (19)	0.000[§]
Postmenopausal	83 (78)	117 (52)	
Age at menopause	47.7 (4.5)	45.6 (5.2)	0.001*
Lifetime use of oral contraceptives (%)	38	61	0.000[‡]
No of years taking oral contraceptives	3.0 (5.4)	4.2 (5.0)	0.065[§]
No of months breastfeeding	($n = 90$)	($n = 195$)	
	7.4 (9.9)	7.4 (12.1)	0.990*
Lifetime use of hormone replacement therapy (%)	29 (27)	78 (35)	0.193[§]
Mean years of hormone replacement therapy	1.6 (3.7)	1.9 (4.0)	0.460*
Family history of ovarian cancer (%)	8 (8)	10 (4)	0.241[§]
History of benign breast disease (%)	15 (15)	105 (47)	0.000[§]
Family history of breast cancer[¶] (%)	16 (15)	35 (16)	0.997[§]
Units of alcohol/week (%):			
0	38 (36)	59 (26)	
0–4	26 (25)	71 (31)	0.927[‡]
5–9	20 (19)	52 (23)	
≥10	22 (21)	44 (20)	
No of cigarettes/day:			
0	83 (78.3)	170 (75.2)	
1–9	8 (7.6)	14 (6.2)	0.383[‡]
≥10	15 (14.2)	42 (18.6)	
Body mass index (kg/m^2)	26.8 (5.5)	24.8 (4.2)	0.001*

*Two sample t test.
[†]Data for one case missing.
[‡]χ^2 test for trend.
[§]χ^2 test.
[¶]No data for one control.

Table 1.7 Patient characteristics from a cross-section study of thrombotic risk during pregnancy. Reproduced with permission from Elsevier (*Obstetrics and Gynaecology*, 1999, Vol. **94**, pages 595–599.

	Thrombosis cases (n = 608)	Controls (n = 114,940)	OR	95% CI
Maternal age (y) (classification 1)				
≤19	26 (4.3)	2817 (2.5)	1.9	1.3, 2.9
20–24	125 (20.6)	23,006 (20.0)	1.1	0.9, 1.4
25–29	216 (35.5)	44,763 (38.9)	1.0	Reference
30–34	151 (24.8)	30,135 (26.2)	1.0	0.8, 1.3
≥35	90 (14.8)	14,219 (12.4)	1.3	1.0, 1.7
Maternal age (y) (classification 2)				
≤19	26 (4.3)	2817 (2.5)	1.8	1.2, 2.7
20–34	492 (80.9)	97,904 (85.2)	1.0	Reference
≥35	90 (14.8)	14,219 (12.4)	1.3	1.0, 1.6
Parity				
Para 0	304 (50.0)	47,425 (41.3)	1.8	1.5, 2.2
Para 1	142 (23.4)	40,734 (35.4)	1.0	Reference
Para 2	93 (15.3)	18,113 (15.8)	1.5	1.1, 1.9
≥Para 3	69 (11.3)	8429 (7.3)	2.4	1.8, 3.1
Missing data	0 (0)	239 (0.2)		
No. of cigarettes daily				
0	423 (69.6)	87,408 (76.0)	1.0	Reference
1–9	80 (13.2)	14,295 (12.4)	1.2	0.9, 1.5
≥10	57 (9.4)	8177 (7.1)	1.4	1.1, 1.9
Missing data	48 (7.9)	5060 (4.4)		
Multiple pregnancy				
No	593 (97.5)	113,330 (98.6)	1.0	Reference
Yes	15 (2.5)	1610 (1.4)	1.8	1.1, 3.0
Preeclampsia				
No	562 (92.4)	111,788 (97.3)	1.0	Reference
Yes	46 (7.6)	3152 (2.7)	2.9	2.1,3.9
Cesarean delivery				
No	420 (69.1)	102,181 (88.9)	1.0	Reference
Yes	188 (30.9)	12,759 (11.1)	3.6	3.0,4.3

OR = odds ratio; CI = confidence interval.
Data presented as *n* (%).

Table 1.8 Basic characteristics of two groups of children in a study to compare two lotions in the treatment of head lice. One group (95 children) were given Malathion lotion, the second group (98 children), d-phenothrin. Reprinted courtesy of Elsevier (*The Lancet*, 1994, **344**, 1724–26)

Characteristic	Malathion ($n = 95$)	d-phenothrin ($n = 98$)
Age at randomisation (yr)	8.6 (1.6)	8.9 (1.6)
Sex—no of children (%)		
Male	31 (33)	41 (42)
Female	64 (67)	57 (58)
Home no (mean)		
Number of rooms	3.3 (1.2)	3.3 (1.8)
Length of hair—no of children (%)*		
Long	37 (39)	20 (21)
Mid-long	23 (24)	33 (34)
Short	35 (37)	44 (46)
Colour of hair—no of children (%)		
Blond	15 (16)	18 (18)
Brown	49 (52)	55 (56)
Red	4 (4)	4 (4)
Dark	27 (28)	21 (22)
Texture of hair—no of children (%)		
Straight	67 (71)	69 (70)
Curly	19 (20)	25 (26)
Frizzy/kinky	9 (9)	4 (4)
Pruritus—no of children (%)	54 (57)	65 (66)
Excoriations—no of children (%)	25 (26)	39 (40)
Evaluation of infestation		
Live lice-no of children (%)		
0	18 (19)	24 (24)
+	45 (47)	35 (36)
++	9 (9)	15 (15)
+++	12 (13)	15 (15)
++++	11 (12)	9 (9)
Viable nits-no of children (%)*		
0	19 (20)	8 (8)
+	32 (34)	41 (45)
++	22 (23)	24 (25)
+++	18 (19)	20 (21)
++++	4 (4)	4 (4)

The 2 groups were similar at baseline except for a significant difference for the length of hair ($p = 0.02$; chi-square).
*One value missing in the d-phenothrin group.
Baseline characteristics of the *P Humanus capitis*-infested schoolchildren assigned to receive malathion or d-phenothrin lotion*

II

Descriptive Statistics

2

Describing data with tables

Learning objectives

When you have finished this chapter you should be able to:

- Explain what a frequency distribution is.

- Construct a frequency table from raw data.

- Construct relative frequency, cumulative frequency and relative cumulative frequency tables.

- Construct grouped frequency tables.

- Construct a cross-tabulation table.

- Explain what a contingency table is.

- Rank data.

What is descriptive statistics?

The next four chapters of the book are about the processes of *descriptive statistics*. What does this mean? When we first collect data for some project, it will usually be in a 'raw' form. That is, not organised in any way, making it difficult to see what's going on. Descriptive statistics is a series of procedures designed to illuminate the data, so that its principal characteristics and

Medical Statistics from Scratch, Second Edition   David Bowers
© 2008 John Wiley & Sons, Ltd

main features are revealed. This may mean sorting the data by size; perhaps putting it into a table, maybe presenting it in an appropriate chart, or summarising it numerically; and so on.

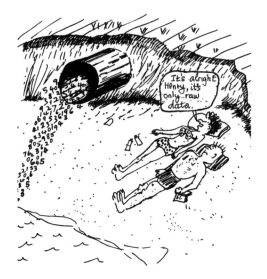

An important consideration in this process is the type of variable concerned. The data from some variables are best described with a table, some with a chart, some, perhaps, with both. With other variables, a numeric summary is more appropriate. In this chapter, I am going to focus on putting the data into an appropriate table. In subsequent chapters, I will look at the use of charts and of numeric summaries.

The frequency table

We'll begin with another look the *frequency table,* which you first encountered in the previous chapter. Let's start with an example using nominal data.

Nominal variables - organising the data into non-ordered categories

In Table 1.8 we had data from the nit lotion study comparing two types of treatment for nits, Malathion or *d-phenothrin*, using a sample of 95 children, and for each child information was collected on nine variables (Chosidow *et al.* 1994). The raw data thus consisted of 95 questionnaires, each containing data on the nine variables, one being the child's hair colour blonde, brown, red and dark.

The resulting *frequency table* for the four colour categories is shown in Table 2.1. As you know, the ordering of nominal categories is arbitrary, and in this example they are shown by the number of children in each – largest first. Notice that total frequency ($n = 95$), is shown at the top of the frequency column. This is helpful to any reader and is good practice. Table 2.1 tells us how the hair colour of each of the 95 children is *distributed* across the four colour categories. In other words, Table 2.1 describes the *frequency distribution* of the variable 'hair colour'.

Table 2.1 Frequency table showing the distribution of hair colour of each of 95 children in a study of Malathion versus *d*-phenothrin for the treatment of nits

Category (hair colour)	Frequency (number of children) $n = 95$
Brown	49
Dark	27
Blonde	15
Red	4

Relative frequency

Often of more use than the actual *number* of subjects in each category are the *percentages*. Tables with this information are called *relative* or *percentage* frequency tables. The third column of Table 2.2 shows the percentage of children in each hair-colour category.

Table 2.2 Relative frequency table, showing the *percentage* of children in each hair-colour category

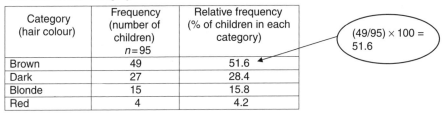

Category (hair colour)	Frequency (number of children) $n=95$	Relative frequency (% of children in each category)
Brown	49	51.6
Dark	27	28.4
Blonde	15	15.8
Red	4	4.2

$(49/95) \times 100 = 51.6$

Exercise 2.1 Table 2.3 shows the frequency distribution for cause of blunt injury to limbs in 75 patients (Rainer *et al.* 2000). Calculate a column of relative frequencies. What percentage of patients had crush injuries?

Table 2.3 Frequency table showing causes of blunt injury to limbs in 75 patients. Reproduced from *BMJ*, **321**, 1247–51, courtesy of BMJ Publishing Group

Cause of injury	Frequency (number of patients) $n = 75$
Falls	46
Crush	20
Motor vehicle crash	6
Other	3

Table 2.4 The frequency distributions for the ordinal variable *'level of satisfaction'*, with nursing care by 475 psychiatric in-patients. Reproduced from *Brit J Nursing*, **3**, 16–17, courtesy of MA Healthcare Limited

Satisfaction with nursing care	Frequency (number of patients) $n = 475$
Very satisfied	121
Satisfied	161
Neutral	90
Dissatisfied	51
Very dissatisfied	52

Ordinal variables – organising the data into ordered categories

When the variable in question is ordinal, we can allocate the data into ordered categories. As an example, Table 2.4 shows the frequency distribution for the variable, *level of satisfaction*, with their psychiatric nursing care, by 475 psychiatric in-patients (Rodgers and Pilgim 1991). The variable has five categories as shown.

'Level of satisfaction' is clearly an ordinal variable. 'Satisfaction' cannot be properly measured, and has no units. But the categories can be meaningfully ordered, as they have been here. The frequency values indicate that more than half of the patients were happy with their psychiatric nursing care, 282 patients ($121 + 161$), out of 475. Much smaller numbers expressed dissatisfaction.

Exercise 2.2   Calculate the relative frequencies for the frequency data in Table 2.4. What percentage of patients were 'very dissatisfied' with their care?

Continuous metric variables – organising the data by value

Organising raw metric *continuous* data into a frequency table is usually impractical, because there are such a large number of possible values. Indeed, there may well be no value that occurs more than once. This means that the corresponding frequency table is likely to have a large, and thus unhelpful, number of rows. Not of much help in uncovering any pattern in the data. The most useful approach with metric continuous data is to *group* them first, and then construct a frequency distribution of the grouped data. Let's see how this works.

Grouping metric continuous data

As an illustration, consider the data in the first two columns of Table 2.5, which shows the birthweight (g) of 30 infants. Birthweight is a metric continuous variable, although it is shown

Table 2.5 Raw data showing a number of characteristics associated with 30 infants, including birthweight (g)

Infant I/D ($n = 30$)	Birthweight (g)	Apgar score[a]	Sex	Mother smoked during pregnancy	Mother's parity
1	3710	8	M	no	1
2	3650	7	F	no	1
3	4490	8	M	no	0
4	3421	6	F	yes	1
5	3399	6	F	no	2
6	4094	9	M	no	3
7	4006	8	M	no	0
8	3287	5	F	yes	5
9	3594	7	F	no	2
10	4206	9	M	no	4
11	3508	7	F	no	0
12	4010	8	M	no	2
13	3896	8	M	no	0
14	3800	8	F	no	0
15	2860	4	M	no	6
16	3798	8	F	no	2
17	3666	7	F	no	0
18	4200	9	M	yes	2
19	3615	7	M	no	1
20	3193	4	F	yes	1
21	2994	5	F	yes	1
22	3266	5	M	yes	1
23	3400	6	F	no	0
24	4090	8	M	no	3
25	3303	6	F	yes	0
26	3447	6	M	yes	1
27	3388	6	F	yes	1
28	3613	7	M	no	1
29	3541	7	M	no	1
30	3886	8	M	yes	1

[a]The Apgar Scale is a measure of the well-being of new-born infants. It can vary between 0 and 10 (low scores bad).

here to the nearest integer value, greater precision not being necessary. Among the 30 infants there are *none* with the same birthweight, and a frequency table with 30 rows and a frequency of 1 in every row would add very little to what you already know from the raw data (apart from telling you what the minimum and maximum birthweights are). One solution is to *group* the data into (if possible) groups of equal width, to produce a *grouped frequency distribution*. This is only be worthwhile, however, if you have enough data values, the 30 here is barely enough, but in practice there will, hopefully, be more.

The resulting grouped frequency table for birthweight is shown in Table 2.6. This gives us a much better idea of the data's main features than did the raw data. For example, you can now

Table 2.6 Grouped frequency distribution for birthweight of 30 infants (data in Table 2.5)

Birthweight (g)	No of infants (frequency) $n = 30$
2700–2999	2
3000–3299	3
3300–3599	9
3600–3899	9
3900–4199	4
4200–4499	3

see that most of the infants had a birthweight around the middle of the range of values, about 3600g, with progressively fewer values above and below this.

Exercise 2.3   The data in Table 2.7 is from a study to ascertain the extent of variation in the case-mix of adult admissions to intensive care units (ICUs) in Britain and Ireland, and its impact on outcomes (Rowan 1993). The table records the percentage mortality in 26 intensive care units. Construct a grouped frequency table of percentage mortality. What do you observe?

Table 2.7   Percentage mortality in 26 intensive care units. Reproduced from *BMJ*, 1992, **307**, 972–981, by permission of BMJ Publishing Group

ICU	1	2	3	4	5	6	7	8	9	10	11	12	13
% mortality	15.2	31.3	14.9	16.3	19.3	18.2	20.2	12.8	14.7	29.4	21.1	20.4	13.6

ICU	14	15	16	17	18	19	20	21	22	23	24	25	26
% mortality	22.4	14.0	14.3	22.8	26.7	18.9	13.7	17.7	27.2	19.3	16.1	13.5	11.2

Open-ended groups

One problem arises when one or two values are a long way from the general mass of the data, either much lower or much higher. These values are called *outliers*. Their presence can mean having lots of empty or near-empty rows at one or both ends of the frequency table. For example, one infant with a birthweight of 6050 g would mean having five empty cells before this value appears. One favoured solution is to use *open-ended* groups. If you define a new last group as ≥ 5000 g, you can record a frequency of 1 in this row,[1] and thus incorporate all of the intervening empty groups into one. As an example, the grouped age distribution at the top of Table 1.7 on p. 12 uses open-ended groups at both ends, i.e. ≤ 19 y, and ≥ 35 y.

---

[1] $\geq$ means greater than or equal to; $\leq$ means less than or equal to.

Table 2.8 Frequency table for discrete metric data
showing number of times that inhaler used in past
24 hours by 53 children with asthma

Number of times inhaler used in past 24 hours	Frequency (number of children) $n = 53$
0	6
1	16
2	12
3	8
4	5
≥ 5	6

Frequency tables with discrete metric variables

Constructing frequency tables for metric *discrete* data is often less of a problem than with continuous metric data, because the number of possible values which the variable can take is often limited (although, if necessary, the data can be grouped in just the same way). As an example, Table 2.8 is a frequency table showing the number of times in the past 24 hours that 53 asthmatic children used their inhaler. We can easily see that most used their inhaler once or twice. Notice the open-ended row showing that six children had used their inhaler five or more times.

Exercise 2.4 The data below are the *parity* (the number of previous live births) of 40 women chosen at random from the 332 women in the stress and breast cancer study referred to in Table 1.6. (a) Construct frequency and relative frequency tables for this parity data. (b) Describe briefly what is revealed about the principal features of parity in these women.

4 0 2 3 2 2 3 3 0 3 1 2 8 3 4 2 1 2 2 2 2 2 3 2
2 3 0 3 2 4 0 1 3 5 1 1 0 3 2 1

Cumulative frequency

The data in Table 2.9 shows the frequency distribution of Glasgow Coma Scale score (GCS) for the last 154 patients admitted to an emergency department with head injury following a road traffic accident (RTA).

Suppose you are asked, 'How many patients had a GCS score of 7 *or less*?'. You could answer this question by looking at Table 2.9 and adding up all of the values in the first five rows. But, if questions like this are likely to come up frequently, it may pay to calculate the *cumulative frequencies*. To do this we successively add, or *cumulate*, the frequency values one by one, starting at the top of the column. The results are shown in the third column of Table 2.10.

Table 2.9 The Glasgow Coma Scale scores of 154 road traffic accident patients

GCS score	Frequency (number of patients) $n = 154$
3	10
4	5
5	6
6	2
7	12
8	15
9	18
10	14
11	15
12	21
13	13
14	17
15	6

The cumulative frequency for each category tells us how many subjects there are in that category, *and* in all the lesser-valued categories in the table. For example, 35 of the total of 154 patients had a GCS score of 7 *or less*.

A cumulative frequency table provides us with a somewhat different view of the data. More-over it allows us to draw a useful chart, as you will see in Chapter 3. Note that although you can legitimately calculate cumulative frequencies for both metric and ordinal data, it makes no sense to do so for nominal data, because of the arbitrary category order.

Exercise 2.5 (a) Add relative and cumulative relative frequency columns to Table 2.10. (b) What percentage of subjects had a GCS score of 10 or less?

Table 2.10 The Glasgow Coma Scale scores of Table 2.9 showing the cumulative frequency values

GCS score	Frequency (number of patients)	Cumulative frequency (cumulative number of patients)
3	10	10
4	5	15
5	6	21
6	2	23
7	12	35
8	15	50
9	18	68
10	14	82
11	15	97
12	21	118
13	13	131
14	17	148
15	6	154

Cumulative frequency is found by adding successive frequencies, i.e. $10 + 5 = 15$ $15 + 6 = 21$, and so on, ...

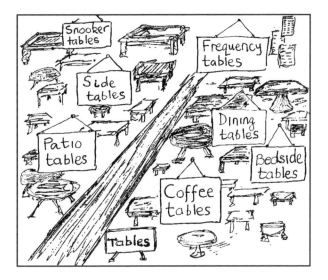

Cross-tabulation

Each of the frequency tables above provides us with a description of the frequency distribution of a *single* variable. Sometimes, however, you will want to examine the association between *two* variables, within a *single* group of individuals. You can do this by putting the data into a table of *cross-tabulations*, where the rows represent the categories of one variable, and the columns represent the categories of a second variable. These tables can provide some insights into *sub-group* structures.[2]

To illustrate the idea, let's return to the 30 infants whose data is recorded in Table 2.5. Suppose you are particularly interested in a possible association between infants whose Apgar score is less than 7 (since this is an indicator for potential problems in the infant's well-being), and whether during pregnancy the mother smoked or not. Notice that we have only one group here, the 30 infants, but two sub-groups, those with an Apgar score of less than 7, and those with a score of 7 or more.

We have two nominal variables each with two categories, and we will thus need a cross-tab table with two rows and two columns, giving us four *cells* in total. We then need to go through the raw data in Table 2.5 and count the number of infants to be allocated to each cell. The final result is shown in Table 2.11.[3]

Obviously Table 2.11 is much more informative than the raw data in Table 2.5. You can see immediately that 11 out of 30 babies had Apgar scores <7, and of these 11 babies, the number with mothers who smoked (8) is almost nearly three times as large as those with non-smoking

---

[2] A 'sub-group' is a smaller identifiable group within the overall group, such as male infants and female infants, among all infants.

[3] We tend to refer to cross-tabulation tables like Table 2.12 as *contingency tables* rather than frequency tables (although they are the same thing). A contingency table represents the *frequency* values for *one* group of individuals, but separated into *sub-groups*, as here for the smoking and non-smoking mothers.

Table 2.11 A cross-tabulation of the variables *'Mother smoked during pregnancy? (Y/N)'* and *'Apgar score <7? (Y/N)'*, for 30 newborn infants (see Table 2.5)

		Apgar < 7	
		Yes	No
Mother smoked?	Yes	8	2
	No	3	17

Table 2.12 The same cross-tabulation as Table 2.11, but with values expressed as percentages of the *column* totals

		Apgar < 7 (%)	
		Yes	No
Mother smoked?	Yes	72.7	10.5
	No	27.3	89.5

mothers (3). More helpful would be a cross-tabulation with *percentage* values, like that in Table 2.12, which shows the data in Table 2.11 expressed as percentages of the *column* totals.[4]

You can see that 72.7 per cent of infants with low Apgar scores had mothers who had smoked, compared to only 27.3 per cent with mothers who hadn't. These results might provoke you into thinking that maybe there's a link of some sort between these two variables. Note that when appropriate you can also express the cross-tabulation with values as percentages of the *row* totals.

Exercise 2.6 The diagnosis (breast lump benign = 0; breast lump malignant = 1), for the same 40 women (in the same order), as in Exercise 2.4, is shown below. (a) Cross-tabulate *diagnosis* against *parity* (with categories, 'two or fewer children', and 'more than two children'). (b) Repeat expressing the values as percentages. (c) Does the cross-tabulation suggest any possible association between diagnosis and parity?

```
0  0  0  0  0  1  0  0  0  0  0  1  1  1  0  0  1  0  0  1  0  0  0  0
0  0  0  1  0  0  0  0  0  1  0  0  0  0  0  0
```

Exercise 2.7 Using data from Table 1.6, the life stress and breast cancer study, construct a suitable 2-by-2 table, in percentage terms, with the columns being *cases* (breast cancer), and *controls* (no breast cancer), and the rows *lifetime use of oral contraceptives, OCP (yes or no)*. Comment on any patterns you can see in the table. Is this a contingency table? Explain your answer.

---

[4] Note that tables with percentage values are not contingency tables.

Ranking data

As you will see later in the book, some statistical techniques require the data to be *ranked,* before any analysis takes place. Ranking means first arranging the data by size, and then giving the largest value a rank of 1, the second largest value a rank of 2, and so on.[5] Any values which are the same, i.e. which are *tied,* are given the average rank. For example, the seven values: 2, 3, 5, 5, 5, 6, 8, could be ranked as: 1, 2, 4 = , 4 = , 4 = , 6, 7, because the three 5 values have the original ranks of 3, 4, 5, the average of which is 4. SPSS and Minitab will both rank data for you if necessary.

---

[5] Or you could give the smallest a rank of 1, the next smallest a rank of 2, and so on.

3

Describing data with charts

Learning objectives

When you have finished this chapter you should be able to:

- Choose the most appropriate chart for a given data type.

- Draw pie charts; and simple, clustered and stacked, bar charts.

- Draw histograms.

- Draw step charts and ogives.

- Draw time series charts.

- Interpret and explain what a chart reveals.

Picture it!

In terms of describing data, of seeing 'what's going on', an appropriate chart is almost always a good idea. What 'appropriate' means depends primarily on the *type* of data, as well as on what particular features of it you want to explore. In addition, if you are writing a report, a chart will always give you an 'impact' factor. Finally, a chart can often be used to illustrate or explain a complex situation for which a form of words or a table might be clumsy, lengthy or otherwise

---

Medical Statistics from Scratch, Second Edition   David Bowers
© 2008 John Wiley & Sons, Ltd

Children receiving Malathion - % by hair colour

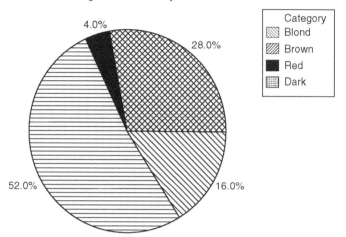

Figure 3.1   Pie chart: children receiving Malathion in nit lotion study, percentage by hair colour. Data in Table 2.1

inadequate. In this chapter I am going to examine some of the commonest charts available for describing data, and indicate which charts are appropriate for each type of data.

Charting nominal and ordinal data

The pie chart

You will all know what a pie chart is, so just a few comments here. Each segment (slice) of a pie chart should be proportional to the frequency of the category it represents. For example, Figure 3.1 is a pie chart of hair colour for the children receiving Malathion in the nit lotion study in Table 2.1. I have chosen to display the percentage values, which are often more helpful. A disadvantage of a pie chart is that it can only represent *one* variable (in Figure 3.1, hair colour). You will therefore need a separate pie chart for each variable you want to chart. Moreover a pie chart can lose clarity if it is used to represent more than four or five categories.

Exercise 3.1   The two pie charts in Figure 3.2 are from a study to investigate the types of stroke in patients with asymptotic internal-carotid-artery stenosis (Inzitari *et al.* 2000). They show the types (in percentages) of disabling and non-disabling ipsilateral strokes, among two categories of patients: those with < 60 per cent stenosis, and those with 60–99 per cent stenosis. What is the most common type of stroke in each of the two categories of stenosis? What is the second most common type?

Exercise 3.2   Sketch a pie chart for the patient satisfaction data in Table 2.4.

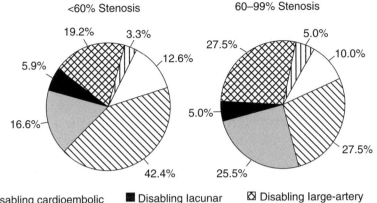

Figure 3.2 Pie charts showing the types (by percentages) of disabling and non-disabling ipsilateral strokes, among two categories of patients, those with < 60 per cent stenosis, and those with 60–99 per cent stenosis. Reproduced from *NEJM*, **342**, 1693–9, by permission of New England Journal of Medicine

The simple bar chart

An alternative to the pie chart for nominal data is the *bar chart*. This is a chart with frequency on the vertical axis and category on the horizontal axis. The *simple bar chart* is appropriate if only one variable is to be shown. Figure 3.3 is a simple bar chart of hair colour for the group of children receiving Malathion in the nit lotion study. Note that the bars should all be the same *width*, and there should be (equal) spaces between bars. These spaces emphasise the categorical nature of the data.

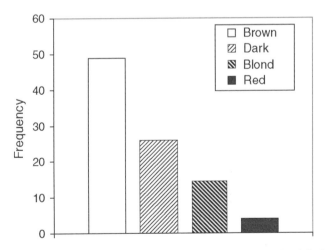

Figure 3.3 Simple bar chart of hair colour of children receiving Malathion in nit lotion study (data in Table 2.1)

Exercise 3.3 Use the data in Table 1.8 to sketch a simple bar chart, showing the hair colour of the children receiving *d*-phenothrin.

Exercise 3.4 Draw a simple bar chart for the patient satisfaction data in Table 2.4. In Exercise 3.2, you drew a pie chart for this data. Which chart do you think works best? Why?

The clustered bar chart

If you have more than one group you can use the *clustered* bar chart. Suppose you also know the *sex* of the children receiving Malathion in the above example. This gives us two sub-groups, boys and girls, with the data shown in Table 3.1.

There are two ways of presenting a clustered bar chart. Figure 3.4 shows one possibility, with hair colour categories on the horizontal axis. This arrangement is helpful if you want to compare the relative sizes of the groups *within each category* (e.g. redheaded boys versus redheaded girls).

Table 3.1 Frequency distribution of hair colour by sex of Malathion children in nit lotion study

Hair colour	Frequency	
	Boys	Girls
Blonde	4	11
Brown	29	20
Red	1	3
Dark	14	13

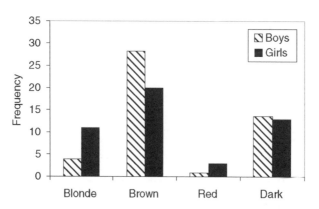

Figure 3.4 Clustered bar chart of hair colour by sex for children in Table 3.1

Alternatively, the chart could have been drawn with the categories *boys* and *girls*, on the horizontal axis. This format would be more useful if you wanted to compare category sizes *within each group*. For example, red haired girls compared to dark haired girls. Which chart is more appropriate depends on what aspect of the data you want to examine.

> **Exercise 3.5** Use the data in Table 3.1 to sketch a clustered percentage bar chart showing the hair colour of children receiving Malathion and *d*-phenothrin. There are two possible formats. Explain why you chose the one you did.

An example from practice

The clustered bar chart in Figure 3.5 is from a study describing the development of the APACHE II scale, used to assess risk of death, and used mainly in ICUs (Knaus *et al.* 1985). APACHE II has a range of 0 (least risk of death) to 71 (greatest risk). Data was available on two groups of patients, one group admitted to ICU for medical emergencies, the second admitted directly to ICU following surgery. The bar chart shows the percentage death rate (vertical axis), against

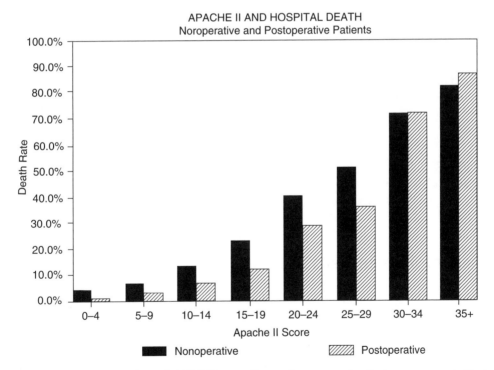

Figure 3.5 Clustered bar chart of APACHE II scores. Data on two groups of patients, one group admitted to ICU for medical emergencies, the second admitted directly to ICU following surgery. The vertical axis is death rate (per cent). Reproduced from *Critical Care Medicine*, **13**, 818–29, courtesy of Lippincott Williams Wilkins

bands of the APACHE II score. Quite clearly, for those less severely ill, percentage mortality among the medical emergency group is noticeably higher than among the post-operative group. For those patients classified as the most severely ill (scores of 35+), the situation is reversed.

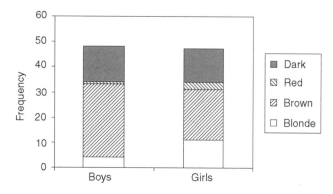

Figure 3.6   A stacked bar chart of hair colour by sex

The stacked bar chart

Figure 3.6 shows a *stacked* bar chart for the same hair colour and sex data shown in Table 3.1. Instead of appearing side by side, as in the clustered bar chart of Figure 3.5, the bars are now stacked on top of each other.[1] Stacked bar charts are appropriate if you want to compare the *total* number of subjects in each group (total number of boys and girls for example), but not so good if you want to compare category sizes *between* groups, e.g. redheaded girls with redheaded boys.

> **Exercise 3.6**   Draw a stacked bar chart showing the same data as in Figure 3.6, but grouped by hair colour (i.e. hair colour on the horizontal axis).

Charting discrete metric data

We can use bar charts to graph discrete metric data in the same way as with ordinal data.[2]

---

[1] We could, alternatively, have used four columns for the four colour categories, with two groups per column (boys and girls). As with the clustered bar chart, the most appropriate arrangement depends on what aspects of the data you want to compare.

[2] In theory we should represent the discrete metric values with vertical lines and not bars, since they are 'point' values, but most common computer statistics packages don't offer this facility.

Number of schools (n=37)

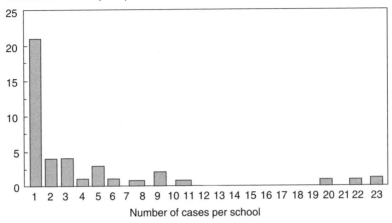

Figure 3.7   Bar chart used to represent discrete metric data on numbers of measles cases in 37 schools. Reproduced from *Amer. J. Epid.*, **146**, 881–2, courtesy of OUP

An example from practice

Figure 3.7 is an example of a bar chart used to present numbers of measles cases (discrete metric data), in 37 schools in Kentucky in a school year (Prevots *et al.* 1997).

> **Exercise 3.7**   What does Figure 3.7 tell you about the distribution of measles cases in these 37 schools?

Charting continuous metric data

The histogram

A continuous metric variable can take a very large number of values, so it is usually impractical to plot them without first grouping the values. The *grouped* data is plotted using a *frequency histogram*, which has frequency plotted on the vertical axis and group size on the horizontal axis.

A histogram looks like a bar chart but without any gaps between adjacent bars. This emphasises the continuous nature of the underlying variable. If the groups in the frequency table are all of the same width, then the bars in the histogram will also all be of the same width.[3] Figure 3.8 shows a histogram of the grouped birthweight data in Table 2.6.

One limitation of the histogram is that it can represent only one variable at a time (like the pie chart), and this can make comparisons between two histograms difficult, because, if you try to plot more than one histogram on the same axes, invariably parts of one chart will overlap the other.

---

[3] But if one group is twice as wide as the others then the frequency must be halved, etc.

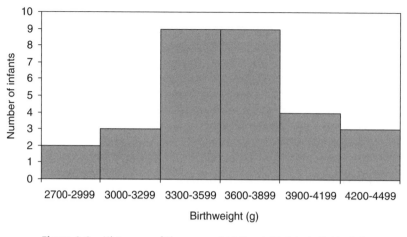

Figure 3.8   Histogram of the grouped birthweight data in Table 2.6

Exercise 3.8   The histogram in Figure 3.9 is from the British Regional Heart Study and shows the serum potassium levels (mmol/l) of 7262 men aged 40–59 *not* receiving treatment for hypertension (Wannamethee *et al.* 1997). Comment on what the histogram reveals about serum potassium levels in this sample of 7262 British men.

Exercise 3.9   The grouped age data in Table 3.2 is from a study to identify predictive factors for suicide, and shows the age distribution by sex of 974 subjects who attempted suicide unsuccessfully, and those among them who were later successful (Nordentoft *et al.* 1993). Sketch separate histograms of percentage age for the *male* attempters and for the later succeeders. Comment on what the charts show.

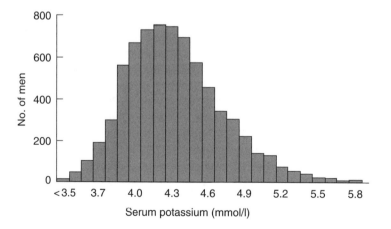

Figure 3.9   Histogram of the serum potassium levels of 7262 British men aged 40–59 years. Reproduced from *Amer. J. Epid.*, **145**, 598–607, courtesy of OUP

Table 3.2 Grouped age data from a follow-up cohort study to identify predictive factors for suicide. Reproduced from *BMJ*, 1993, **306**, 1637–1641, by permission of BMJ Publishing Group

	No (%) attempting suicide		No (%) later successful	
	Men (n = 412)	Women (n = 562)	Men (n = 48)	Women (n = 55)
Age (years)				
15–24	57 (13.8)	80 (14.2)	3 (6.3)	3 (5.5)
25–34	131 (31.8)	132 (23.5)	10 (20.8)	12 (21.8)
35–44	103 (25.0)	146 (26.0)	16 (33.3)	16 (29.1)
45–54	62 (15.0)	90 (16.0)	11 (22.9)	9 (16.4)
55–64	38 (9.2)	58 (10.3)	4 (8.3)	4 (7.3)
65–74	18 (4.4)	43 (7.7)	3 (6.3)	8 (14.5)
75–84	1 (0.2)	11 (2.0)	0	2 (3.6)
>85	2 (0.5)	2 (0.4)	1 (2.1)	1 (1.8)
Living alone	96 (23.3)	85 (15.1)	17 (35.4)	14 (25.5)
Employed	139 (33.7)	185 (32.9)	14 (29.2)	13 (23.6)

Charting cumulative data

The step chart

You can chart *cumulative* ordinal data or cumulative discrete metric data (data for both types of variables are integers) with a *step chart*. In a step chart the total height of each step above the horizontal axis represents the cumulative frequency, up to and including that category or value. The height of each individual step is the frequency of the corresponding category or value.

An example from practice

Figure 3.10 is a step chart of the cumulative rate of suicide (number per 1000 of the population), in 152 Swedish municipalities, taken from a study into the use of calcium channel blockers

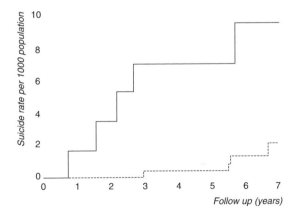

Figure 3.10 A step chart of the cumulative rate of suicide (number per 1000 of the population) in 152 Swedish municipalities. 617 users (continuous line) and 2780 non-users (dotted line). Reproduced from *BMJ*, **316**, 741–5, courtesy of BMJ Publishing Group

(prescribed for hypertension) and the risk of suicide (Lindberg *et al.* 1998). So for example, in year 4 the suicide rate per 1000 of the population was $(7 - 5.2) = 1.8$ (the approximate height of the step). And over the course of the first four years, the suicide rate had risen to seven per thousand. You can produce step charts for numeric ordinal data, such as cumulative Apgar scores in exactly the same way, although not, as far as I am aware, with Word or Excel, or with SPSS or Minitab.

Table 3.3 Cumulative and relative cumulative frequency for the grouped birthweight from the data in Table 2.6

Birthweight (g)	No of infants (frequency)	Cumulative frequency	% cumulative frequency
2700–2999	2	2	6.67
3000–3299	3	5	16.67
3300–3599	9	14	46.67
3600–3899	9	23	76.67
3900–4199	4	27	90.00
4200–4499	3	30	100.00

Exercise 3.10 Draw a step chart for the percentage cumulative Apgar scores in Table 3.3.

The cumulative frequency curve or ogive

With *continuous* metric data, there is assumed to be a smooth *continuum* of values, so you can chart cumulative frequency with a correspondingly smooth curve, known as a *cumulative frequency curve*, or *ogive*.[4] If you add columns for cumulative and relative cumulative frequency to the grouped birthweight data in Table 2.6, you get Table 3.3.

If you want to draw an ogive by hand, you plot, for each group or class, the group cumulative frequency value against the *lower* limit of the next *higher* group. So, for example, 16.67 is plotted against 3300, 46.67 against 3600, and so on. The points should be joined with a smooth curve.[5] The result is shown in Figure 3.11. Notice that I have put a percentage cumulative frequency of zero in the imaginary group 2400–2699 g. This enables me to close the ogive at the left-hand end.

The ogive can be very useful if you want to estimate the cumulative frequency for any value on the horizontal axis, which is not one of the original group values. For example, suppose you want to know what percentage of infants had a birthweight of 3750 g or less. By drawing a line vertically upwards from a value of 3750 g on the horizontal axis to the ogive, and then horizontally to the vertical axis, you can see that about 63 per cent of the infants weighed 3750 g or less. You can of course ask such questions in reverse, for example, what birthweight marks the lowest 50 per cent of birthweights? This time you would start with a value of 50 per cent

---

[4] The 'g' in ogive is pronounced as the j in 'jive'.
[5] Unfortunately, I couldn't find a program that would allow me to join the points with a smooth curve.

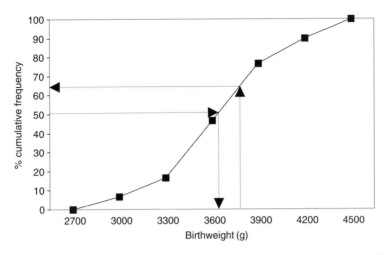

Figure 3.11   The relative cumulative frequency curve (or ogive) for the percentage cumulative birth-weight data in Table 3.3

on the vertical axis, move right to the ogive, then down to the value of about 3700 g on the horizontal axis.

An example from practice

Figure 3.12 shows two per cent ogives for total cholesterol concentration in two groups taken from a study into the effectiveness of health checks conducted by nurses in primary care (Imperial Cancer Fund OXCHECK Study Group 1995)

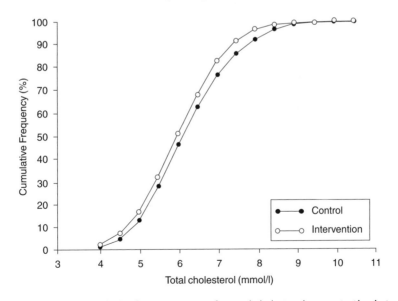

Figure 3.12   Percentage cumulative frequency curves for total cholesterol concentration in two groups. Reproduced from *BMJ*, **310**, 1099–104, courtesy of BMJ

Exercise 3.11 (a) Comment on what Figure 3.12 reveals about the cholesterol levels in the two groups. (b) Sketch percentage cumulative frequency curves for the age of the male suicide attempters and later succeeders, shown in Table 3.2. For each of the two groups, half of the subjects are older than what age?

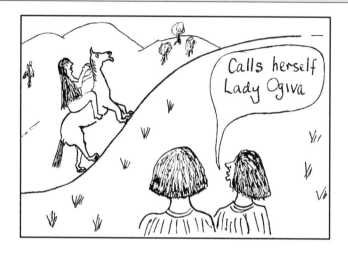

Charting time-based data – the time series chart

If the data you have collected are from measurements made at regular intervals of time (minutes, weeks, years, etc.), you can present the data with a *time series chart*. Usually these charts are used with metric data, but may also be appropriate for ordinal data. Time is always plotted on the horizontal axis, and data values on the vertical axis.

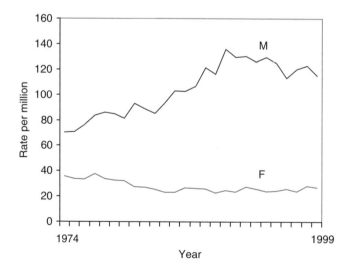

Figure 3.13 Suicide rates for males and females aged 15–29 years in England and Wales

Table 3.4 Choosing an appropriate chart

Data type	Pie chart	Bar chart	Histogram (if grouped)	Step chart	Ogive
Nominal	yes	yes	no	no	no
Ordinal	no	yes	no	yes (cumulative)	no
Metric discrete	no	yes	yes	yes (cumulative)	yes (cumulative)
Metric continuous	no	no	yes	no	yes (cumulative)

An example from practice

Figure 3.13 shows the suicide rates (number of suicides per one million of population), for males and females aged 15–29 years in England and Wales, between 1974 and 1999. The contrasting patterns in the male/female rates are noticeable, more perhaps in this chart form than if shown in a table.

There is one other useful chart, the *boxplot*, but that will have to wait until we meet some new ideas in the next two chapters. Meanwhile Table 3.4 may help you to decide on the most appropriate chart for any given set of data.

4

Describing data from its shape

Learning objectives

When you have finished this chapter you should be able to:

- Explain what is meant by the 'shape' of a frequency distribution.

- Sketch and explain: negatively skewed, symmetric and positively skewed distributions.

- Sketch and explain a bimodal distribution.

- Describe the approximate shape of a frequency distribution from a frequency table or chart.

- Sketch and describe a Normal distribution.

The shape of things to come

I have said previously that the choice of the most appropriate procedures for summarising and analysing data will depend on the type of variable involved. Variable type is the most important consideration. In addition, however, the way the data are distributed – the *shape of the distribution*, can also be influential. By 'shape' I mean:

- Are the values fairly evenly spread throughout their possible range? This is a *uniform* distribution.

- Are most of the values concentrated towards the bottom of the range, with progressively fewer values towards the top of the range? This is a *right or positively skewed* distribution...

- ... or towards the top of the range, with progressively fewer values towards the bottom of the range? This is a *left or negatively skewed* distribution.

- Do most of the values clump together around *one* particular value, with progressively fewer values both below and above this value? This is a *symmetric* or *mound-shaped* distribution.

- Do most of the values clump around *two* or more particular values? This is a *bimodal* or multimodal distribution.

One simple way to assess the shape of a frequency distribution is to plot a bar chart, or a histogram. Here are some examples of the shapes described above.

Negative skew[1]

Figure 4.1 shows age distribution of 2454 patients with acute pulmonary embolism and is drawn from 52 hospitals in seven countries (Goldhaber *et al.* 1999). You can see that most values lie towards the top end of the range, with progressively fewer lower values. This distribution is *negatively skewed.*

> **Exercise 4.1** In Figure 4.1, which age group has: (a) the highest number of patients? (b) the lowest number?

Positive skew

The histogram in Figure 4.2 shows serum E_2 levels from a study of hormone replacement therapy for osteoporosis prevention (Rodgers and Miller 1999). This distribution has most of its values in the lower end of the range with progressively fewer towards the upper end. There is a single high valued *outlier*. This distribution is *positively skewed.*

> **Exercise 4.2** In Figure 4.2, if the outlier was removed, would the distribution be less or more skewed?

---

[1] *Skewness* is the primary measure used to describe the asymmetry of frequency distributions, and many computer programs will calculate a skewness *coefficient* for you. This can vary between −1 (strong negative skew), and +1 (strong positive skew). Values of zero or close to it, indicate lower levels of skew, but do *not* necessarily mean that the distribution is symmetric.

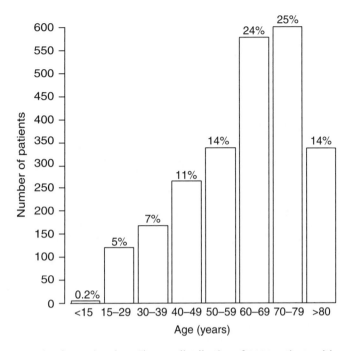

Figure 4.1 An example of negative skew. The age distribution of 2454 patients with acute pulmonary embolism. Reproduced with permission from Elsevier (*The Lancet*, 1999, Vol No. **353**, pp. 1386–9)

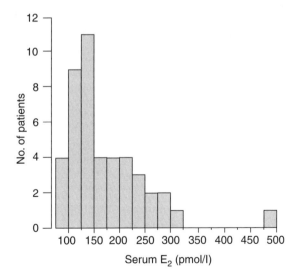

Figure 4.2 An example of positive skew. Serum E2 levels in 45 patients in a study of HRT for the prevention of osteoporosis. Reproduced with permission of the *British Journal of General Practice* (1997, Vol. **47**, pages 161–165)

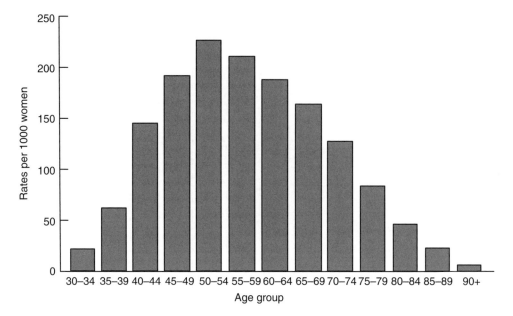

Figure 4.3   Histogram of mammography utilisations rate (per 1000 women), by broad age group, in 33 health districts in Ontario. Reproduced from *J. Epid. Comm. Health*, **51**, 378–82, courtesy of BMJ Publishing Group

Symmetric or mound-shaped distributions

The bar chart in Figure 4.3 is from a study into the use of the mammography service by women in the 33 health districts of Ontario, from mid-1990 to end-1991 (Goel *et al.* 1997). It shows the variation in the utilisation rates[2] by women for a number of age groups. You can see that the distribution is reasonably symmetric and mound shaped, and has only one peak.

Exercise 4.3   (a) What sort of skew is exhibited by the Apache scores in Figure 3.5? (b) The simple bar chart in Figure 4.4 is from a study describing the development of a new scale to measure psychiatric anxiety, called the Psychiatric Symptom Frequency scale (PSF) (Lindelow *et al.*), Describe the shape of the distribution of PSF in terms of symmetry, skewness, etc. Does this chart tell the whole story?

Exercise 4.4   Comment on the shapes of the age distributions shown in Table 3.2, for male and female suicide attempters, and later succeeders (you may also want to look at the histograms you drew in Exercise 3.9).

---

[2] The utilisation rate is the number of consultations per 1000 women.

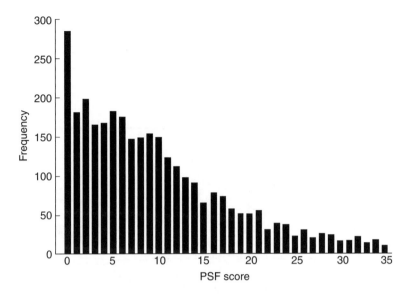

Figure 4.4 Simple bar chart showing the lowest 95 per cent of values of the Psychiatric Symptom Frequency scale. Reproduced from *J. Epid. Comm. Health*, **51**, 549–57, courtesy of BMJ Publishing Group

Bimodal distributions

A bimodal distribution is one with two distinct humps. These are less common than the shapes described above, and are sometimes the result of two separate distributions, which have not been disentangled. Figure 4.5 shows a hypothetical bimodal distribution of systolic blood pressure. The upper peak could be due to a sub-group of hypertensive patients, but whose presence in the group has not been separately identified.

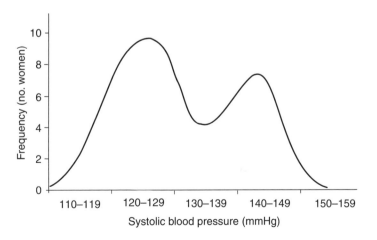

Figure 4.5 A bimodal frequency distribution

Normal-ness

There is one particular symmetric bell-shaped distribution, known as the *Normal distribution*, which has a special place in the heart of statisticians.[3] Many human clinical features are distributed Normally, and the Normal distribution has a very important role to play in what is to come later in this book.

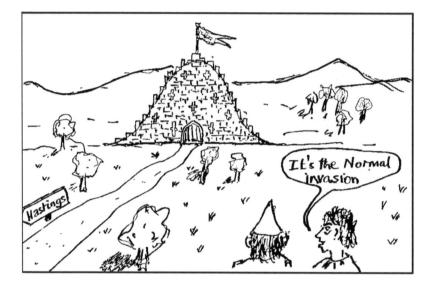

An example from practice

Figure 4.6 shows a histogram for the distribution of the cord platelet count (10^9/l), in 4382 Finnish infants, from a study of the prevalence and causes of thrombocytopenia[4] in full-term infants (Sainio *et al.* 2000). You can see, even without the help of the Normal curve superimposed upon it, that the distribution has a very regular bell-shaped symmetric distribution – in fact is pretty well as Normal as it gets with real data.

Although the Normal distribution is one of the most important in a health context, you may also encounter the *binomial* and *Poisson* distributions. As an example of the former, suppose you need to choose a sample of 20 patients from a very large list of patients, which contains *equal* numbers of males and females. The chance of choosing a male patient is thus 1 in 2. Provided that the probability of picking a male patient each time remains fixed at 1 in 2, the binomial equation will tell you the probability of getting any given number of males (or females), in your 20 selected patients. For example, the probability of getting eight males in a sample of 20 patients is 0.1201 – about 12 chances in a 100.

---

[3] Note the capitalised, 'N', to distinguish this statistical usage from that of the word 'normal' meaning usual, ordinary, etc.

[4] Thrombocytopenia is deemed to exist when the cord platelet count is less than 150×10^9/l. It is a risk factor for intraventricular haemorrhage and contributes to the high neurological morbidity in infants affected.

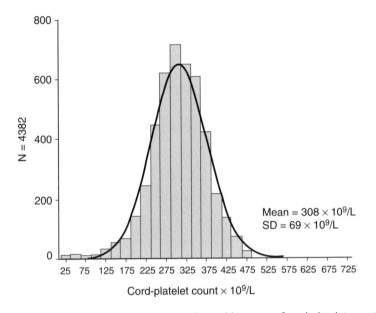

Figure 4.6 A Normal frequency curve superimposed on a histogram of cord platelet count (10^9/l) in 4382 infants. Reproduced from *Obstetrics and Gynecology*, **95**, 441–4, courtesy of Lippincott Williams Wilkins

The Poisson distribution is appropriate for calculating chance or probability when events occur in a seemingly random and unpredictable fashion. It describes the probability of a given number of events occurring in a fixed period of time. For example, suppose that the average number of children with burns arriving at an Emergency Department in any given 24-hour period is 12. Then the Poisson equation indicates that the probability of one child with burns arriving in the next hour is 30 in 100, the probability of two is about 7 in a 100.

To sum up so far. You have seen that you can describe the principal features of a set of data using tables and charts. A description of the shape of the distribution is also an important part of the picture. In the next chapter you will meet a way of describing data using *numeric summary values*.

5

Describing data with numeric summary values

Learning objectives

When you have finished this chapter, you should be able to:

- Explain what prevalence and incidence are.

- Explain what a summary measure of location is, and show that you understand the meaning of, and the difference between, the mode, the median and the mean.

- Be able to calculate the mode, median and mean for a set of values.

- Demonstrate that you understand the role of data type and distributional shape in choosing the most appropriate measure of location.

- Explain what a percentile is, and calculate any given percentile value.

- Explain what a summary measure of spread is, and show that you understand the difference between, and can calculate, the range, the interquartile range and the standard deviation.

- Show that you can estimate percentile values from an ogive.

- Demonstrate that you understand the role of data type and distributional shape in choosing the most appropriate measure of spread.

Medical Statistics from Scratch, Second Edition   David Bowers
© 2008 John Wiley & Sons, Ltd

- Draw a boxplot and explain how it works.

- Show that you understand the area properties of the Normal distribution, and how these relate to standard deviation.

Numbers R us

As you saw in the previous two chapters, we can 'describe' a mass of raw data by charting it, or arranging it in table form. In addition, we can examine its shape. These procedures will help us to make some sense of what initially might be a confusing picture, and hopefully to see patterns in the data. As you are about to see, however, it is often more useful to summarise the data *numerically*. There are two principal features of a set of data that can be summarised with a single numeric value:

- First, a value around which the data has a tendency to congregate or cluster. This is called a *summary measure of location*.[1]

- Second, a value which measures the degree to which the data are, or are not, spread out, called a *summary measure of spread or dispersion*.

With these two summary values you can then compare different sets of data *quantitatively*. Before I discuss these two measures, however, I want to look first at a number of simpler numeric summary measures.

Numbers, percentages and proportions

When you present the results of an investigation, you will almost certainly need to give the *numbers* of the subjects involved; and perhaps also provide values for *percentages*. In Table 1.6, the authors give the percentage of subjects who are in each 'social class' category. For example, 26 per cent, i.e. $(28/106) \times 100$, and 32 per cent, i.e. $(72/226) \times 100$, of the cases and controls respectively, are in the category, 'III non-manual'. As in this example, it is usually categorical data that are summarised with a value for percentage or proportion.

> **Exercise 5.1**   The data in Table 5.1 are taken from a study of duration of breast feeding and arterial distensibility leading to cardiovascular disease (Leeson *et al.* 2001). The table describes the basic characteristics of two groups, 149 subjects who were breast-fed as infants, and 182 who were bottle-fed. Using the values in the first row of the table in Table 3.2, calculate both the proportion and the percentage of men, among those subjects who were: (a) breastfed; (b) bottle-fed.

---

[1] Also known as measures of central tendency.

Table 5.1 Basic characteristics of two groups of individuals, breast-fed and bottle fed, from a study of duration of breast feeding and arterial distensibility leading to cardiovascular disease. Reproduced from *BMJ*, **322**, 643–7, courtesy of BMJ Publishing Group

Variable	Breast fed	Bottle fed	P value for difference between groups
No of participants (men/women)	149 (67/82)	182 (93/89)	—
Age (years)	23 (20 to 28)	23 (20 to 27)	0.07
Height (cm)	170 (10)	168 (9)	0.03
Weight (kg)	70.4 (14.5)	68.7 (13.1)	0.28
Body mass index (kg/m^2)	24.2 (4.1)	24.3 (3.7)	0.83
Length of breast feeding (months)	3.33 (0 to 18)	—	—
Resting arterial diameter (mm)	3.32 (0.59)	3.28 (0.59)	0.45
Distensibility coefficient (mm/Hg^{-1})	0.133 (0.07)	0.140 (0.08)	0.38
Cholesterol (mmol/l)	4.43 (0.99)	4.61 (1.01)	0.11
LDL cholesterol (mmol/l)	2.71 (0.88)	2.90 (0.93)	0.07
HDL cholesterol (mmol/l)	1.18 (0.25)	1.18 (0.31)	0.96
Systolic blood pressure (mm Hg)	128 (14)	128 (14)	0.93
Diastolic blood pressure (mm Hg)	70 (9)	71 (8)	0.31
Smoking history (No (%)):			
Smokers	49 (33)	64 (35)	
Former smokers	25 (17)	22 (12)	0.78
Non-smokers	75 (50)	96 (53)	
No (%) in social class:			
I	12 (8)	13 (7)	
II	36 (24)	33 (18)	
IIINM	51 (34)	62 (34)	
IIIM	24 (16)	36 (20)	0.19
IV	22 (15)	33 (18)	
V	4 (3)	5 (3)	

LDL = Low density lipoprotein, HDL = High density lipoprotein.

Prevalence and the incidence rate

If appropriate we can also summarise data by providing a value for the *prevalence* or the *incidence rate* of some condition. The *point prevalence* of a disease is the number of *existing* cases in some population at a given time. In practice, the *period prevalence* is more often used. We might typically report it as, 'the prevalence of genital chlamydia in single women in England in 1996 was 3.1 per cent'. The prevalence figure will include existing cases, i.e. those who contracted the disease before 1996, and still had it, *as well as* those first getting the disease in 1996. The *incidence* or inception rate of a disease is the number of *new* cases occurring per 1000, or per 10 000, of the population,[2] during some period, usually 12 months.

---

[2] Or whatever base is arithmetically appropriate.

Exercise 5.2 (a) When a group of 890 women was tested for genital chlamydia with a ligase chain reaction test, 23 of the women had a positive response. Assuming the test is always 100 per cent efficient, what is the prevalence of genital chlamydia among women in this group? (b) Suppose in a certain city that there were 10 000 live births in 2002. Ten of the infants died of sudden infant death syndrome. What is the incidence rate for sudden infant death syndrome in this city?

Summary measures of location

A summary measure of location is a value around which most of the data values tend to congregate or centre. I am going to discuss three measures of location: the mode; the median; and the mean. As you will see, the choice of the most appropriate measure depends crucially on the type of data involved. I will summarise which measure(s) you can most appropriately use with which type of data, later in the chapter

The mode

The *mode* is that category or value in the data that has the highest frequency (i.e. occurs the most often). In this sense, the mode is a measure of *common-ness* or *typical-ness*. As an example, the modal Apgar score in Table 2.5 is 8, this being the category with the highest frequency (of 9 infants), i.e. is the most commonly occurring. The mode is not particularly useful with metric continuous data where no two values may be the same. The other shortcoming of this measure is that there may be more than one mode in a set of data.

Exercise 5.3 Determine the modal category for: (a) Social class for both cases and controls, in the stress and breast cancer study shown in Table 1.6. (b) The level of satisfaction with nursing care, from the data in Table 2.4. (c) The PSF score in Figure 4.4.

Exercise 5.4 What is the modal cause of injury in Table 2.3?

The median

If we arrange the data in ascending order of size, the *median* is the middle value. Thus, half of the values will be equal to or less than the median value, and half equal to or above it. The median is thus a measure of *central-ness*. As an example of the calculation of the median, suppose you had the following data on age (in ascending order of years), for five individuals: 30 31 **32** 33 35. The middle value is 32, so the median age for these five people is 32 years. If you have an *even* number of values, the median is the average of the two values either side of the 'middle'.

An advantage of the median is that it is not much affected by skewness in the distribution, or by the presence of outliers. However, it discards a lot of information, because it ignores most of the values, apart from those in the centre of the distribution.

There is another, quite easy way, of determining the value of the median, which will also come in useful a bit later on. If you have n values arranged in ascending order, then:

$$\text{the median} = \tfrac{1}{2}(n+1)^{\text{th}} \text{ value.}$$

So, for example, if the ages of six people are: 30 31 32 33 35 36, then $n = 6$, therefore:

$$\tfrac{1}{2}(n+1) = \tfrac{1}{2} \times (6+1) = \tfrac{1}{2} \times 7 = 3.5.$$

Therefore the median is the 3.5th value. That is, it is the value half way between the 3rd value of 32, and the 4th value of 33, or 32.5 years, which is the same result as before.

Exercise 5.5   (a) Determine the median percentage mortality of the 26 ICUs in Table 2.7 (see also Exercise 2.3). (b) From the data in Table 3.2, determine which age group contains the median age for (i) men, and (ii) women, both for those attempting suicide, and for later successful suicides.

The mean

The mean, or the *arithmetic mean* to give it its full name, is more commonly known as the average. One advantage of the mean over the median is that it uses all of the information in the data set. However, it is affected by skewness in the distribution, and by the presence of outliers in the data. This may, on occasion, produce a mean that is not very representative of the general mass of the data. Moreover, it cannot be used with ordinal data (recall from Chapter 1 that ordinal data are not real numbers, so they cannot be added or divided).

Exercise 5.6   Comment on the likely relative sizes of the mean and median in the distributions of (a) serum potassium and (b) serum E_2, shown in the histograms in Figure 3.9 and Figure 4.2.

Exercise 5.7   Determine the mean percentage mortality in the 26 ICUs in Table 2.7, and compare with the median value you determined in Exercise 5.5(a).

Exercise 5.8   The histogram of red blood cell thioguanine nucleotide concentration (RBCTNC), in *pmol/8 × 10^8 red blood cells,* in 49 children, shown in Figure 5.1, is from a study into the potential causes of high incidence of secondary brain tumours in children after radiotherapy (Relling *et al.* 1999). (a) Using the information in the figure, calculate median and mean RBCTNC for the 49 children. (b) Remove the two outlier values of 3300, and re-calculate the mean and median. Compare and comment on the two sets of results.

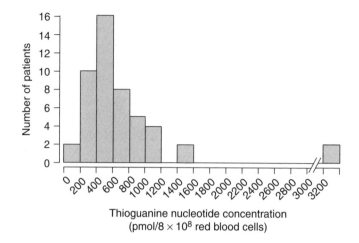

Figure 5.1   Histogram of red blood cell thioguanine nucleotide concentration (RBCTNC), in *pmol/8 ×* 10^8 *red blood cells,* in 49 children. Reprinted courtesy of Elsevier (*The Lancet* 2002, **354**, 34–9)

Percentiles

Percentiles are the values which divide an ordered set of data into 100 equal-sized groups. As an illustration, suppose you have birthweights for 1200 infants, which you've put in ascending order. If you identify the birthweight that has 1 per cent (i.e. 12) of the birthweight values below it, and 99 per cent (1188) above it, then this value is the *1st percentile*. Similarly, the birthweight which has 2 per cent of the birthweight values below it, and 98 per cent above it is the 2nd percentile. You could repeat this process until you reached the 99th percentile, which would have 99 per cent (1188) of birthweight values below it and only 1 per cent above. Notice that this makes the median the *50th percentile*, since it divides the data values into two equal halves, 50 per cent above the median and 50 per cent below.

Calculating a percentile value

How do you determine any particular percentile value? Take the example of the 30 birthweights in Table 2.5, which we reproduce below, but now in ascending order, along with their position in the order:

2860	2994	3193	3266	3287	3303	3388	3399	3400	3421	3447	3508	3541	3594	3613
1	2	3	4	5	6	7	8	9	10	11	12	13	14	15

3615	3650	3666	3710	3798	3800	3886	3896	4006	4010	4090	4094	4200	4206	4490
16	17	18	19	20	21	22	23	24	25	26	27	28	29	30

The *p*th percentile is the value in the $p/100(n+1)$th position. For example, the 20th percentile is the $20/100(n+1)$th value. With the 30 birthweight values, the 20th percentile is therefore the $20/100(30+1)$th value $= 0.2 \times$ 31st value $= 6.2$th value. The 6th value is 3303 g and the

7th value is 3388g, a difference of 85g, so the 20th percentile is 3303g plus 0.2 of 85g, which is $3303g + 0.2 \times 85g = 3303g + 17g = 3320g$.

You might be thinking, this all seems a bit messy, but a computer will perform these calculations effortlessly. As well as percentiles, you might also encounter *deciles*, which sub-divide the data values into 10, not 100, equal divisions, and *quintiles*, which sub-divide the values into five equal-sized groups. Collectively, we call percentiles, deciles and quintiles, *n-tiles*.

Exercise 5.9   Calculate the 25th and 75th percentiles for the ICU per cent mortality values in Table 2.7, and explain your results.

Choosing the most appropriate measure

How do you choose the most appropriate measure of location for some given set of data? The main thing to remember is that the mean *cannot* be used with ordinal data (because they are not real numbers), and that the median can be used for both ordinal and metric data (particularly when the latter is skewed).

As an illustration of the last point, look again at Figure 3.7 which shows the distribution of the number of measles cases in 37 schools. Not only is this distribution positively skewed, it has a single high-valued outlier. The median number of measles cases is 1.00, but the mean number is 2.91, almost three times as many! The problem is that the long positive tail and the outlier are dragging the mean to the right. In this case, the median value of 1 seems to be more representative of the data than the mean. I have summarised the choices of a measure of location in Table 5.2.

Table 5.2   A guide to choosing an appropriate measure of location

		Summary measure of location	
Type of variable	mode	median	mean
Nominal	yes	no	no
Ordinal	yes	yes	no
Metric discrete	yes	yes, if distribution	yes
Metric continuous	no	is markedly skewed	yes

Summary measures of spread

As well as a summary measure of location, a summary measure of spread or dispersion can also be very useful. There are three main measures in common use, and once again, as you will see, the type of data influences the choice of an appropriate measure.

The range

The *range* is the distance from the smallest value to the largest. The range is not affected by skewness, but is sensitive to the addition or removal of an outlier value. As an example, the range of the 30 birthweights in Table 2.5 is (2860.0 to 4490.0) g. The range is best written like this, rather than as the single-valued difference, i.e. as 1630 g, in this example, which is much less informative.

> **Exercise 5.10**   What are the ranges for age among those infants breast-fed, and those bottle-fed in Table 5.1?

The interquartile range (iqr)

One solution to the problem of the sensitivity of the range to extreme value (outliers) is to chop a quarter (25 per cent) of the values off both ends of the distribution (which removes any troublesome outliers), and then measure the range of the remaining values. This distance is called the *interquartile range,* or *iqr*. The interquartile range is not affected either by outliers or skewness, but it does not use all of the information in the data set since it ignores the bottom and top quarter of values.

Calculating interquartile range by hand (avoid if possible!)

To calculate the interquartile range by hand, you need first to determine two values:

- The value which cuts off the bottom 25 per cent of values; this is known as the *first quartile* and denoted *Q1*.

- The value which cuts off the top 25 per cent of values, known as the *third quartile* and denoted *Q3*.[3]

The interquartile range is then written as (Q1 to Q3). With the birthweight data: Q1 = 3396.25 g, and Q3 = 3923.50 g. Therefore: interquartile range = (3396.25 to 3923.50) g. This result tells you that the middle 50 per cent of infants (by weight) weighed between 3396.25 g and 3923.50 g.

An example from practice

Table 5.3 describes the baseline characteristics of 56 patients in an investigation into the use of analgesics in the prevention of stump and phantom pain in lower-limb amputation (Nikolajsen

---

[3] The median is sometimes denoted as Q2.

et al. 1997). The 'blockade' group of patients were given bupivacaine and morphine, the control (comparison) group, were given an identically administered saline placebo.

As you can see, two variables, 'pain in week before amputation', and 'daily opioid consumption at admission (mg)', were summarised with median and interquartile range values. Pain was measured using a visual analogue scale (VAS[4]), which of course produces ordinal data, so the mean is not appropriate, and the authors have used the median and interquartile range as their summary measures of location and spread.

The median level of pain in the blockade group is 51, with an iqr of (23.8 to 87.8).[5] This means that 25 per cent of this group had a pain level of less than 23.8, and 25 per cent a pain level greater than 87.8. The middle 50 per cent had a pain level between 23.8 and 87.8. I'll return to the opioid consumption variable shortly.

Table 5.3   The baseline characteristics of 56 patients in an investigation into the use of analgesics in the prevention of stump and phantom pain in lower-limb amputation. Reproduced from *The Lancet*, 1994, **344**, 1724–26, courtesy of Elsevier

Characteristics of patients	Blockade group (n = 27)	Control group (n = 29)
Men/women	15/12	18/11
Mean (SD) age in years	72.8 (13.2)	70.8 (11.4)
Diabetes	10	14
Concurrent treatment because of cardiovascular disease	18	19
Previous stroke	3	2
Previous contralateral amputation	7	3
Median (IQR) pain in week before amputation (VAS, 0–100 mm)	51 (23.8–8–78)	44 (25.3–68)
Median (IQR) daily opioid consumption at admission (mg)	50 (20–68.8)	30 (5–62.5)
Level of amputation		
Below knee	15	16
Through knee-joint	5	2
Above knee	7	11
Reamputations during follow-up	3	2
Died during follow-up	10	10

Exercise 5.11   Calculate the iqr for the ICU percentage mortality values in Table 2.7. (You have already calculated the 25th and 75th percentiles in Exercise 5.9).

Exercise 5.12   Interpret the median and interquartile range values for pain in the week before amputation, for the control group in Table 5.3.

---

[4] See Chapter 1.
[5] The table contains a typographical error, recording 87.8 as '8–78'.

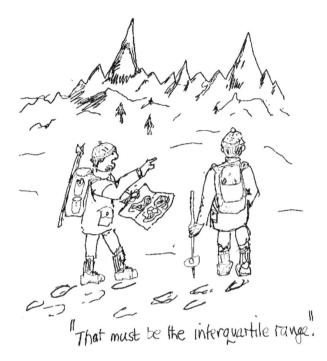

"That must be the interquartile range."

Estimating the median and interquartile range from the ogive

As I indicated earlier, you can estimate the median and the interquartile range from the cumulative frequency curve (the ogive). Figure 5.2 shows the ogive for the cumulative birthweight
data in Table 3.3.

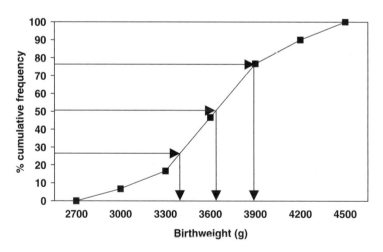

Figure 5.2   Using the relative cumulative frequency curve (or ogive) of birthweight to estimate the
median and interquartile range values (Note that this *should* be a smooth curve)

If you draw horizontal lines from the values 25 per cent, 50 per cent and 75 per cent on the *y* axis, to the ogive, and then down to the *x* axis, the points of intersection on the *x* axis approximate values for Q1, Q2 (the median), and Q3, of 3400 g, 3650 g and 3900 g. Thus, if you happen to have an ogive handy, these approximations can be helpful. I plotted *per cent* cumulative frequency because it makes it slightly easier to do find the percentage values. Notice that you can also use the ogive to answer questions like, 'What percentage of infants weighed less than, say, 4000 g?' The answer is that a value of 4000 g on the *x* axis produces a value of 80 per cent for cumulative frequency on the *y* axis.

Exercise 5.13 Estimate the median and iqr for total blood cholesterol for the control group from the ogive in Figure 3.12.

The boxplot

Now that we have discussed the median and interquartile range, I can introduce the *boxplot* as I promised in Chapter 3. The general discussion on measures of spread continues overleaf if you want to continue with this and come back to consider the boxplot later. Boxplots provide a graphical summary of the three quartile values, the minimum and maximum values, and any outliers. They are usually plotted with value on the vertical axis. Like the pie chart, the boxplot can only represent one variable at a time, but a number of boxplots can be set alongside each other.

An example from practice

Figure 5.3 is from the same study as Figure 4.3, into the use of the mammography service in the 33 health districts of Ontario, in which investigators were interested in the variation in the mammography utilisation rate across age groups (Goel *et al.* 1997). They supplemented their

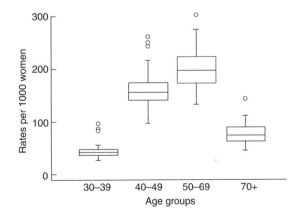

Figure 5.3 Boxplots of the rate of use of mammography services in 33 health districts in Ontario. Reproduced from *J. Epid. Comm. Health*, **51**, 378–82, courtesy of BMJ Publishing Group

results with the boxplots shown in the figure, for the age groups: (30–39); (40–49); (50–59); and 70+ years. The vertical axis is the mammography utilisation rate (visits per 1000 women), in the 33 health districts. Outliers are denoted by the small open circles.

Let's look at the third boxplot, that for the women aged 50–69:

- The bottom end of the lower 'whisker' (the line sticking out of the bottom of the box), corresponds to the minimum value – about 125 visits per 1000 women.

- The bottom of the box is the 1st quartile value, Q1. So about 25 per cent of women had a utilisation rate of 175 or less visits per 1000 women.

- The line across the inside of the box (it won't always be half-way up), is the median, Q2. So half of the women had a utilisation rate of less than about 200 consultations per 1000 women, and half a rate of more than 200. The more asymmetric (skewed) the distributional shape, the further away from the middle of the box will be the median line, closer to the top of the box is indicative of negative skew, closer to the bottom of the box – positive skew.

- The top of the box is the third quartile Q3. That is, about a quarter of women had a consultation rate of 225 or more per 1000.

- The top end of the upper whisker is the 'maximum' mammography utilisation rate – about 275 consultations per 1000 women. This is the maximum value that can be considered still to be part of the general mass of the data. Because. . .

- . . .there is one outlier. One of the health districts reported a utilisation rate of about 300 per 1000 women.[6] This is, of course, the actual maximum value in the data.

Exercise 5.14   Sketch the box plot for the percentage mortality in ICUs shown in Table 2.7. (Note that you have already calculated the median and iqr values in Exercises 5.6 and 5.10). What can you glean from the boxplot about the shape of the distribution of the ICU percentage mortality rate?

Exercise 5.15   The boxplots in Figure 5.4 are from a study of sperm integrity in adult survivors of childhood cancer compared to a control group of non-cancer individuals (Thomson *et al.* 2002). What do the two boxplots tell you?

Standard deviation

The limitation of the interquartile range as a summary measure of spread is that (like the median) it doesn't use all of the information in the data, since it omits the top and bottom

---

[6] Outliers are defined in various ways by different computer programs. Outliers are here defined as any value more than thee halves of the interquartile range greater than the third quartile, or less than the first quartile.

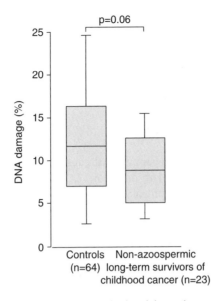

Figure 5.4 Boxplots from a study of sperm integrity in adult survivors of childhood cancer, compared to a control group of non-cancer individuals. Reprinted from *The Lancet* 2002, **360**, 361–6, Fig. 2, p. 364, courtesy of Elsevier

quarter of values. An alternative approach uses the idea of summarising spread by measuring the mean (average) distance of all the data values from the *overall* mean of all of the values. The smaller this mean distance is, the narrower the spread of values must be, and vice versa. This idea is the basis for what is known as the *standard deviation*, or s.d. The following way of calculating the sample standard deviation by hand illustrates this idea:[7]

- Subtract the mean of the sample from each of the *n* sample values in the sample, to give the *difference* values.

- Square each of these differences.

- Add these squared values together (called the *sum of squares*).

- Divide the sum of squares by $(n-1)$; i.e. divide by 1 less than the sample size.[8]

- Take the square root. This is the standard deviation.

One advantage of the standard deviation is that, unlike the interquartile range, it uses all of the information in the data.

---

[7] This is a very tedious procedure. If you have an s.d. key on your calculator use that. Better still, use a computer!
[8] If we divide by *n*, as we normally would do to find a mean, we get a result which is slightly too small. Dividing by $(n-1)$ adjusts for this. Technically, the sample s.d. is said to be a biased estimator of population s.d. See Chapter 7 for the meaning of sample and population.

Exercise 5.16 In Figure 4.6 the authors tell us that the mean cord platelet count is 308×10^9/l, and the standard deviation is 69×10^9/l (notice the two measures have the same units).[1] Explain what this value means.

An example from practice

In Table 5.3, the analgesic/amputation pain study, the authors summarise the age of the patients in the study with the mean and standard deviation. As you can see, the spread of ages in the blockade group is wider than in the control group, 13.2 years around a blockade group's mean of 72.8 years, compared to 11.4 years around a control group's mean of 70.8 years.

The authors could also have used the mean and standard deviation for daily opioid consumption (mg), since this is a metric variable, but instead used the median and interquartile range; there are a number of possible reasons for this. First, the data may be noticeably skewed and/or contained outliers, perhaps making the mean a little too unrepresentative of the general mass of data. Or the investigators may have specifically wanted a summary measure of central-ness, which the median provides. Third, they may have felt that asking people to recall their opioid consumption last week was likely to lead to fuzzy, imprecise, values, and so have preferred to treat them as if they were ordinal.

Exercise 5.17 Calculate and interpret the standard deviation for the ICU percentage mortality values in Table 2.7. (You have already calculated the mean percentage mortality in Exercise 5.7). I would hesitate to do this without a calculator with a standard deviation function.

To sum up summary measures of spread: with ordinal data use either the range or the interquartile range. The standard deviation is not appropriate because of the non-numeric nature of ordinal data. With metric data use either the standard deviation, which uses all of the information in the data, or the interquartile range. The latter if the distribution is skewed, and/or you have already selected the median as your preferred measure of location. Don't mix-and-match measures – standard deviation goes with the mean, and iqr with the median. These points are summarised in Table 5.4.

Table 5.4 Choosing an appropriate measure of spread

	Summary measure of spread		
Type of variable	Range	Interquartile range	Standard deviation
Nominal	No	No	No
Ordinal	Yes	Yes	No
Metric	Yes	Yes, if skewed	Yes

---

[1] 10^9 means 1000 000 000.

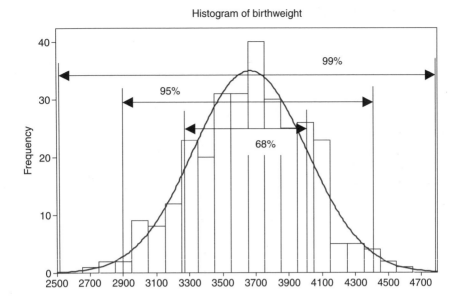

Figure 5.5   The area properties of the Normal distribution illustrated with the birthweight data

Standard deviation and the Normal distribution

If you are working with metric data which is distributed Normally, the standard deviation has one very useful property that relates to the percentage of data between certain values. These *area properties of the Normal distribution* are illustrated in Figure 5.5 for the histogram of birthweight data from Table 2.5,[9] through which a Normal curve is drawn. Minitab calculates these birthweights to have a mean of 3644 g, and a standard deviation of 377 g. In words, the area properties are as follows:

- About 68 per cent of the birthweights will lie within one standard deviation either side of the mean. That is, from 3644 g − 377 g to 3644 g + 377 g, or from 3267 g to 4021 g.

- About 95 per cent of the birthweights will lie within two standard deviations either side of the mean. That is, from 3644 g − 754 g to 3644 g + 754 g, or from 2890 g to 4398 g.

- About 99 per cent of the birthweights will lie within three standard deviations either side of the mean. That is, from 3644 g − 1131 g to 3644 g + 1131 g, or from 2513 g to 4775 g.

So, if you have some data that you know is Normally distributed, and you also know the values of the mean and standard deviation, then you can make statements such as, 'I know that 95 per cent of the values must lie between so-and-so and so-and-so.'

---

[9] Which is reasonably Normally distributed.

An example from practice

To illustrate the usefulness of the Normal area properties, look again at the histogram of the cord platelet count for 4382 infants in Figure 4.6, which appears to be reasonably Normal, and has a mean of $308 \times 10^9/l$, and a standard deviation of $69 \times 10^9/l$. You can therefore say that about two-thirds (67 per cent) of the 4382 infants, i.e. 2936 infants, had a cord platelet count between $308 - 69$ and $308 + 69$, which is between 239 and 377 $10^9/l$.

Table 5.5 Output measures from a study of the effectiveness of lisinopril as a prophylactic for acute migraine. Figures are means (SD). Reproduced from *BMJ*, **322**, 19–22, courtesy of BMJ Publishing Group

	Lisinopril	Placebo	Mean % reduction (95% Cl)
Primary efficacy parameter			
Hours with headache	129 (125)	162 (142)	20 (5 to 36)
Days with headache	19.7 (14)	23.7 (11)	17 (5 to 30)
Days with migraine	14.5 (11)	18.5 (10)	21 (9 to 34)
Secondary efficacy parameter			
Headache severity index	297 (325)	370 (310)	20 (3 to 37)
Triptan doses	15.7 (15)	20.2 (17)	22 (7 to 38)
Doses of analgesics	14.5 (23)	16.2 (20)	11 (−16 to 37)
Days with sick leave	2.30 (4.32)	2.09 (2.50)	−10 (−64 to 37)
Bodily pain*	63.7 (29)	53.8 (23)	−18 (−35 to −1)
General health*	73.6 (20)	74.1 (21)	1 (−6 to 7)
Vitality*	61.1 (24)	58.2 (21)	−5 (−18 to 8)
Social functioning*	81.4 (25)	79.5 (23)	−2 (−11 to 6)

* From SF-36.

Exercise 5.18   Table 5.5 is from a study of the effectiveness of lisinopril as a prophylactic for acute migraine, in which one group of patients was given lisinopril, and a second group a placebo (Schrader *et al.* 2001). Outcome measures included, 'hours with headache', 'days with headache' and 'days with migraine', all metric continuous variables. The mean and standard deviation for each of these variables for both groups is shown in the figure. Do you think they can be Normally or symmetrically distributed? Explain your answer.

Transforming data

Later in the book you will meet some procedures which require the data to be Normally distributed. But what if it isn't? Happily some non-Normal data can be *transformed* to make the distribution more Normal (or at least more Normal than it was to start with). The most popular approach is to take the *log* of the data (to base 10); first because it works more often than other procedures, and second because the back-transformation (i.e. anti-logging the results at the end of the analysis) can be meaningfully interpreted.

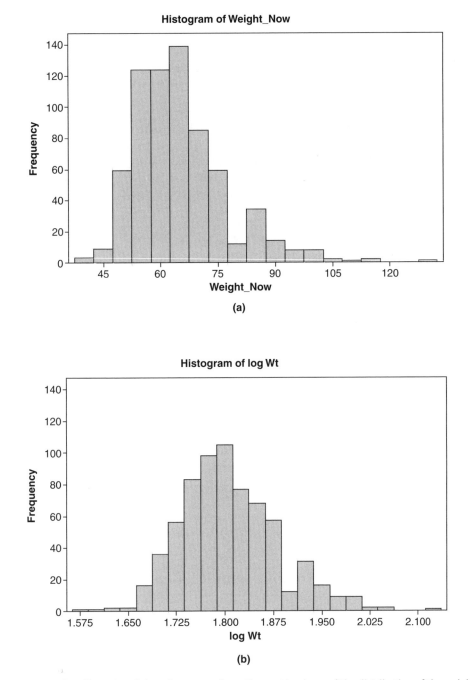

Figure 5.6 The effect of applying a $\log_{10}$ transformation on the shape of the distribution of the weight of 658 women

An example from practice

Figure 5.6 shows histograms for the original and transformed data on the weight (kg) of 685 women in a diet and health cohort study.[10] The original data is positively skewed, Figure 5.6a. If we transform the data by taking $logs_{10}$, you can see that the transformed data has a more Normal-ish shape, Figure 5.6b.

In Part II, I have discussed ways of looking at sample data – with tables, with charts, from its shape, and with numeric summary measures. Collectively these various procedures are labelled *descriptive statistics*. However, in all of the above, I assumed that you *already* had the data that you were describing, and I've said nothing so far about how you might collect the data in the first place. This is the question I will address in the following chapter.

---

[10]This data was kindly supplied by Professor Janet Cade of Leeds University Medical School.

III

Getting the Data

6

Doing it right first time – designing a study

Learning objectives

When you have finished this chapter you should be able to:

- Explain what a sample is, and what the difference between study and target populations is.

- Explain why it is important for a sample to be as representative of the population from which it is taken as possible.

- Define a random sample, and explain what a sampling frame is.

- Briefly outline what is meant by a contact sample, and by stratified and systematic samples.

- Explain the difference between observational and experimental studies.

- Explain the difference between matched and independent groups.

- Briefly describe case-series, cross-section, cohort and case-control studies, and their limitations and advantages.

- Explain the problem of confounding.

Medical Statistics from Scratch, Second Edition   David Bowers
© 2008 John Wiley & Sons, Ltd

- Outline the general idea of the clinical trial.

- Explain the concept of randomisation, and why it is important, and demonstrate that you can use a random number table to perform a simple block randomisation.

- Describe the concept of blinding, and what it is intended to achieve.

- Outline and compare the design of the parallel and cross-over randomised controlled trials, and summarise their respective advantages and shortcomings.

- Explain what intention-to-treat means.

- Be able to choose an appropriate study design to answer some given research question.

Hey ho! Hey ho! It's off to work we go

There are two main threads here. First, the *study design* question, and second, the *data collection* question. Study design embraces issues like:

- What is the research question? What are we hypothesising?

- Which variables do we need to measure?

- Which is our main *outcome variable* (the variable we are most interested in)?

- How many subjects need to be included in the study?

- Who exactly are the subjects? How should we select them?

- How many groups do we need?

- Are we going to make some form of clinical intervention or simply observe?

- Do we need a comparison group?

- At what stage are we going to take measurements? Before, during, after, etc.?

- How long will the study take? And so on.

Study design is a systematic way of dealing with these issues, and offers a good-practice blueprint that is applicable in almost all research situations.

Second, the *data collection* question. Having decided an appropriate study design, we then have to consider the following:

- How are we going collect the data from the subjects?

- How do we ensure that the sample is as representative as possible?

I want to start with the data collection question. First, though, a brief mention of what we mean by a *population*.

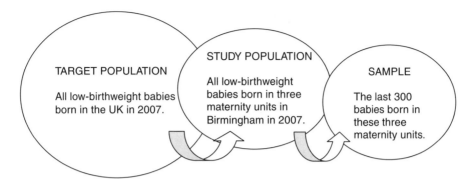

Figure 6.1 The target population, the study population and the sample

Samples and populations

In clinical research, we usually study a sample of individuals who are assumed to be representative of a wider group, to whom (with a good research design and appropriate sampling) the research might apply. This wider group is known as the *target population*, for example 'all low-birthweight babies born in the UK in 2007'.

It would be impossible to study every single baby in such a large target population (or every member of *any* population). So instead, we might choose to take a sample from a (hopefully) more accessible group. For example, 'all low-birthweight babies born in three maternity units in Birmingham in 2007'. This more restricted group is the *study population*. Suppose we take as our sample the last 300 babies born in these three maternity units. What we find out from this sample we hope will also be true of the study population, and ultimately of the target population. The degree to which this will be the case depends largely on the representativeness of our sample. These ideas are shown schematically in Figure 6.1. I'll have more to say about this process in Chapter 7.

> **Exercise 6.1** Explain the differences between a target population, a study population and a sample. Explain, with an example, why it is almost never possible to study every member of a population.

Sampling error

Needless to say, samples are never perfect replicas of their populations, so when we draw a conclusion about a population based on a sample, there will always be what is known as *sampling error*. For example, if the percentage of women in the UK population with genital chlamydia is 3.50 per cent (we wouldn't know this of course), and a sample produces a sample percentage of 2.90 per cent, then the difference between these two values, 0.60 per cent, is the sampling error. We can never completely eliminate sampling error, since this is an inherent feature of any sample.

Collecting the data – types of sample

Now the data collection question. There are many books wholly dedicated to the various methods of collecting sample data. I am going to do little more than mention a couple of these methods by name. Those interested in more details of the methods referred to should consult other readily available sources.

The simple random sample and its offspring

The most important consideration is that any sample should be *representative* of the population from which it is taken. For example, if your population has equal numbers of male and female babies, but your sample consists of twice as many male babies as female, then any conclusions you draw are likely to be, at least, misleading. Generally, the most representative sample is a *simple random sample*. The only way that a simple random sample will differ from the population will be *due to chance* alone.

For a sample to be truly random, every member of the population must have an equal chance of being included in the sample. Unfortunately, this is rarely possible in practice, since this would require a complete and up-to-date list (name and contact details) of, for example, *every* low-birthweight baby born in the UK in 2007. Such a list is called a *sampling frame*. In practice, compiling an accurate sampling frame for any population is hardly ever going to be feasible!

This same problem applies also to two close relatives of simple random sampling – *systematic* random sampling, and *stratified* random sampling. In the former, some fixed fraction of the sampling frame is selected, say every 10th or every 50th member, until a sample of the required size is obtained. Provided there are no hidden patterns in the sampling frame, this method will produce samples as representative as a random sample. In stratified sampling, the sampling frame is first broken down into strata relevant to the study, for example men and women; or non-smokers, ex-smokers and smokers. Then each separate stratum is sampled using a systematic sampling approach, and finally these strata samples are combined. But both methods require a sampling frame.

Contact or consecutive samples

The need for an accurate sampling frame makes random sampling impractical in any realistic clinical setting. One common alternative is to take as a sample, individuals in current or recent *contact* with the clinical services, such as consecutive attendees at a clinic. For example, in the study of stress as a risk factor for breast cancer (Table 1.6), the researchers took as their sample 332 women attending a clinic at Leeds General Infirmary for a breast lump biopsy.

Alternatively, researchers may study a group of subjects *in situ*, for example on a ward, or in some other setting. In the nit lotion study (Table 2.1), researchers took as their sample all infested children from a number of Parisian primary schools, based on the high rates of infestation in those same schools the previous year.

If your sample is not a random sample, then the obvious question is, 'How representative is it of the population?' And, moreover, which population are we talking about here? In the breast cancer study, if the researchers were confident that their sample of 332 women was reasonably representative of *all such women* in the Leeds area (their study population), then they would perhaps have felt justified in generalising their findings to this population, and maybe to all women in the UK (a possible target population). But if they knew that the women in their sample were all from a particularly deprived (or particularly affluent) part of the city, or if some ethnic minority formed a noticeably large proportion of the women, then such a generalisation would be more risky.

> **Exercise 6.2** What is the principal advantage of random sampling? What is the principal drawback of this approach? Describe another method of getting samples that is used in clinical research.

Types of study

With this brief look at the data collection problem, I want to return now to the study design question. Study design divides into two main types. Some alternative ways of classifying these are:

- Observational versus experimental studies.
- Prospective versus retrospective studies.
- Longitudinal versus cross-sectional studies.

I am going to use the first classification, although I will explain the other terms along the way. Broadly speaking, an *observational* study is one in which researchers *actively* observe the subjects involved, perhaps asking questions, or taking some measurements, or looking at clinical records, but they *don't* control, change or effect in any way, their selection, treatment or care. An *experimental* study, on the other hand, does involve some sort of *active* intervention with the subjects. I will first discuss a number of types of observational study designs.

> **Exercise 6.3** What is the fundamental difference between an observational study and an experimental study?

Observational studies

There are four principal types of observational study:

- Case-series.
- Cross-section studies.
- Cohort studies.
- Case-control studies.

Case-series studies

A health carer may see a series of patients (cases) with similar but unusual symptoms or outcomes, find something interesting and write it up as a study. This is a *case-series*.

An example from practice

In 1981 a drug technician at the Centre for Disease Control in the USA, noticed an unusually high number of requests for the drug pentamidine, used to treat Pneumocystis carinii pneumonia (PCP). This led to a scientific report, in effect a case-series study, of PCP occurring unusually in five gay men in Los Angeles. At the same time a similar outbreak of Kaposi's Sarcoma (previously rare except in elderly men) in a small number of young gay men in New York, also began to raise questions. These events signalled the arrival of HIV in the USA.

In the same way, new variant CJD was also first suspected from an unusual series of deaths of young people in the UK, from an apparent dementia-like illness, a disease normally associated with the elderly. Case-series studies often point to a need for further investigations, as was the case in each one of these quoted examples.

Cross-section studies

A cross-section study aims to take a 'snapshot' of some situation at some particular point in time,[1] but notably data on one or more variables from each subject in the study is collected only once.

An example from practice

The following extract is from a cross-section study carried out in 1993 on 2542 rural Chinese subjects, into the relationship between body mass index[2] and cardiovascular disease, in a rural Chinese population (1st paragraph in text below) (Hu *et al.* 2000). The population of this region of China was about 6 million, and the 2542 individuals included in the sample were selected using a two-stage sampling process, as the 2nd paragraph explains. Each subject was then interviewed and the necessary measurements were taken (3rd paragraph).

> A total of 2 542 subjects aged 20–70 years from a rural area of Anqing, China, participated in a **cross-sectional survey**, and 1 610 provided blood samples in 1993. Mean BMI (kg/m^2) was 20.7 for men and 20.9 for women. . .

---

[1] In practice this 'point' in time may in fact be a short-ish period of time.
[2] Body mass index, used to measure obesity, is equal to a person's weight (kg) divided by their height squared (m)^2. A bmi of between 20 to 25 is considered 'normal', 25 to 30 indicates a degree of obesity. Higher scores indicate greater levels of obesity.

...These participants were selected from 20 townships in four counties based on a two-stage sampling approach. The sampling unit is a village in the first stage and a nuclear family in the second stage, based on the following criteria: 1) both parents are alive; and 2) there are at least two children in the family. We limited the analysis to 2 542 participants aged 20 years or older from 776 families...

...Trained interviewers administered questionnaires to gather information on each participant's date of birth, occupation, education level, current cigarette smoking, and alcohol use... measurements, including height and weight, were taken using standard protocols, with subjects not wearing shoes or outer-wear. BMI was calculated as weight (kg)/height (m^2). Blood pressure measurements were obtained by trained nurses after subjects had been seated for 10 minutes by using a mercury manometer and appropriately sized cuffs, according to standard protocols.

Note that there is no intervention by the researchers into any aspect of the subjects' care or treatment – the observers only take measurements, ask some questions or study records. The results from the above study showed that subjects in the sample with higher body mass index values were also likely to have higher blood pressures. The researchers might reasonably claim that this link would also exist in the province's population of 6 million – that's their *inference* – but the truth of this would depend on how representative the sample was of the whole Anqing population. Whether or not the finding could be extended to the rest of the diverse Chinese population is more questionable. To sum up, cross-section studies:

- Take only one measurement from each subject at one moment in, or during one period of, time. Data from one or more than one variable may be collected.

- Can be used to investigate a link between two or more variables, but not the *direction* of any causal relationship. The Anqing study does not reveal whether a higher body mass index leads to higher blood pressures (more strain on the heart, for example), or whether higher blood pressures lead to higher body mass index (maybe higher blood pressures increase appetite), it simply establishes some sort of association.

- Are not particularly helpful if the condition being investigated is rare. If, for example, only 0.1 per cent of a population has some particular disease, then a very large sample would be needed to provide any reliable results. Too small a sample might lead you to conclude that nobody in the population had the disease!

- Can be more limited in scope and aim only to *describe* some existing state of affairs, such as the *prevalence* of some condition – for example, the percentage of 16+ UK individuals who have taken ecstasy. Only one variable is measured – use of ecstasy, yes or no. Since this is the only variable measured, no link with any other variable can be explored.

- That aim to uncover attitudes, opinions or behaviours, are often referred to as *surveys*. For example, the views of clinical staff towards having patients' relatives in Emergency Department trauma rooms.

Exercise 6.4   Give two examples of the application of the cross-section design in a clinical setting.

From here to eternity – cohort studies

The main objective of a cohort study is to identify risk factors causing a particular outcome, for example death, or lung cancer, or stroke, or low-birthweight babies and so on. The principle structure of a cohort study (also known as a *follow-up*, *prospective*, or *longitudinal* study) is as follows:

- A group of individuals is selected at random from the general population, for example all women living in Manchester. . .

- . . .or from a particular population, for example all call-centre workers. . .

- . . .or via a clinical setting, for example women diagnosed with breast cancer.

- The group is followed forward over a period of time,[3] and the subjects monitored on their exposure to suspected risk factors, or to different clinical interventions.

- At the end of the study, a comparison is made between groups with and without the outcome of interest (say cardio-vascular disease), in terms of their exposure over the course of the study to a suspected risk factor (e.g. smoking, lack of exercise, diet, etc.).

- A reasoned conclusion is drawn about the relationship between the outcome of interest and the suspected risk factor or intervention.

A well-known prospective cohort study was that conducted by Doll and Hill into a possible connection between mortality and cigarette smoking. They recruited about 60 per cent of the doctors in the UK, determined their age and smoking status (among other things), and then followed them up over the ensuing years, recording deaths as they arose. Very quickly the data began to show significantly higher mortality among doctors who smoked.

In some cohort studies, the data may be collected from existing historical records, and subjects followed from some time starting in the past, as the following example demonstrates.

An example from practice

An investigation of the relationship between weight in infancy and the prevalence of coronary heart disease (CHD) in adult life used a sample of 290 men born between 1911 and 1930, and living in Hertfordshire, whose birthweights and weights at one year were on record. In 1994

---

[3] Note that 'forward' doesn't necessarily mean from *today*, although *prospective* cohort studies *do* follow subjects forward from the time the study is initiated.

various measurements were made on the 290 men, including the presence or not of CHD (Fall *et al.* 1995). So 'forward' here means from each birth year between 1911 and 1930, up to 1944.

The researchers found that 42 men had CHD, a prevalence of 14 per cent, (42/290) × 100. But weight at *birth* was not influential on adult CHD. However, men who weighed 18 lbs (8.2kg) or less, at *one year*, had almost twice the risk of CHD as men who weighed more than 18 lbs. This of course is only the sample evidence. Whether this finding applies to the population of *all* men born in Hertfordshire during this period, or today, or indeed in the UK, depends on how representative this sample is of either of these populations.

Table 6.1 shows this cohort study expressed as a contingency table (see Chapter 2). The subjects are grouped according to their exposure or non-exposure to the risk factor (in this case weighing 18 lbs or less at one year is taken to be the risk factor), and these groups form the columns of the table. The rows identify the presence or otherwise of the *outcome*, CHD. Clearly this design does suggest (but certainly does not prove) a cause and effect – low weight at one year seems to lead to coronary heart disease in adult life. Cohort studies suffer a number of drawbacks, among which are the following:

- Selection of appropriate subjects may cause difficulties. If subjects are chosen using a contact sample, for example attendees at a clinic, then the outcomes for these individuals may be different from those in the general population.

- If the condition is rare in the population, i.e. has low prevalence, it may require a very large cohort to capture enough cases to make the exercise worthwhile.

- The subjects will have to be followed-up for a long time, possibly many years, before any worthwhile results are obtained. This can be expensive as well as frustrating, and not good if a quick answer is needed. Moreover, this long time-period allows for considerable losses, as subjects drop out for a variety of reasons - they move away, they die from other non-related causes, and so on.

- Over a long period a significant proportion of the subjects may change their habits, quit smoking, for example, or take up regular exercise. However, this problem can be monitored with frequent checks of the state of the cohort.

Table 6.1 The cohort study of weight at one year and its effect on the presence of coronary heart disease (CHD) in adult life, expressed in the form of a contingency table

| | | Group by exposure to risk factor – weighed ≤ 18 lbs at 1 year | | Totals |
		Yes	No	
Has CHD	Yes	4	38	42
	No	11	237	248
	Totals	15	275	290

Finally, note again that the selection of the groups in the cohort contingency table is based on *whether individuals have or have not been exposed to the risk factor*, for example weighing 18 lbs or less at one year (or smoking, or exposure to asbestos, or whatever).

Back to the future – case-control studies

A number of the limitations of the cohort design are addressed by the *case-control* design, although it is itself far from perfect, as you will see. In a cohort study, a group of subjects is followed up to see if they develop an outcome (a condition) of interest. In contrast, in a case-control study the groups are selected on the basis of having or not having the outcome or condition. The objective is the same in both types of study – can the outcome of interest be related to the candidate risk factor? The structure of a case-control study (also known as a *longitudinal* or *retrospective* study) is as follows:

- Two groups of subjects are selected on the basis of whether they have or do not have some condition of interest (for example, sudden infant death, or stroke, or depression, etc.).

- One group, the *cases*, will *have* the condition of interest.

- The other group, the *controls*, will *not* have the condition, but will be as similar to the cases as possible in all other ways.

- Individuals in both groups are then questioned about past exposure to possible risk factors.

- A reasoned conclusion is then drawn about the relationship between the condition in question and exposure to the suspected risk factor.

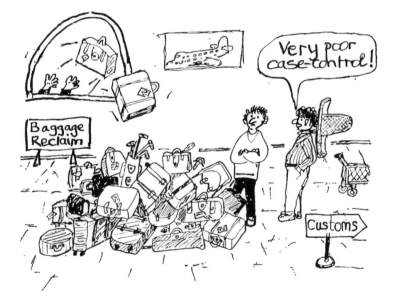

It was the outcome from such a case-control study by Doll and Hill that led them to conduct the later cohort study referred to above. Before I discuss the case-control design in more detail, there are a couple of important ideas to be dealt with first.

Confounding

Why do we want to ensure that the cases and controls are broadly similar (on age and sex, if nothing else). The reason is that it would be very difficult to identify smoking, say, as a risk factor for lung cancer in the cases, if these were on average twice as old as the controls. Who is to say that it is not increased age that causes a corresponding increased risk of lung cancer and not smoking. Consider the following situation.

Researchers noticed that mothers who smoke more have fewer Down syndrome babies than mothers who smoke less (or don't smoke at all) (Chi-Ling *et al.*1999). So at first glance smoking less seems to be a risk factor for Down syndrome. It would appear that if a mother wants to reduce the risk of having a baby with Down syndrome she should smoke a lot! However, the fact is that younger mothers have fewer Down syndrome babies but smoke more, while older mothers have more Down syndrome babies but smoke less. Thus the apparent connection between smoking and Down syndrome babies is a mirage. It disappears when we take age into account. We say that age is confounding the relationship between smoking and Down syndrome, i.e. age is a *confounder*.

To be a confounder, a variable must be associated with *both* the risk factor (smoking) *and* the outcome of interest (Down syndrome). Age satisfies this condition since smoking is connected with age, and having a Down syndrome baby is also connected with age. Age is commonly found to be a confounder, as is sex. When we allow for the effects of possible confounders, we are said to be *controlling* or *adjusting* for confounders. Results which are based on unadjusted data are said to be 'crude' results. I'll have more to say about confounding later in the book.

Matching

One way to make cases and controls more similar is to *match* them. How we match cases and controls divides case-control studies into two types – the matched and the unmatched designs. To qualify as a *matched case-control* each control must be *individually* matched (or paired), *person-to-person*, with a case. If cases and controls are independently selected, or are only *broadly* matched (for example, the same *broad mix* of ages, same *proportions* of males and females – known as *frequency matching*), then this is an *unmatched case-control* design. Finally, bear in mind that variables on which the subjects are matched cannot be used to shed any light on the relationship between outcome and risk. For example, if we are interested in coffee as one possible risk factor for people with pancreatic cancer (the cases), we should certainly not match cases and controls so that *both* groups drink lots of coffee.

Unmatched case-control design – an example from practice

In the following extract, from a frequency-matched case-control study into the possible connection between lifelong exercise and stroke (Shinton and Sagar 1993), the authors describe the selection of the cases and the controls.

SUBJECTS

Between 1 October 1989 and 30 September 1990 we recruited men and women who had just had their first stroke and were aged 35–74. The patients were assessed by one of us using the standard criteria (for stroke) of the World Health Organisation.

Control subjects were randomly selected from the general practice population to broadly match the distribution of age and sex among the patients with stroke (frequency matching). All those on the register of the 11 participating practices aged 35–74 were eligible for inclusion. The controls were each sent a letter signed by their general practitioner, which was followed up by a telephone call or visit to arrange an appointment for assessment, usually at their practice surgery.

Table 6.2   Outcome from the exercise and stroke unmatched case-control study for those subjects who had and who had not exercised between the ages of 15 and 25

		Group by disease or condition	
		Cases (stroke)	Controls
Risk factor: exercise	Yes	55	130
undertaken when aged 15–25	No	70	68

The researchers came up with 125 cases with stroke and 198 controls, broadly matched by age and sex. Notice that the numbers of cases and controls need not be the same (and usually aren't). All subjects (or their relatives if necessary), were interviewed and asked about their history of regular vigorous exercise at various times in the past. Table 6.2 shows the results for those subjects who had, and had not, taken exercise between the ages of 15 and 25.

In contrast to cohort studies, in case-control study tables you group by 'has outcome (e.g. disease) or not', for the columns. The rows correspond to whether or not subjects were exposed to the risk factor. From these results you can calculate (you'll see how later) that among those who had had a stroke, the chance that they had exercised in their youth was only about half the chance that somebody without a stroke had exercised. Notice that Table 6.2 is not a contingency table since you now have more than one group, the cases and the controls.

Matched case-control studies

With individuals matched person-to person, you have matched or paired data, which means that the groups of cases and controls are necessarily the same size. Otherwise, the matched design has the same underlying principle as the unmatched design. With individual matching the problem of confounding variables is much reduced. However, one practical difficulty is that it is sometimes quite hard to find a suitable control to match each of the cases on anything more than age and sex.

Comparing cohort and case-control designs

The case-control design has a number of advantages over the cohort study:

- With a cohort study, as you saw above, rare conditions require large samples, but with a case-control study, the availability of potential cases is much greater and sample size can be smaller. Cases will often be contact samples, i.e. selected from patients attending particular clinics.

- Case-control studies are cheaper and easier to conduct.

- Case-control studies give results much more quickly.

But they do have a number of limitations:

- Problems with the selection of suitable control subjects. You want subjects who, apart from not having the condition in question, are otherwise similar to the cases. But such individuals are often not easily found.

- Problems with the selection of cases. One problem is that many conditions vary in their type and nature and it is thus difficult to decide which cases should be included.

- The problem of recall bias. In case-control studies you are asking people to recall events in their past. Memories are not always reliable. Moreover cases may have a better recall of relevant past events than controls – over the years their illness may provide more easily remembered signposts, and they have a better motive for remembering – to get better!

Because of these various difficulties, case-control studies often provide results which seem to conflict with findings of other apparently similar case-control studies. For reliable conclusions, cohort studies are generally preferred – but are not always a practical alternative.

Exercise 6.5   (a) What advantages does a case-control study have over a cohort study?
(b) What are the principal shortcomings of a case-control study?

Getting stuck in – experimental studies

We can now turn to designs, where, in contrast to observational studies, the investigators actively participate in some aspect of the recruitment, treatment or care of the subjects in the study.

Clinical trials

Clinical trials are *experiments* to compare two or more clinical treatments. I use the word 'treatment' here, to mean any sort of clinical intervention, from kind words to new drugs. Many books have been written wholly on clinical trials, and I can only touch briefly upon some of the more important aspects of this design. Consider the following imaginary scenario. A new drug, *Arabarb*, has been developed for treating hypertension. You want to investigate its efficacy compared to the existing drug of choice. Here's what you need to do:

- Decide on an outcome measure – diastolic blood pressure seems a good candidate.

- Select a sample of individuals with hypertension. Divide into two groups (we'll see how below)

- Ensure that the two groups are as similar as possible. Similar, not only for the obvious variables, such as sex and age, but similar also for other variables whose existence you're aware of but can't easily measure. For example, emotional state of mind, lifestyles, genetic differences and so on. But also similar in terms of other variables whose existence you are *not* even aware of.

- Give one group the new drug, Arabarb. This is the *treatment* group.

- Give the other group the existing drug. This is the comparison or *control group*. A control group is imperative. If you have only one group of people, and you measure their diastolic blood pressure before and after they get the Arabarb, you cannot conclude that any decrease in diastolic blood pressure is caused necessarily by the drug. Being in a calm, quiet clinical setting, or having someone fussing over them, might reduce diastolic blood pressure.

- Group similarity is a possible answer to the *confounding* problem. If the groups were *identical* in every respect, the only difference being that one group got Arabarb, while the other got the existing drug, then any *greater* reduction in diastolic blood pressure in the treatment group is likely to be due to the new drug. We know it can't be due to the fact that the subjects in one group were slightly older, or contained more people who lived alone, or had a greater proportion of males, etc. because we have set out to make the groups identical with respect to these variables. So how do we do this?

Randomisation

The solution is to allocate subjects to one group or the other, using some random procedure. We could toss a coin – heads they go to the treatment group, tails to the control group. This method has the added virtue, not only of making the groups similar, but also of taking the allocation process out of the hands of the researcher. He or she might unconsciously introduce *selection bias* in the allocation, for example by choosing the least well patients for the treatment group. If the *randomisation* is successful, and the original sample is large enough, then the two groups should be more or less identical, differing *only by chance*. This design is thus called the *randomised controlled trial* (RCT).

Coin tossing is a little impractical of course, and instead a table of *random numbers* (there's one in the Appendix) can be used for the allocation process. Let's see how we might use this method to randomly allocate 12 patients.

You decide to allocate a patient to the treatment group (T), if the random number is *even*, say, and to the control group (C), if *odd*. You then need to determine a starting point in the random number table, maybe by sticking a pin in the table and identifying a start number. Suppose, to keep things simple, you start at the top of column 1 and go down the column; the first six rows contain the values: 23157, 05545, 14871, 38976, 97312, 11742. Combining these three rows gives:

The numbers: 2 3 1 5 7 0 5 5 4 5 1 4

The allocations: T C C C T C C T C C T

This gives you four treatment group subjects and eight control group subjects. This is a problem because if possible you want your groups to be the same size. You can fix this with *block randomisation*.

Block randomisation

Here's how it works. You decide on a block size, let's say blocks of four, and write down all combinations that contain *equal* numbers of Cs and Ts. Since there are six such possible combinations, you will have six blocks:

Block1 : CCTT

Block2 : CTCT

Block3 : CTTC

Block4 : TCTC

Block5 : TCCT

Block6 : TTCC

With the same random numbers as before, the first number was 2, so the first four subjects are allocated according to Block 2, i.e. CTCT. The next number was 3, so the next four subjects are allocated as Block 3, i.e. CTTC. The next number was 1, giving the allocation CCTT, and so on. Obviously random numbers greater than 6 are ignored. You will end up with the allocation:

CTCT   CTTC   CCTT

which gives equal numbers, six, in both groups.

Blinding

If at all possible, you don't want the patients to know whether they are in the treatment group or the control groups. This is to avoid the possibility of *response* or *placebo bias*. If a patient knows, or thinks they know, that they are getting the active drug, their psychological response to this knowledge may cause a physical, i.e. a biochemical, response, which conceivably might in turn affect their diastolic blood pressure. In the Arabarb trial, you could achieve this 'blinding' of the patients to their treatment, for example, by giving them all identical tablets, one containing the Arabarb, the other a placebo. This blinding is not always possible. For example, you might be testing out a new walking frame for elderly infirm patients. It will be difficult to disguise this from the older existing frame with which they are all familiar.

A further desirable precaution is also to blind the investigator to the allocation process. If the investigator doesn't know which subject is receiving the drug and which the placebo, their treatment of the subjects will remain impartial and even-handed. Human nature being what it is, there may be an unconscious inclination to treat a patient who is known to be in the treatment group differently to one in the control group. This effect is known as *treatment bias*, and can be avoided by blinding the investigator. We can do this by entrusting a disinterested third party to obtain the random numbers and decide on the allocation rules. Only this person will know which group any given subject is in, and will not reveal this until after the treatment is complete and the results collected and analysed.

Assessment bias can also be overcome by blinding the investigator. This applies to where an *assessment* of some condition after treatment, is required. For example, in trials of a drug to control agitation or anxiety, where proper *measurement* is not possible, then an investigator, knowing that a patient got the active drug, might then judge a patient's condition to be more 'improved', than would an uninvolved outsider, who should thus be involved in the process.

When both subject and investigator are blinded, we refer to the design as a *double-blind randomised controlled trial* – the gold standard among experimental designs. Without blinding the trial is referred to as being *open*. Compared to other designs, the RCT gives the most robust and dependable results.

The design described above, in which two groups receive identical treatment (except for the difference in drugs) throughout the period of the trial, is known as a *parallel* design.

The cross-over randomised controlled trial

A variation on the parallel design is the *cross-over* design, shown schematically in Figure 6.2. In this design one group gets drug A, say, for some fixed period of time and the second group get drug B (or placebo). Then, after a *wash-out* period to prevent drug effect carry-over, the groups are reversed. The group which got drug A now gets drug B, and vice versa, and for the same period of time. Which group gets which treatment first is decided randomly.

The advantage of this method is that each subject gets both treatments, and thus acts as his or her own control. 'Same-subject' matching, if you like. As a consequence of the matched-pair feature, this design requires smaller samples to achieve the same degree of efficiency. Unfortunately, there are a number of problems with this approach.

- A subject may undergo changes between the first treatment period and the second.

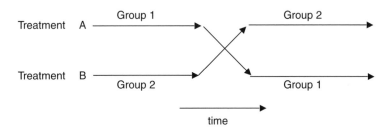

Figure 6.2 Schematic of a cross-over randomised controlled trial

- The method doesn't work well if the drug or treatment to be investigated requires a long time to become effective - for practical reasons cross-over trials are generally of relatively short duration (one reason is to avoid excessive drop out).

- Despite a wash-out interval, there may still be a drug carry-over effect. If carry-over is detected the second half of the trial has to be abandoned.

- The cross-over design is also inappropriate for conditions which can be cured – most of the subjects in the active drug half of the study might be cured by the end of the first period!

An example from practice

The following extract describes the design of a randomised cross-over trial of regular versus as-needed salbutamol in asthma control (Chapman *et al.* 1994).

> If inclusion criteria were met at the first clinic visit, patients were enrolled in a four-week randomised crossover assessment of regular vs. as-needed salbutamol. Patients took either 2 puffs (200 mg) metered dose salbutamol from a coded inhaler or matching placebo four times daily for two weeks. On return to the clinic, diary cards were reviewed and patients assigned to receive the crossover treatment for two weeks. During both treatment arms patients carried a salbutamol inhaler for relief of episodic asthma symptoms. Thus, the placebo treatment arm constituted as-needed salbutamol.
>
> Patients were instructed to record their peak expiratory flow rate (PEFR) twice daily: in the early morning and late at night, before inhaler use. Patients also recorded in a diary the number of daytime and night-time asthma episodes suffered and the number of as-needed salbutamol puffs used for symptom relief.

Data from the last eight days of each treatment period were analysed; the first six acted as an active run-in or washout period. Two investigators, blinded to the treatment assignment, examined these comparisons for each patient, and categorised each patient as: showing no difference in asthma control between treatment periods; greater control during the first treatment period; greater control during the second treatment period; or differences between treatment periods that did not indicate control to be clearly better during either.

Selection of subjects

Just a brief word about selecting subjects for the RCT. Essentially you want a sample of subjects (and they will usually be patients of some sort), who represent a cohesive and clearly defined population. Thus you might want to exclude subjects who, although they have the condition of interest, have a complicated or more advanced form of it, or simultaneously have other significant illnesses or conditions, or are taking drugs for another condition – indeed anything which you feel makes them untypical of the population you have in mind. If your sample is not truly representative of the population you are investigating (a problem known as *selection bias*), then any conclusions you arrive at about your target population are unlikely to be at all reliable.

An example from practice

The following extract is from a RCT to compare the efficacy of having midwives solely manage the care of pregnant Glasgow women, with the more usual arrangements of care being shared between midwife, hospital doctors, and GPs (Turnbull *et al.* 1996). Outcomes were the number of interventions and complications, maternal and fetal outcomes, and maternal satisfaction with the care received. The first paragraph details the selection criteria, the second and third paragraphs describe the random allocation and the blinding processes.

Methods
Design and participants
The study was carried out at Glasgow Royal Maternity Hospital, a major urban teaching hospital with around 5000 deliveries per year, serving a largely disadvantaged community. Between Jan 11, 1993, and Feb 25, 1994, all women booking for routine care at hospital-based consultant clinics were screened for eligibility; the criteria were residence within the hospital's catchment area, booking for antenatal care within 16 completed weeks of pregnancy, and absence of medical or obstetric complications (based on criteria developed by members of the clinical midwifery management team in consultation with obstetricians; available from the MDU).

The women were randomly assigned equally between the two types of care without stratification. A restricted randomisation scheme (random permutated blocks of ten) by random number tables was prepared for each clinic by a clerical officer who was not involved in determining eligibility, administering care, or assessing outcome. The research team telephoned a clerical officer in a separate office for care allocation for each woman.

Women in the control group had no identifying mark on their records, and clinical staff were unaware whether a particular woman was in the control group or was not in the study. We decided not to identify control women. . .because of concern that the identification of the control group would prompt clinical staff to treat these women differently (i.e., the Hawthorne effect).

Intention-to-treat

One problem that often arises in an RCT, after the randomisation process has taken place, is the loss of subjects, principally through drop-out (moving away, refusing further treatment, dying from non-related causes, etc.), and withdrawal for clinical reasons (perhaps they cannot tolerate the treatment). Unfortunately, such losses may adversely affect the balance of the two groups achieved through randomisation. In these circumstances it is good practice to analyse the data as if the lost subjects were still in the study, as you originally intended – even if all of their measurements are not complete. This is known as *intention-to-treat* analysis. It does, however, require that you have information on the outcome variable for all participants who were originally randomised, even if they didn't complete the course of treatment in the trial. Unfortunately this information is not always available, and in many studies therefore intention–to-treat may be more an aspiration than a reality.

> **Exercise 6.6** Explain how the possibility of treatment and assessment bias, and response bias, is overcome in the design of a RCT.
>
> **Exercise 6.7** (a) What is the principle purpose of randomisation in clinical trials? (b) Using block randomisation, with blocks of four, and a random number table, allocate 40 subjects into two groups, each with 20 individuals.
>
> **Exercise 6.8** The following paragraphs contain the stated objective or hypothesis (the wording might have been changed slightly in some cases), in each of a number of recently published clinical research papers. In each case: (a) suggest a suitable outcome variable; (b) suggest an appropriate study design or designs (there's usually more than one way to skin a cat), which would enable the investigators to achieve their stated objective(s); (c) identify possible confounders (if appropriate); (d) comment on the appropriateness of the designs and methods actually chosen by the researchers.

(a) To determine whether a child's tendency to atopic diseases (asthma, hay fever, eczema, etc.), is affected by the number of siblings that child has.

(b) To compare two drugs, ciprofoloxacin (CF) and pivmecillinam (PM), for the treatment of childhood shigellosis (dysentery).

(c) To study the effect of maternal chronic hypertension on the risk of small-for-gestational age birthweight.

(d) To evaluate a possible association between maternal smoking and the birth of a Down syndrome child.

(e) To compare a community-based service (patients living and treated at home), with a hospital-based service (patients admitted to and treated in hospital), for patients with acute, severe psychiatric illness, with reference to psychiatric outcomes, the burden on relatives and relatives' satisfaction with the service.

(f) To compare regular with as-needed inhaled salbutamol in asthma control.

(g) To evaluate the impact of counselling on: client symptomatology, self-esteem and quality of life; drug prescribing; referrals to other mental health professionals; and client and GP satisfaction.

IV

From Little to Large – Statistical Inference

7

From samples to populations – making inferences

Learning objectives

When you have finished this chapter you should be able to:

- Show that you understand the difference, and the connection, between a population parameter and a sample statistic.

- Explain what statistical inference is.

- Explain what an estimate is and why this is unlikely to be exactly the same as the population parameter being estimated.

Statistical inference

You saw in the previous chapter, that when we want to discover things that interest us about a population, we take a sample. We then hope to generalise our sample findings, first to the study population and ultimately to the target population. Statisticians call this process, of generalising from a sample to a population, *statistical inference* or *inferential statistics*.

To take an example (Grun *et al.* 1997): researchers were interested in comparing two methods of screening for genital chlamydia in women attending general practice. Their target population was, 'all asymptomatic women attending general practice'.[1] Their study population was four

---

[1] They don't say whether this is all such women in London, or England, or Wales, or the UK!

Medical Statistics from Scratch, Second Edition   David Bowers
© 2008 John Wiley & Sons, Ltd

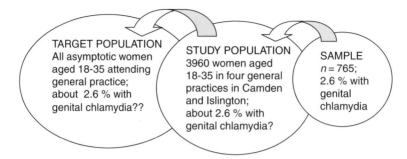

Figure 7.1   The process of statistical inference – from sample to population

general practices in the London Boroughs of Camden and Islington, with a total of 37 000 patients. All women aged between 18 and 35 were invited to take part in the study. A total study population of 3960 women were eligible for inclusion. After exclusions for various reasons, a total sample of 765 women were finally included. As well as the results of their cervical smear for genital chlamydia, data from a brief questionnaire on demographic details, history of urogenital problems and information on sexual history, was also included in the sample data.

The prevalence of genital chlamydia in the sample was found to be 2.6 per cent. The authors might then have inferred from this sample result that the prevalence of genital chlamydia in the study population of 3960 women in the four practices, was also *about* 2.6 per cent. And by extension, was also true of the target population of all asymptotic women attending general practice.

The accuracy of this *estimate* would depend on how typical the 765 women in the sample were of all the 3960 women in the study population, and in turn how typical these women were of all the women in the target population – all women 18–35 in the UK attending GP practice. This particular statistical inference process is illustrated in Figure 7.1.

I have used the word 'estimate' [2] here deliberately, because the value you get from your sample (from *any* sample) is never going to be exactly the same as the population value. You have to accept that the percentage with genital chlamydia in the population is probably *around* 2.6 per cent, *give or take a bit*. The size of the 'bit' depends on how similar your sample is to its population – and on sampling error. I'll have a lot more to say on this later in the book.

For the moment, the meaning of a few terms. The feature or characteristic of a population whose value you want to determine is known as a *population parameter*. For example, the mean or the median of some variable in a population are both population parameters. In the genital chlamydia example, the population parameter you want to estimate is the *percentage* with genital chlamydia.

The value that you get from your sample, in this case the *sample percentage* with genital chlamydia (on which you are going to base your estimate of the population value) is called the *sample statistic*. This is why we are so interested in the summary descriptive measures, such as the sample mean and the sample median, described in Chapter 6. In other words, you can use the sample mean, for example, to estimate the population mean, the sample median to estimate the population median and so on.

---

[2] An *estimate* is just a fancy word for an informed guess.

Actually, estimation is not the only way of making inferences about population parameter values. An alternative approach is to hypothesise that a population parameter has a particular value, and then see if the value of the corresponding sample statistic is compatible with your hypothesis. This approach is called hypothesis testing. In Chapters 9 to 11, I am going to discuss some common estimation procedures and in Chapters 12 to 14, I will discuss the alternative hypothesis test approach. First, however, I need to say a few words on probability, and some other related stuff; this I will do in the next chapter.

Exercise 7.1   (a) Explain the meaning of and the difference between a population parameter and a sample statistic. (b) Why is a sample, however well chosen, never going to be *exactly* representative of the sampled population? (c) Give a couple of examples that illustrate the difference between a target and a study population?

Exercise 7.2   Give a few reasons why women aged 18–35 in the London boroughs of Camden and Islington may not be typical of all women in London, or of all women in the UK.

8

Probability, risk and odds

Learning objectives

When you have finished this chapter you should be able to:

- Define probability, explain what an event is and calculate simple probabilities.

- Explain the proportional frequency approach to calculating probability.

- Explain how probability can be used with the area properties of the Normal distribution.

- Define and explain the idea of risk and its relationship with probability.

- Calculate the risk of some outcome from a contingency table and interpret the result.

- Define and explain the idea of odds.

- Calculate odds from a case-control 2 × 2 table and interpret the result.

- State the equation linking probability and odds and be able to calculate one given the other.

- Explain what the risk ratio of some outcome is, calculate a risk ratio and interpret the result.

- Explain what the odds ratio for some outcome is, calculate an odds ratio and interpret the result.

Medical Statistics from Scratch, Second Edition   David Bowers
© 2008 John Wiley & Sons, Ltd

- Explain why it's not possible to calculate a risk ratio in a case-control study.

- Define number needed to treat, explain its use and calculate NNT in a simple example.

Chance would be a fine thing – the idea of probability

Probability is a measure of the chance of getting some outcome of interest from some event. The event might be rolling a dice and the outcome of interest might be getting a six; or the event might be performing a biopsy with the outcome of interest being evidence of malignancy and so on. Some basic ideas about probability:

- The probability of a particular outcome from an event will lie between zero and one.

- The probability of an event that is certain to happen is equal to one. For example, the probability that everybody dies eventually.

- The probability of an event that is impossible is zero. For example, throwing a seven with a normal dice.

- If an event has as much chance of happening as of not happening (like tossing a coin and getting a head), then it has a probability of $^1/_2$ or 0.5.

- If the probability of an event happening is p, then the probability of the event *not* happening is $1 - p$.

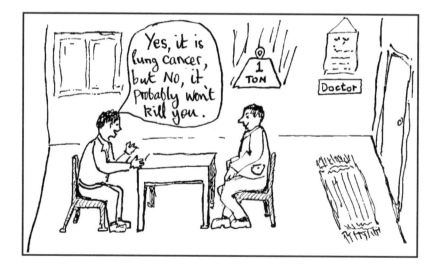

Table 8.1 Frequency table showing causes of blunt injury to limbs in 75 patients

Cause of injury	Frequency (number of patients) $n = 75$	Proportional frequency	
Falls	46	0.613	46/75 = 0.613
Crush	20	0.267	
Motor vehicle crash	6	0.080	
Other	3	0.040	

Calculating probability

You can calculate the probability of a particular outcome from an event with the following expression:

The probability of a particular outcome from an event is equal to the number of outcomes that favour that event, divided by the *total* number of possible outcomes.

To take a simple example: What is the probability of getting an even number when you roll a dice?

Total number of possible outcomes = 6 (1 or 2 or 3 or 4 or 5 or 6)

Total number of outcomes favouring the event 'an even number' = 3 (i.e. 2 or 4 or 6)

So probability of getting an even number = 3/6 = ½ = 0.5

The above method for determining probability works well with experiments where all of the outcomes have the same probability, e.g. rolling dice, tossing a coin, etc. In the real world you will often have to use what is called the *proportional frequency* approach, which uses existing frequency data as the basis for probability calculations.

As an example, look at Table 8.1 (which is Table 2.3 reproduced for convenience) which shows the causes of blunt injury to limbs. I have added an extra column showing the *proportional* frequency (category frequency divided by total frequency). Notice that the proportional frequencies sum to one.

Exercise 8.1   Table 1.6 shows the basic characteristics of the two groups of women receiving a breast lump diagnosis in the stress and breast cancer study. What is the probability that a woman chosen at random: (a) will have had her breast lump diagnosed as (i) benign? (ii) malignant?; (b) will be post-menopausal?; (c) will have had three or more children?

Exercise 8.2   Table 1.7 is from a study of thrombotic risk during pregnancy. What is the probability (under classification 1) that a subject chosen at random will be aged: (a) less than 30?; (b) more than 29?

Now ask the question, 'What is the probability that if you chose one of these 75 patients at random their injury will have been caused by a fall?'. The answer is the proportional frequency for the 'fall' category, i.e. 0.613. In other words, we can interpret proportions as equivalent to probabilities. Probability is a huge subject with many textbooks devoted to it, but for our purposes in this book we don't really need to know any more.

Probability and the Normal distribution

We know that if data is Normally distributed then about 95 per cent of the values will lie no further than two standard deviations from the mean (see Figure 5.5). In probability terms, we can say that there is a probability of 0.95 that a single value chosen at random will lie no further than two standard deviations from the mean. In the case of the Normally distributed birthweight data, this means that there is a probability of 0.95 that the birthweight of one of these infants chosen at random will be between 2890 g and 4398 g.

Exercise 8.3   Using the information on cord platelet count in Figure 4.6, determine the probability that one infant chosen at random from this sample will have a cord platelet count: (a) between $101 \times 10^9/l$ and $515 \times 10^9/l$; (b) less than $239 \times 10^9/l$.

Risk

As I mentioned earlier a *risk* is the same as a probability, but the former word tends to be favoured in the clinical arena. So the definition of probability given earlier applies equally here to risk. In other words, the risk of any particular outcome from an event is equal to the number of favourable outcomes divided by the total number of outcomes. Risk accordingly can vary between zero and one.

As an example, and also to re-visit the contingency table, look again at the table in Table 6.1 from the cohort study of coronary heart disease (CHD) in adult life and the risk factor 'weighing 18 lbs or less at one year'. The risk (or probability) that those adults who as infants weighed 18 lbs or less at one year will have CHD, is equal to the number who weighed 18 lbs or less at one year and had CHD, divided by the total number who weighed 18 lbs or less. This is equal to 4/15 = 0.2667.

Similarly, the risk (or probability) for those who weighed more than 18 lbs at one year will have CHD equals the number who weighed more than 18 lbs at one year and had CHD, divided by the total number who weighed more than 18 lbs. This is equal to 38/275 = 0.1382 and thus is only half the risk of those weighing 18 lbs or less.

The risk for a single group, as it is described it above, is also known as the *absolute risk*, mainly to distinguish it from *relative risk*, which is the risk for one group *compared* to the risk for some other group (which we'll come to shortly).

Table 8.2 The distribution of alcohol intake and deaths by sex and level of alcohol intake. Reproduced from *BMJ*, **308**, 302–6, courtesy of BMJ Publishing Group

Alcohol intake (beverages a week)*	Men		Women	
	No of subjects	No (%) of deaths	No of subjects	No (%) of deaths
<1	625	195 (31.2)	2472	394 (15.9)
1–6	1183	252 (21.3)	3079	283 (9.2)
7–13	1825	383 (21.0)	1019	96 (9.4)
14–27	1234	285 (23.1)	543	46 (8.5)
28–41	585	118 (20.2)	72	6 (8.3)
42–69	388	99 (25.5)	29	5 (17.2)
> 69	211	66 (31.3)	20	1 (5.0)
Total	6051	1398 (23.1)	7234	831 (11.5)

*One beverage contains 9–13 g alcohol.

Exercise 8.4 Table 8.2 is from a cohort study into the influence of sex, age, body mass index and smoking on alcohol intake and mortality in Danish men and women aged between 30 and 79 years (Gronbaek *et al.* 1994). The table shows the distribution of alcohol intake and deaths by sex and level of alcohol intake. Use the information in the table to construct an appropriate contingency table for: (a) men; (b) women. Calculate the absolute risk of death among those subjects who consume: (i) less than one beverage a week; (ii) more than 69 beverages a week. Interpret your results.

Odds

The *odds* for a particular outcome from an event is closely related to probability, is perhaps a more difficult concept, but important in medical statistics, and we will meet it again later in the book. As you saw above, the probability (or risk) of a particular outcome from an event is the number of outcomes favourable to the event divided by the *total* number of outcomes. But:

> The *odds* for an event is equal to the number of outcomes favourable to the event divided by the number of outcomes not favourable to the event.

Notice that:

- The value of the odds for an outcome can vary from zero to infinity.

- When the odds for an outcome are less than one, the odds are *unfavourable* to the outcome; the outcome is *less* likely to happen than it is *to* happen.

- When the odds are equal to one, the outcome is as likely to happen as not.

- When the odds are greater than one, the odds are *favourable* to the outcome; the outcome is *more* likely to happen than not.

Let's go back to the dice rolling game. The *odds* in favour of the outcome 'an even number', is the number of outcomes favourable to the event (the number of *even* numbers, i.e. 2, 4, 6), divided by the number of outcomes not favourable to the event (the number of *not* even numbers, i.e. 1, 3, 5), which is $3/3 = 1/1$ or one to one.

So the odds of getting an even number are the same as the odds of getting an odd number. Nearly all the odds in health statistics are expressed as 'something' to one. We call this value of one the *reference value*.

As a further more relevant example, we can also calculate odds from a table such as that for the exercise and stroke case-control study in Table 6.2. For instance:

- Among those patients who'd *had* a stroke, 55 had exercised (been exposed to the 'risk' of exercising) and 70 had not, so the odds that those with a stroke had exercised is $55/70 = 0.7857$.

- Among those patients who *hadn't* had a stroke, 130 had exercised and 68 had not, so the odds that they had exercised is $130/68 = 1.9118$.

In other words, among those who'd had a stroke, the odds that they had exercised was less than half the odds ($0.7857/1.9118$) of those who hadn't had a stroke. We can conclude on the basis of this sample that exercise when young seems to confer protection against a stroke.

Exercise 8.5   Table 8.3 is from a matched case-control study into maternal smoking during pregnancy and Down syndrome (Chi-Ling *et al.* 1999). It shows the basic characteristics of mothers giving birth to babies with Down syndrome (cases), and without Down syndrome (controls). Use the information in the table to construct appropriate separate 2×2 contingency tables for women: (a) aged under 35; (b) aged 35 and over. Hence calculate the odds that they had smoked during pregnancy among mothers giving birth to: (i) a Down syndrome baby; (ii) a healthy baby. What do you conclude?

Why you can't calculate risk in a case-control study

For most people the *risk* of an event, being akin to probability, makes more sense and is easier to interpret than the odds for that same event. That being so, maybe it would be more helpful to express the stroke/exercise result as a risk rather than as odds. Unfortunately we can't, and here's why.

To calculate the risk that those with a stroke had exercised, you need to know two things: the total number who'd had a stroke, and the number of these who had been exposed to the risk (of exercise). You then divide the latter by the former. In a cohort study you would select the groups on this basis – whether they had been exposed to the risk (of exercising) or not. So one group would contain individuals exposed to the risk and the other those not exposed.

Table 8.3 Basic characteristics of mothers in a case-control study of maternal smoking and Down syndrome. Reproduced from *Amer. J. Epid.*, **149**, 442–6, courtesy of Oxford University Press

Selected characteristics of Down syndrome cases and birth-matched controls. Washington State, 1984–1994

	Cases (n = 775)		Controls (n = 7750)	
	No.	%	No.	%
Smoking during pregnancy				
Age < 35 years				
Yes	112	20.0	1411	20.2
No	421	75.0	5214	74.6
Unknown	28	5.0	363	5.2
Aged ≥ 35 years				
Yes	15	7.0	108	14.2
No	186	86.9	611	80.2
Unknown	13	6.1	43	5.6

But in a case-control study you don't select on the basis of whether people have been exposed to the risk or not, but on the basis of whether they have some condition (a stroke) or not. So you have one group composed of individuals who have had a stroke, and one group who haven't, but *both* groups will contain individuals who were and were not exposed to the risk (of exercising). Moreover, you can select whatever number of cases and controls you want. You could for example halve the number of cases and double the number of controls. This means the column totals, which you would otherwise need for your risk calculation, are meaningless.

The link between probability and odds

The connection between probability (risk) and odds means that it is possible to derive one from another:

risk or probability = odds/(1 + odds)

odds = probability/(1 − probability)

Exercise 8.6 Following on from Exercise 8.5, what is the probability that a mother chosen at random from those aged ≥ 35, will have smoked during pregnancy if they are: (a) mothers of Down syndrome babies; (b) mothers of healthy babies?

Table 8.4 Generalised contingency table for risk ratio calculations in a cohort study

		Group by exposed to risk factor		
		Yes	No	Totals
Outcome: has disease	Yes	a	b	$(a+b)$
	No	c	d	$(c+d)$
	Totals	$(a+c)$	$(b+d)$	

The risk ratio

In practice, risks and odds for a single group are not nearly as interesting as a *comparison* of risks and odds between *two* groups. For risk you can make these comparisons by dividing the risk for one group (usually the group exposed to the risk factor) by the risk for the second, non-exposed, group. This gives us the *risk ratio*.[1] Let's calculate the risk ratio for the data in Table 6.1, from the cohort study of coronary heart disease (CHD) in adult life and weighing 18 lbs or less at one year, using the results obtained on page 100:

Among those weighing 18 lbs or less at one year, the risk of CHD = 0.2667

Among those weighing more than 18 lbs at one year, the risk of CHD = 0.1382

So the risk *ratio* for CHD among those weighing 18 lbs or less at one year compared to those weighing more than 18 lbs = 0.2667/0.1382 = 1.9298. We interpret this result as follows: adults who weighed 18 lbs or less at one year old have nearly twice the risk of CHD as those who weighed more than 18 lbs.

We can generalise the risk ratio calculation with the help of the contingency table as in Table 8.4, where the cell values are represented as a, b, c and d.

- Among those exposed to the risk factor, the risk of disease $= a/(a+c)$.

- Among those not exposed, the risk of disease $= b/(b+d)$.

- Therefore : risk ratio $= \frac{a}{(a+c)} / \frac{b}{(b+d)} = \frac{a(b+d)}{b(a+c)}$

Exercise 8.7 Use the results you obtained in Exercise 8.4 to calculate the risk ratio of death for those who consumed more than 69 beverages a week, compared to those who consumed less than one beverage per week (which we'll define as the reference group), for: (a) men; (b) women. Interpret your results.

---

[1] Risk ratio is also commonly known as *relative risk*.

Table 8.5 Generalised 2 × 2 table for odds ratio calculations in a case-control study

		Group by outcome (e.g. disease)	
		Cases	Controls
Exposed to risk factor?	Yes	*a*	*b*
	No	*c*	*d*

The odds ratio

With a case-control study you can compare the odds that those with a disease will have been exposed to the risk factor, with the odds that those who don't have the disease will have been exposed. If you divide the former by the latter you get the *odds ratio*.

On p. 102 you calculated the following odds for the stroke and exercise study (where we are treating exercise as the risk factor): the odds that those with a stroke had exercised = 55/70 = 0.7857; and the odds that those without a stroke had exercised = 130/68 = 1.9118. Diving the former by the latter, you get the odds ratio = 0.7857/1.9118 = 0.4110. This result suggests that those with a stroke are less than half as likely to have exercised when young as the healthy controls. It would seem that exercise is a *beneficial* 'risk' factor. We can generalise the odds ratio calculation with the help of the 2 × 2 table in Table 8.5.

- The odds of exposure to the risk factor among those with the disease = a/c,

- The odds of exposure to the risk factor among the healthy controls = b/d.

- Therefore: odds ratio = $\frac{a/c}{b/d} = ad/bc$.

Exercise 8.8 Use the results from Exercise 8.5 to calculate the odds ratio for smoking among the mothers of Down syndrome babies compared to mothers of healthy babies, for: (a) mothers aged under 35; (b) mothers aged 35 and over. Interpret your results.

Remember that the risk ratios and odds ratios in the coronary heart disease and in the stroke examples above are *sample* risk and odds ratios. For instance, from the *sample* risk ratio of 1.928 in the CHD/weight at one year study, you can infer that the *population* risk ratio is also *about* 1.93 ± a 'bit'. But how big is this 'bit', how precise is your estimate? This is a question I'll address in Chapter 11.

Finally, I mentioned earlier that most people are happier with the concept of 'risk' than with 'odds', but that you can't calculate risk in a case-control study. However, there is a happy ending. The odds ratio in a case-control study is a reasonably good estimator of the equivalent risk ratio, so you can at least approximate its value with the corresponding odds ratio.

Number needed to treat (NNT)

This seems as good a time as any to discuss a measure of the effectiveness of a clinical procedure which is related to risk; more precisely, to absolute risk. This is the *number needed to treat*, or NNT. NNT is the number of patients who would need to be treated with the active procedure, rather than a placebo (or alternative procedure), in order to reduce by one the number of patients experiencing the condition.

To explain NNT let's go back to the example for weighing 18 lbs or less at one year as a risk factor for coronary heart disease (CHD). The absolute risk of CHD among those weighing 18 lbs or less was 0.2667. The absolute risk of CHD for those weighing more than 18 lbs was 0.1382.

We need now to define the *absolute risk reduction or ARR* as the difference between two absolute risks. So in this example, the absolute risk reduction is the difference in these two absolute risks – the reduction in risk gained by weighing more than 18 lbs at one year rather than weighing 18 lbs or less. In this case:

$$ARR = 0.2667 - 0.1382 = 0.1285$$

Now the number needed to treat is defined as follows: NNT = 1/ARR
   Thus in this case: NNT = 1/0.1285 = 7.78

In other words, if you had some treatment (infant-care advice for vulnerable parents, for example), which would cause infants who would otherwise have weighed less than 18 lbs at one year to weigh 18 lbs or more, then you would need to 'treat' eight infants (or their parents) to ensure that one of these infants did not develop coronary heart disease when an adult.[2] NNT is often used to give a familiar and practical meaning to outcomes from clinical trials and systematic reviews,[3] where measures of risk, and risk ratios, may be difficult to translate into the potential benefit to patients.

An example from practice

Table 8.6 is from the follow-up (cohort) study into the effectiveness of carotid endarterectomy in ipsilateral stroke prevention first referred to in Figure 3.2 (Inzitari *et al.* 2000). The table shows that for any stroke, the (absolute) risk if treated medically is 0.110 (11.0 per cent), and if treated surgically is 0.051 (5.1 per cent). The reduction in absolute risk, ARR = 0.110 - 0.051 = 0.059 (5.9 per cent). So NNT = 1/0.059 = 16.95 or 17, at five years. In other words, 17 patients would have to be treated with carotid endarterectomy to prevent one patient from having a stroke within five years who, without the treatment, would otherwise have done so.

---

[2] The number must always be rounded up.
[3] Systematic review is the systematic collection of all the results from as many similarly-designed studies as possible dealing with the same clinical problem. I discuss this procedure in Chapter 20.

Table 8.6 Example of numbers needed to treat (NNT), at five years and two years from a follow-up (cohort) study into the effectiveness of carotid endarterectomy in stroke prevention. Reproduced from *NEJM*, **342**, 1693–9, by permission of Massachusetts Medical Society

Cause	Medically Treated Group	Surgically Treated Group	Reduction in Risk	Absolute Difference in Risk	No. Needed to Treat*	
					at 5 yr	at 2 yr
Any stroke[†]	11.0	5.1	54	5.9	17	67
Large-artery stroke[‡]	6.6	3.1	54	3.5	29	111

*The number needed to treat is calculated as the reciprocal of the difference in risk. At two years, the number needed to treat is based on estimated differences in risk of 1.5 percent for stroke of any cause and 0.9 percent for large-artery stroke.

[†]The risk of stroke from any cause in the medical and surgical groups in the Asymptomatic Carotid Atherosclerosis Study is shown.

[‡]The estimates of the risk of large-artery stroke were based on the observations that for subjects in the NASCET with 60 to 99 percent stenosis, the ratio of the risk of large-artery stroke to the risk of stroke from any cause in the territory of a symptomatic artery was similar in the medically and surgically treated subjects, and the risk of large-artery stroke was approximately 60 percent of the risk of stroke from any cause in the territory of an asymptomatic artery (i.e., 6.6 percent = 60 percent of 11.0 percent, and 3.1 percent = 60 percent of 5.1 percent).

Exercise 8.9 In a cohort study of a possible connection between dental disease and coronary heart disease (CHD), subjects were tracked for 14 years (deStefano *et al.*). Of 3542 subjects with no dental disease, 92 died from CHD, while of 1786 subjects with periodontitis, 151 died from CHD. How many people must be successfully treated for periodontitis to prevent one person dying from CHD?

V

The Informed Guess – Confidence Interval Estimation

9

Estimating the value of a *single* population parameter – the idea of confidence intervals

Learning objectives

When you have finished this chapter you should be able to:

- Describe the sampling distribution of the sample mean and the characteristics of its distribution.

- Explain what the standard error of the sample mean is and calculate its value.

- Explain how you can use the probability properties of the Normal distribution to measure the preciseness of the sample mean as an estimator of the population mean.

- Derive an expression for the confidence interval of the population mean.

- Calculate and interpret a 95 per cent confidence interval for a population mean.

- Calculate and interpret a 95 per cent confidence interval for a population proportion.

- Explain and interpret a 95 per cent confidence interval for a population median.

Medical Statistics from Scratch, Second Edition   David Bowers
© 2008 John Wiley & Sons, Ltd

Confidence interval estimation for a population mean

You saw at the beginning of Chapter 6 that we can use a sample statistic to make an informed guess, or *estimate,* of the value of the corresponding *population* parameter. For example, the sample mean birthweight for the 30 infants in Table 2.5 was 3644.4 g, so you can estimate the population mean birthweight of *all* infants of whom this sample is representative, also to be *about* 3644 g,[1] plus or minus some (hopefully) small random or *sampling error*. The obvious questions are:

- How small is this 'plus or minus' bit?

- Can it be *quantified?*

- Can we establish how *precise* our *sample* mean birthweight is as an estimate of population mean birthweight?

- How close to a population mean can you expect any given sample mean to be?

As you can see these are all essentially the same question, 'How big an *error* might we be making when we use the sample mean as an estimate of the population mean?'. This question can be answered with what is known as a *confidence interval estimator,* which is a numeric expression that quantifies the likely size of the sampling error. But to get a confidence interval we need first to introduce an important concept in statistical inference – the *standard error*.

The standard error of the mean

Our sample of 30 infants produced a sample mean birthweight of 3644.4 g. You could take a second, different, sample of 30 infants from the same population, and this sample would produce a different value for the sample mean. And a third sample, and a fourth and so on. In fact from any realistic population you could (*in theory*), take a huge number of different same-size samples, each of which would produce a different sample mean. You would end up with a large number of sample means, and if you were to arrange all of these sample means into a frequency curve, you would find:

- That it was Normal. This Normal-ness of the distribution of sample means is a very useful quality (to say the least); we will depend on it a lot in what is to come.

- That it was centred around the true population mean. In other words, the mean of all possible sample means is the same as the population mean.

This is very re-assuring. It means that, *on average,* the sample mean estimates the population mean exactly. But note the 'on average'. A particular *single* sample mean may still be some distance from the true mean.

---

[1] The value of the sample mean of 3644.4g is known as the *point estimate* of the population mean. It's the *single best guess* you could make as to the value of the population mean.

We can measure the spread of all of these different sample means in the usual way - with the standard deviation. However, to distinguish it from the spread of values in a *single* sample, we call it the *standard error*.[2] It is usually abbreviated as s.e.($\bar{x}$), where the symbol $\bar{x}$ stands for the sample mean. Remember that the standard deviation is a measure of the spread of the data in a *single* sample. The standard error is a measure of the spread in *all* (same-size) sample means from a population.

We can very easily *estimate* the standard error with the equation: s.e.($\bar{x}$) = $s/\sqrt{n}$. Here s is the sample standard deviation and n is the sample size. Notice that as the sample size n increases, the standard error decreases. In other words, the bigger the sample, the smaller the error in our estimate of population mean. Intuitively this feels right.

For example, if we took a sample of size $n = 100$ from a population, and measured systolic blood pressure, and obtained a sample mean of 135 mmHg and a sample standard deviation of 3 mmHg, then the estimated standard error would be:

$$s.e.(\bar{X}) = 3/\sqrt{100} = 3/10 = 0.33 \, mmHg$$

Since the distribution of sample means is Normal, we can make use of the area properties of the Normal distribution (see Figure 5.5). If the sample standard deviation is 3 mmHg and sample size $n = 100$, then the standard error = 0.33 mmHg. Because the distribution of sample means is Normal, this means that about 95 per cent of sample means will lie within plus or minus two standard errors of the population mean. That is within plus or minus 0.66 mmHg of the population mean. In other words there's a pretty good chance (a probability of 0.95 in fact) that any single sample mean will be no further than 0.66 mmHg from the (unknown) population mean.

The above discussion about taking lots of different samples from a population is entirely theoretical. In practice, you will usually only get to take *one* sample from a population, the value of whose mean you will never know. To sum up, the standard error is a measure of the preciseness of the sample mean as an estimator of the population mean. Smaller is better. If you are comparing the precision of two different sample means as estimates of a population mean, the sample mean with the smallest standard error is likely to be the more precise.

Exercise 9.1   A team of researchers used a cohort study to investigate the intake of vitamins E and C and the risk of lung cancer, 19 years into the study (Yong *et al.* 1997). They calculated the mean (and the standard error) intake of vitamins E and C, of individuals with and without lung cancer (cases and non-cases respectively). These were:

Vitamin E.   Cases: 6.03 mg (0.35 mg);   non-cases: 6.30 mg (0.05 mg).
Vitamin C.   Cases: 64.18 mg (5.06 mg);   non-cases: 82.21 mg (0.80 mg).

How would you interpret these results in terms of the likely precision of each of the sample means as estimators of their respective population means?

---

[2] To give it its full name, the *standard error of the sampling distribution of the sample mean* (quite a mouthful), but thankfully, it is usually just called the *standard error*.

How we use the standard error of the mean to calculate a confidence interval for a population mean

With the standard error under our belt we can now get to grips with the confidence interval. You have seen that we can be 95 per cent confident that any sample mean is going to be within plus or minus two standard errors of the population mean.[3] From this we can show that:

$$\text{Population mean} = \text{sample mean} \pm 2 \times \text{standard error}$$

That is:

- We can be 95 per cent confident that the interval, from the sample mean $- 2 \times$ standard error, to the sample mean $+ 2 \times$ standard error, will include the population mean.

- Or in probability terms, there is a probability of 0.95 that the interval from the sample mean $- 2 \times$ standard error, to the sample mean $+ 2 \times$ standard error, will contain the population mean.

In other words, if you pick one out of all the possible sample means at random, there is a probability of 0.95 that it will lie within two standard errors of the population mean. We call the distance from the sample mean $- 2 \times$ s.e.$(\bar{x})$, to the sample mean $+ 2 \times$ s.e.$(\bar{x})$, the *confidence interval.*

   The above result means that you now quantify just how close a sample mean is likely to be to the population mean. For obvious reasons the value you get when you put some figures into this expression is known as the *95 per cent confidence interval estimate* of the population mean. A 95 per cent *confidence level* is most common, but 99 per cent confidence intervals are also used on occasion. Note that the confidence interval is sometimes said to represent a *plausible range of values* for the population parameter.

A worked example from practice

In the cord-platelet count histogram in Figure 4.6, the mean cord platelet count in a sample of 4382 infants is 306×10^9/l, and the standard deviation is 69×10^9/l, so the standard error of the mean is:

$$\text{s.e.}(\bar{X}) = 69 \times 10^9 / \sqrt{4382} = 1.042 \times 10^9 / l$$

---

[3] I have used the value two in all of these expressions as a convenient *approximation* to the exact value (which in any case will be very close to two, when the probability is 0.95). The exact value comes from what is known as the *t distribution*. The *t* distribution is similar to the Normal distribution, but for small sample sizes is slightly wider and flatter. It is used instead of the Normal distribution for reasons connected to inferences about the population standard deviation, which we don't need to go into here. Anyway, in practice you will use a computer to obtain your confidence interval result. This will use the proper value.

Therefore the 95 per cent confidence interval for the population mean cord platelet count is:

$$(306 - 2 \times 1.042 \text{ to } 306 + 2 \times 1.042) \text{ g or } (303.916 \text{ to } 308.084) \times 10^9/l$$

Which we can interpret as follows: we can be 95 per cent confident that the population mean cord platelet count is between $303.916 \times 10^9/l$ and $308.084 \times 10^9/l$, or alternatively that there's a probability of 0.95 that the interval from 303.916 to 308.084 will contain the population mean value. Of course there's also a 5 per cent chance (or a 0.05 probability), that it will not!

Alternatively we can say that the interval (303.916 to 308.084) $\times 10^9/l$ represents a *plausible range of values* for the population mean cord platelet count. The narrower the confidence interval the more precise is the estimator. In the cord platelet example, the small width, and therefore high precision of the confidence interval, is due to the large sample. By the way, it's good practice to put the confidence interval in brackets and use the 'to' in the middle and not a '–' sign, since this may be confusing if the confidence interval has a negative value(s).

Exercise 9.2   Use the summary age measures given in Table 1.6 for the life events and breast cancer study, to calculate the standard error and the 95 per cent confidence intervals for population mean age of: (a) the cases; (b) the controls. Interpret your confidence intervals. What do you make of the fact that the two confidence intervals don't overlap?

An example from practice

The results in Table 9.1 are from a randomised trial to evaluate the use of an integrated care scheme for asthma patients, in which care is shared between the GP and a specialist chest physician (Grampian Asthma Study 1994). The treatment group patients each received this integrated care, the control group received conventional care from their GP only. The researchers were interested in the differences between the groups, if any, in a number of outcomes, shown in the figure (ignore the last column for now). The target population they have in mind is, perhaps, all asthma patients in the UK.

Table 9.1   Means and 95 per cent confidence intervals for a number of clinical outcomes over 12 months, for asthma patients. The treatment group patients received integrated care, the control group conventional GP care. Reproduced from *BMJ*, **308**, 559–64, courtesy of BMJ Publishing Group

Clinical outcome	Integrated care ($n \geq 296$)	Conventional care ($n \geq 277$)	Ratio of means
No of bronchodilators prescribed	10.1 (9.2 to 11.1)	10.6 (9.7 to 11.7)	0.95 (0.83 to 1.09)
No of inhaled steroids prescribed	6.4 (5.9 to 6.9)	6.5 (6.1 to 7.1)	0.98 (0.88 to 1.09)
No of courses of oral steroids used	1.6 (1.4 to 1.8)	1.6 (1.4 to 1.9)	0.97 (0.79 to 1.20)
No of general practice asthma consultations	2.7 (2.4 to 3.1)	2.5 (2.2 to 2.8)	1.11 (0.95 to 1.31)
No of hospital admissions for asthma	0.15 (0.11 to 0.19)	0.11 (0.08 to 0.15)	1.31 (0.87 to 1.96)

Means and 95% confidence interval are estimated from Poisson regression models after controlling for initial peak flow, forced expiratory volume (as % of predicted), and duration af asthma.

You can see that in the integrated care group of 296 subjects, the *sample* mean number of bronchodilators prescribed over 12 months was 10.1, with a 95 per cent confidence interval for the *population* mean of (9.2 to 11.1). So you can be 95 per cent confident that the population mean number of bronchodilators prescribed for this group is somewhere between 9.2 and 11.1. In the control group, the sample mean is 10.6 with a 95 per cent confidence interval for the population mean (9.7 to 11.7), which can be similarly interpreted.

Exercise 9.3   Interpret and compare the sample mean number of hospital admissions, and their corresponding confidence intervals, for the two groups in Table 9.1.

Confidence intervals as described above can also be applied to a population *percentage,* provided that the values are percentages of a metric variable, for example percentage mortality across a number of hospitals following some procedure (see, for example, Table 2.7). However, if the data is a proportion or percentage of a nominal or ordinal variable, say the proportion of patients with a pressure sore, or the proportion of mothers with an Edinburgh Maternal Depression Scale score of more than 8, then a different approach, described next, is needed.

Confidence interval for a population proportion

We start with an expression for the standard error of the sample proportion:

$$\text{s.e.} = (p)\sqrt{\frac{p(1-p)}{n}}$$

where p is the sample proportion, and n is sample size. Incidentally, the sampling distribution of sample proportions has a binomial distribution, which is quite different from the Normal distribution if the sample is small, but becomes more Normal as sample size increases. The 95 per cent confidence interval for the population proportion is equal to the sample proportion plus or minus 1.96 [4] standard errors:

$$\{[p - 1.96 \times \text{s.e.}(p)] \text{ to } [p + 1.96 \times \text{s.e.}(p)]\}$$

For example, from Table 1.6, 14 of the 106 women with a malignant diagnosis are premenopausal giving a sample proportion p of 14/106 or 0.13. The standard error of p is thus:

$$\text{s.e.}(p) = \sqrt{\frac{0.13(1-0.13)}{106}} = 0.033$$

Therefore the 95 per cent confidence interval for the population proportion who are

---

[4] When we are dealing with proportions, we use, not the *t* distribution, but the *z*, or *Standard Normal*, distribution. The 95 per cent value for *z* is 1.96.

pre-menopausal is:

$$(0.13 - 1.96 \times 0.033 \text{ to } 0.13 + 1.96 \times 0.033) = (0.065 \text{ to } 0.195)$$

In other words you can be 95 per cent confident that the proportion of cases in this population who are pre-menopausal lies somewhere between 0.065 to 0.195. Or alternatively, that this interval represents a plausible range of values for the population proportion who are menopausal.

Exercise 9.4   Calculate the standard error for the sample proportion of controls in Table 1.6 who are pre-menopausal, and hence calculate the 95 per cent confidence interval for the corresponding population proportion. Interpret your result.

Estimating a confidence interval for the median of a single population

If your data is ordinal then the median rather than the mean is the appropriate measure of location (review Chapter 5 if you're not sure why). Alternatively, if your data is metric but skewed (or your sample is too small to check the distributional shape), you might also prefer the median as a more representative measure. Either way a confidence interval will enable you to assess the likely range of values for the population median. As far as I know, SPSS does not calculate a confidence interval for a single median, but Minitab does, and bases its calculation on the *Wilcoxon signed-rank* test[5] (I'll discuss this in Chapter 12).

Table 9.2   Sample median pain levels, and 95 per cent confidence intervals for the difference between the two groups, at three time periods, in the analgesics/stump pain study. Reproduced courtesy of Elsevier (*The Lancet*, 1994, Vol No. **344**, page 1724–6)

	Median (IQR) pain		
	Blockade group (n = 27)	Control group (n = 29)	95% CI for difference (p)
After epidural bolus	0 (0–0)	38 (17–67)	24 to 43 (p < 0.0001)
After continuous epidural infusion	0 (0–0)	31 (20–51)	24 to 43 (p < 0.0001)
After epidural bolus in operating theatre	0 (0–0)	35 (16–64)	19 to 42 (p < 0.0001)

Pain assessed by visual analogue scale (0–100 mm).

---

[5] We won't deal with tests (i.e. *hypothesis tests*) until we get to Chapter 12, but the confidence intervals that I discuss in this and in the next chapter are based on a number of different hypothesis tests. The alternative would have been for me to introduce hypothesis tests before I dealt with confidence intervals. However, for various pedagogic reasons I didn't think this was appropriate.

An example from practice

Table 9.2 is from the analgesics and stump pain study referred to in Table 5.3, and shows the sample median pain levels and their 95 per cent confidence intervals (assessed using a visual analogue scale), for the treatment and control groups, at three time periods.

> **Exercise 9.5**   In Table 9.2, interpret and compare the differences in median pain levels and their 95 per cent confidence intervals for each of the three time periods.

10

Estimating the difference between two population parameters

Learning objectives

When you have finished this chapter you should be able to:

- Give some examples of situations where there is a need to estimate the difference between two population parameters.

- Very briefly outline the basis of estimation of the difference between two population means using methods based on the two-sample t test[1] (for independent populations) and the matched-pairs t test (for matched populations).

- Very briefly outline the basis of estimation of the difference between two population medians using methods based on the Mann-Whitney test (for independent populations) and the Wilcoxon test (for matched populations).

- Interpret results from studies that estimate the difference between two population means, two percentages or two medians.

- Demonstrate an awareness of any assumptions that must be satisfied when estimating the difference between two population parameters.

---

[1] Throughout this chapter we will be looking at methods of estimation based on various *hypothesis tests*. I will begin to discuss hypothesis tests properly in Chapter 12.

Medical Statistics from Scratch, Second Edition   David Bowers
© 2008 John Wiley & Sons, Ltd

What's the difference?

As you have just seen, it's possible to determine a confidence interval for any single population parameter – a population mean, a median, a percentage and so on. However, by far the most common application of confidence intervals is the *comparison* of *two* population parameters, for example between the means of two populations, such as the mean age of a population of women and the mean age of a population of men; I'll start with this.

Estimating the difference between the means of two independent populations – using a method based on the two-sample *t* test

The procedure here, like that for the single mean (see Chapter 9), is based on the *t* distribution (see the footnote on p. 114). However, with two populations, you need to know if they are *independent* or *matched* (see p. 81 to review matching). I'll start with estimating the difference in the means of two *independent* populations, since this is by far the most common in practice. For this we use a method based on the *two-sample* t *test*. First, there are a number of prerequisites that need to be met:

- Data for both groups must be *metric*. As you know from Chapter 5 the mean is only appropriate with metric data anyway.

- The distribution of the relevant variable in *each* population must be reasonably *Normal*. You can check this assumption from the sample data using a histogram, although with small sample sizes this can be difficult.

- The population standard deviations of the two variables concerned should be *approximately* the same, but this requirement becomes less important as sample sizes get larger. You can check this by examining the two sample standard deviations.[2]

An example using birthweights

Suppose you want to compare (by estimating the difference between them), the population mean birthweights of infants born in a maternity unit with that of infants born at home (sample data in Table 10.1). The two samples were selected independently with no attempt at matching.

Both SPSS and Minitab compute the sample mean birthweight of the home-born infants to be 3726.5 g, with a standard deviation of 385.7 g. Recall that for the infants born in the maternity units, sample mean birthweight was 3644.4 g with a standard deviation of 376.8 g (see p. 112). So there *is* a difference in the *sample* mean birthweights of 82.1 g, (3726.5 g − 3644.4 g), but this does *not* mean that there is a difference in the *population* mean birthweights.

---

[2] This condition is usually stated in terms of the two *variances* being approximately the same. Variance is standard deviation squared.

Table 10.1   Sample data for birthweight (g), Apgar scores and whether mother smoked during pregnancy for 30 infants born in a maternity unit and 30 born at home

Infant	Birthweight (g)		Mother smoked		Apgar score	
	Hospital birth[a]	Home birth	Hospital birth	Home birth	Hospital birth	Home birth
1	3710	3810	0	0	8	10
2	3650	3865	0	0	7	8
3	4490	4578	0	0	8	9
4	3421	3522	1	0	6	6
5	3399	3400	0	1	6	7
6	4094	4156	0	0	9	10
7	4006	4200	0	0	8	9
8	3287	3265	1	0	5	6
9	3594	3599	0	1	7	8
10	4206	4215	0	0	9	10
11	3508	3697	0	0	7	8
12	4010	4209	0	0	8	9
13	3896	3911	0	0	8	8
14	3800	3943	0	0	8	9
15	2860	3000	0	1	4	3
16	3798	3802	0	0	8	9
17	3666	3654	0	0	7	8
18	4200	4295	1	0	9	10
19	3615	3732	0	0	7	8
20	3193	3098	1	1	4	5
21	2994	3105	1	1	5	5
22	3266	3455	1	0	5	6
23	3400	3507	0	0	6	7
24	4090	4103	0	0	8	9
25	3303	3456	1	0	6	7
26	3447	3538	1	0	6	7
27	3388	3400	1	1	6	7
28	3613	3715	0	0	7	7
29	3541	3566	0	0	7	8
30	3886	4000	1	0	8	6

[a] This is the data from Table 2.5.

It is important to remember that a difference between two sample values does not necessarily mean that there is a difference in the two population values. Any difference in these sample birthweight means might simply be due to chance. Now we come to an important point:

> If the 95 per cent confidence interval for the difference between two population parameters includes zero, then you can be 95 per cent confident that there is *no* difference in the two parameter values. If the interval *doesn't* contain zero, then you can be 95 per cent confident that there *is* a statistically significant difference in the means.

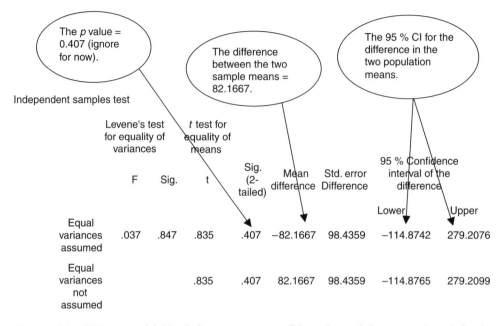

Figure 10.1 SPSS output (abridged) for 95 per cent confidence interval (last two columns) for the difference between two independent population mean birthweights, using samples of 30 infants born in maternity units and 30 at home (data in Table 10.1)

In other words, if you want to know if there is a statistically significant difference between two population means, calculate the 95 per cent confidence interval for the difference and see if it contains zero.

It is possible to calculate these confidence intervals by hand, but the process is time-consuming and tedious. Fortunately, most statistics programs will do it for you. Since difference between independent population means is one of the most commonly used approaches in clinical research, you might find it helpful to see some of the output from SPSS and Minitab for this procedure.

With SPSS

Using the birthweight data in Table 10.1, SPSS produces the results (abridged[3]) shown in Figure 10.1. These tell us that the difference in the two *sample* mean birthweights is −82.17 g. The sign in front of this value depends on which variable you select first in the SPSS dialogue box. SPSS subtracts the second variable selected (home births in this case) from the first (maternity unit births). This result means that the sample mean birthweight was 82.17 g higher in the home birth infants.

SPSS calculates two confidence intervals, one with standard deviations[4] assumed to be equal, and one with them not equal. The 95 per cent confidence interval shown in the last two columns

---

[3] I've removed material that is not relevant.
[4] Both Minitab and SPSS refer to equality of *variances*.

is (−114.9 to 279.2)g, the same in both cases. SPSS tests for equality of the standard deviations (or *variances*), using Levene's test. The assumption is that they are the same. We will discuss tests in Chapter 12.

Since this confidence interval includes zero, you can conclude that there is no statistically significant difference in *population* mean birthweights of infants born in a maternity unit and infants born at home.

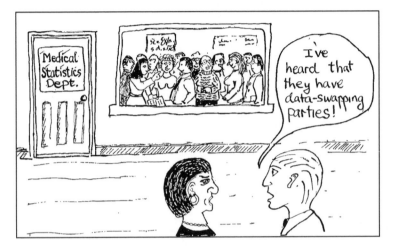

With Minitab   The Minitab output, which confirms that from SPSS, is shown in Figure 10.2. The 95 per cent confidence interval is in the second row up.

An example from practice

Table 10.2 is from a cohort study of maternal smoking during pregnancy and infant growth after birth (Conter *et al* 1995). The subjects were 12 987 babies who were followed up for three years after birth. Of these, 10 238 had non-smoking mothers, 2276 had mothers who had

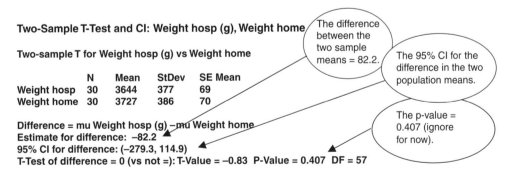

Figure 10.2   Minitab output for 95 per cent confidence interval for the difference between two independent population mean birthweights, using samples of 30 infants born in maternity units and 30 at home. Note that Minitab uses the word 'mu' to denote the population mean, normally designated as Greek μ

Table 10.2 95 per cent confidence intervals for difference in weights according to sex and smoking habits of mothers between independent groups of babies. Reproduced from *BMJ*, **310**, 768–71, courtesy of BMJ Publishing Group

Mother's smoking habit	At birth			At 3 months			At 6 monts		
	No. children	Weight (g)	95%CI for difference	No. children	Weight (g)	95%CI for difference	No. children	Weight (g)	95%CI for difference
Girls									
Non-smokers	4904	3220		4904	5584		4895	7462	
1–9 cigs per day	1072	3132	(−121 to −55)	1071	5550	(−77 to 9)	1072	7471	(−47 to 65)
≥10 per day	228	3052	(−234 to −102)	228	5519	(−152 to 22)	227	7434	(−141 to 85)
Boys									
Non-smokers	5334	3373		5332	6026		5330	8038	
1–9 cigs per day	1204	3266	(−139 to −75)	1204	5958	(−113 to −23)	1204	7974	(−118 to −10)
≥10 cigs per day	245	3126	(−312 to −181)	245	5907	(−212 to −26)	245	8014	(−136 to 88)

smoked one to nine cigarettes a day, and 473 had mothers who had smoked 10 or more cigarettes a day. The figure shows the 95 per cent confidence intervals for differences in mean weight according to sex of baby and smoking habits of mothers: at birth, and at three and six months.

The results show, for example, that at birth, the difference between the sample mean weight of female babies born to non-smoking mothers and those born to mothers smoking 10 or more cigarettes a day, was $(3220 - 3052) = 168$ g. That is, the infants of smoking mothers are on average lighter by 168 g. Is this difference statistically significant in the population, or due simply to chance? The 95 per cent confidence interval of $(-234$ to $-102)$ g, does *not* include zero, so you can be 95 per cent confident that the difference is real, i.e. is statistically significant.

Exercise 10.1   Interpret the sample mean and confidence intervals shown in Table 10.2 for all four differences in weights at six months.

Estimating the difference between two matched population means – using a method based on the matched-pairs *t* test

If the data within each of the two groups whose means you are comparing is widely spread compared to the difference in the spreads between the groups,[5] this can make it more difficult to detect any difference in their means. When data is matched (see Chapter 7 for an explanation of matching), this reduces much of the within-group variation, and, for a given sample size, makes it easier to detect any differences between groups. As a consequence, you can achieve better precision (narrower confidence intervals), without having to increase sample size. The disadvantage of matching is that it is sometimes difficult to find a sufficiently large number of matches (as you saw in the case-control discussion earlier).

In the independent groups case, the mean of each group is computed separately, and then a confidence interval for the difference in these means is calculated. In the matched groups case, we use a method based on the *matched-pairs* t *test*, in which the *difference* between each pair of values is computed first and then a confidence interval for the mean of these differences is calculated.

An example from practice

Table 10.3 shows the 95 per cent confidence intervals for the difference in bone mineral density in two matched groups of women, one group depressed and one 'normal' (Michelson *et al.* 1995). (Ignore the 'SD from expected peak' rows.) Only one of the confidence intervals contains zero, indicating that there is no difference in population mean bone mineral density at the radius, but there is at all of the other five sites.

---

[5] Called 'between-group' variation.

Table 10.3 Confidence intervals for the differences between the population mean bone mineral densities in two individually *matched* groups of women, one group depressed, the other 'normal', using a method based on the matched-pairs t test. Reproduced from *NEJM*, **335**, 1176–81, by permission of Massachusetts Medical Society

Bone Measured[†]	Depressed Women	Normal Women	Mean Difference (95% CI)	P Value
Lumbar spine (anteroposterior)				
Density (g/cm²)	1.00 ± 0.15	1.07 ± 0.09	0.08 (0.02 to 0.14)	0.02
SD from expected peak	-0.42 ± 1.28	0.26 ± 0.82	0.68 (0.13 to 1.33)	
Lumbar spine (lateral)[‡]				
Density (g/cm²)	0.74 ± 0.09	0.79 ± 0.07	0.05 (0.00 to 0.09)	0.03
SD from expected peak	-0.88 ± 1.07	-0.36 ± 0.80	0.50 (0.04 to 1.03)	
Femoral neck				
Density (g/cm²)	0.76 ± 0.11	0.88 ± 0.11	0.11 (0.06 to 0.17)	<0.00
SD from expected peak	-1.30 ± 1.07	-0.22 ± 0.99	1.08 (0.55 to 1.61)	
Ward's triangle				
Density (g/cm²)	0.70 ± 0.14	0.81 ± 0.13	0.11 (0.06 to 0.17)	<0.00
SD from expected peak	-0.93 ± 1.24	0.18 ± 1.22	1.11 (0.60 to 1.62)	
Trochanter				
Density (g/cm²)	0.66 ± 0.11	0.74 ± 0.08	0.08 (0.04 to 0.13)	<0.001
SD from expected peak	-0.70 ± 1.22	0.26 ± 0.91	0.97 (0.46 to 1.47)	
Radius				
Density (g/cm²)	0.68 ± 0.04	0.70 ± 0.04	0.01 (−0.01 to 0.04)	0.25
SD from expected peak	-0.19 ± 0.67	0.03 ± 0.67	0.21 (−0.21 to 0.64)	

[*]Plus-minus values are means ± SD. CI denotes confidence interval.
[†]Values for "SD from expected peak" are the numbers of standard deviations from the expected peak density derived from a population-based study of normal white women.[3]
[‡]This measurement was made in 23 depressed women and 23 normal women.

Exercise 10.2 In Table 10.3, which population difference in bone mineral density is estimated with the greatest precision?

You can also calculate a confidence interval for the difference in two population *percentages* provided they derive from two metric variables. For the difference between two population proportions, however, a different approach is needed. This is an extension of the single proportion case discussed in Chapter 9, as you will now see.

Estimating the difference between two independent population proportions

Suppose you want to calculate a 95 per cent confidence interval for the difference between the population proportion of women having maternity unit births who smoked during pregnancy and the proportion having home births who smoked. The sample data on smoking status for the sample of 60 mothers is shown in Table 10.1.

There are 10 mothers who smoked among the 30 giving birth in the maternity unit and six among the 30 giving birth at home. This gives sample proportions of $10/30 = 0.3333$, and $6/30 = 0.2000$, respectively. You can check whether this difference is statistically significant or likely to be due to chance alone, by calculating a 95 per cent confidence interval for the difference in the corresponding population proportions.[6] To do this by hand is a bit long-winded and you would want to use a computer program to do the calculation for you.

An example from practice

If you look back at Table 9.1, the randomised trial of integrated versus conventional care for asthma patients, the last column shows the 95 per cent confidence intervals for the difference in population percentages between the two groups, for a number of patient perceptions of the scheme. As you can see, none of the confidence intervals include zero, so you can be 95 per cent confident that the difference in population percentages between the groups of patients is statistically significant in each case.

Estimating the difference between two independent population medians – the Mann–Whitney rank-sums method

As you know from Chapter 5, the mean may not be the most representative measure of location if the data is skewed, and is not appropriate anyway if the data is ordinal. In these circumstances, you can compare the population *medians* rather than the means, and in place of the 2-sample t test (a parametric procedure), use a method based on the *Mann–Whitney* test (a non-parametric procedure).

Parametric versus non-parametric methods

A *parametric* procedure can be applied to data which is metric, and also has some particular distribution, most commonly the Normal distribution. A *non-parametric* procedure does not make these distributional requirements. So if you are analysing data that is either metric but not Normal, or is ordinal, then you need to use a non-parametric approach. The Mann–Whitney procedure only requires that the two population distributions have the same approximate shape, but does not require either to be Normal. It is the non-parametric equivalent of the two-sample t test.

Briefly, the Mann–Whitney method starts by combining the data from both groups, which are then ranked. The rank values for each group are then separated and summed. If the medians of the two groups are the same, then the sums of the ranks of the two groups should be

---

[6] The 95 per cent confidence interval is (-0.088 to 0.355). Since this interval includes 0, we conclude that there is no difference in the proportion of mothers who smoked at home and in the maternity unit.

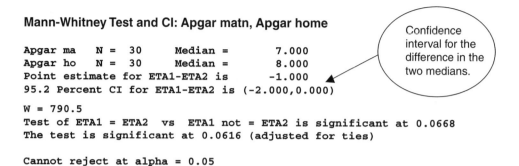

```
Mann-Whitney Test and CI: Apgar matn, Apgar home

Apgar ma    N =  30       Median =        7.000
Apgar ho    N =  30       Median =        8.000
Point estimate for ETA1-ETA2 is       -1.000
95.2 Percent CI for ETA1-ETA2 is (-2.000,0.000)

W = 790.5
Test of ETA1 = ETA2  vs  ETA1 not = ETA2 is significant at 0.0668
The test is significant at 0.0616 (adjusted for ties)

Cannot reject at alpha = 0.05
```

Confidence interval for the difference in the two medians.

Figure 10.3   Minitab's Mann–Whitney output for a 95 per cent confidence interval for the difference between two independent median Apgar scores – for infants born in maternity units and at home (raw data in Table 10.1). Note that Minitab uses Greek 'ETA' to denote the population median

similar. However, if the rank sums are different, you need to know whether this difference could simply be due to chance, or is because there really is a statistically significant difference in the population medians. A Mann–Whitney confidence interval for the difference will help you decide between these alternatives.

As an illustration, let's compare the difference in the population median Apgar scores for the maternity unit and home birth infants, using the sample data in Table 10.1. These are independent groups, but since this data is ordinal, we cannot use the two-sample *t* test, but we can use the Mann–Whitney test of medians. The output from Minitab is shown in Figure 10.3, with the 95 per cent confidence interval in the fourth row.[7] Since the confidence interval of (−2 to 0) contains zero, you must conclude that the difference in the population median Apgar scores is not statistically significant. Notice that the confidence level is given as 95.2 per cent, not 95 per cent. Confidence intervals for medians cannot always achieve the precise confidence level you asked for, because of the way in which a median is calculated.

An example from practice

Table 10.4 is from a randomised controlled double-blind trial to compare the cost effectiveness of two treatments in relieving pain after blunt instrument injury in an A&E department (Rainer *et al.* 2000). It shows the median times spent by two groups of patients in various clinical situations. One group received ketorolac, the other group morphine. The penultimate column contains the 95 per cent confidence intervals for the difference in various median treatment times (minutes), between the groups (ignore the last column). As the footnote to the table indicates, these results were obtained using the Mann–Whitney method.

The only confidence interval not containing zero is that for the difference in median 'time between receiving analgesia and leaving A&E', for which the difference in the sample medians is 20.0 minutes. So this is the only treatment time for which the difference in population median

---

[7] As far as I am aware, SPSS does not appear to calculate a confidence interval for two independent medians.

Table 10.4 Mann–Whitney confidence intervals for the difference between two *independent* groups of patients in their median times spent in several clinical situations. One group received ketorolac, the other morphine median number (interquartile range) of minutes relating to participants treatment. Reproduced from *BMJ*, **321**, 1247–51, courtesy of BMJ Publishing Group

Variable	Ketorolac group (n = 75)	Morphine group (n = 73)	Median difference (95% confidence interval)	P value[*]
Interval between arrival in emergency department and doctor prescribing analgesia	38.0 (30.0 to 54.0)	39.0 (29.0 to 53.0)	1.0 (−5.0 to 7.0)	0.72
Preparation for analgesia	5.0 (5.0 to 10.0)	10.0 (5.5 to 12.5)	2.0 (0 to 5.0)	0.0002
Undergoing radiography	5.0 (5.0 to 10.0)	5.0 (4.0 to 10.0)	0 (−1.0 to 0)	0.75
Total time spent in emergency department	155.0 (112.0 to 198.0)	171.0 (126.0 to 208.5)	15.0 (−4.0 to 33.0)	0.11
Interval between receiving analgesia and leaving emergency department	115.0 (75.0 to 149.0)	130.0 (95.0 to 170.0)	20.0 (4.0 to 39.0)	0.02

[*] Mann–Whitney U test.

Table 10.5 Confidence interval estimates from the Wilcoxon signed-ranks method for the difference in population food intakes per day, for a number of substances, from a study of the dietary habits of schizophrenics. Values are median (range). Reproduced from *BMJ*, **317**, 784–5, courtesy of BMJ Publishing Group

Intake/day	Men		Women		All		Wilcoxon signed ranks test	
	Patients (n=17)	Controls (n=17)	Patients (n=13)	Controls (n=13)	Patients (n=30)	Controls (n=30)	Median difference (95% CI)	P
Energy (MJ)	11.84 (7.67–17.93)	14.19 (6.94–23.22)	8.87 (5.07–13.02)	9.99 (5.25–16.25)	9.71 (5.07–17.94)	11.98 (5.25–23.22)	2.06 (0.26–4.23)	0.04
Protein (g)	92.5 (65.1–157.4)	114.2 (74–633)	68.7 (38.4–104.2)	82.5 (40.5–142.7)	84.5 (38.4–157.4)	96.0 (40.5 to 633.0)	15.9 (−1.1 to 32.8)	0.07
Total fibre (g)	13.0 (8.5–20.8)	22.0 (8.7–86.2)	10.7 (7.3–18.0)	15.5 (10.7–22.9)	12.6 (7.3–20.8)	18.9 (8.7–86.2)	7.0 (3.6 to 10.6)	0.0001
Retinol (μg)	647 (294–1498)	817 (134–12341)	533 (288–7556)	817 (201–11585)	590 (288–7556)	817 (134–12341)	310 (93 to 1269)	0.02
Carotene (μg)	783 (219–3638)	2510 (523–11313)	2048 (550–4657)	3079 (956–6188)	1443 (219–4657)	2798 (523–11313)	1376 (549 to 2452)	0.004
Vitamin C (mg)	41.0 (4.0–204)	81.0 (14.0–262)	40.0 (3–165)	61.0 (27.0–291.0)	40.5 (3.0–204)	80.5 (14.0–219)	33.5 (2.0 to 64.0)	0.03
Vitamin E (mg)	4.8 (3.4–18.0)	10.26 (2.23–32.0)	4.5 (2.3–6.0)	5.38 (3.6–14.7)	4.7 (2.3–18.0)	7.8 (2.2–32.0)	2.9 (1.45 to 5.35)	0.0002
Alcohol (g)	3.8 (0–19.4)	11.7 (0–80)	0 (0–5.6)	1.8 (0–12)	0 (0–19.4)	5.7 (0–80)	5.4 (1.2 to 9.9)	0.009

times is statistically significant, and you can be 95 per cent confident that this difference is between 4 and 39 minutes.

Exercise 10.3   Table 10.4 includes the sample median times and their 95 per cent confidence intervals for each time interval, for both groups separately. Only one pair of confidence intervals don't overlap, those for the only time difference which is statistically significant. Why aren't you surprised by this?

Estimating the difference between two matched population medians – Wilcoxon signed-ranks method

When two groups are *matched*, but either the data is ordinal, or if metric is noticeably skewed, you can obtain confidence intervals for differences in population medians, based on the non-parametric *Wilcoxon test*. The two population distributions, regardless of shape, should be symmetric. This is the non-parametric equivalent of the parametric matched-pairs *t* test, described above. The matching will again reduce the variation within groups, so narrower, and therefore more precise, confidence intervals are available for a given sample size.

Briefly the Wilcoxon method starts by calculating the difference between each pair of values, and these differences are then ranked (ignoring any minus signs). Any negative signs are then restored to the rank values, and the negative and positive ranks are separately summed. If the medians in the two groups are the same, then these two rank sums should be similar. If different, the Wilcoxon method provides a way of determining whether this is due to chance, or represents a statistically significant difference in the population medians.

An example from practice

Table 10.5 contains the results of a case-control study into the dietary intake of schizophrenic patients living in the community in Scotland (McCreadie *et al.* (1998). It shows the daily energy intake of eight dietary substances for the cases (17 men and 13 women diagnosed with schizophrenia), and the controls, each individually matched on sex, age, smoking status and employment status.

If you focus on the penultimate column, in which data for men and women is combined, you can see that only the confidence interval for daily protein intake, $(-1.1$ to $32.8)$ g, contains zero, which implies that there is no difference in population median protein intake between schizophrenics and normal individuals. For all other substances, the difference is statistically significant.

Exercise 10.4   Explain the meaning of the 95 per cent confidence interval for difference in median alcohol intake of the two groups in Table 10.5.

11
Estimating the *ratio* of two population parameters

Estimating ratios

Estimating the ratio of two independent population means

When you compare two population means you usually want to know if they're the same or not, and if not, how big the difference between them is. Sometimes though, you might want to know *how many times bigger* one population mean is than another. The *ratio* of the two means will tell us that.

Medical Statistics from Scratch, Second Edition   David Bowers
© 2008 John Wiley & Sons, Ltd

If two sample means have a ratio of 1, this tells us *only* that the means are the same size in the *sample*. If the sample ratio *is* different from 1, you need to check whether this is simply due to chance, or if the difference is statistically significant – one mean *is* bigger than the other. You can do this with a 95 per cent confidence interval for the ratio of population means. And here's the rule:

> If the confidence interval for the *ratio* of two population parameters does *not* contain the value 1, then you can be 95 per cent confident that any difference in the size of the two measures is statistically significant.

Compare this with the rule for the *difference* between two population parameters, where that rule is that if the confidence interval does *not* contain zero, then any difference between the two parameters *is* statistically significant.

An example from practice

Look again at the last column in Table 9.1, which shows a number of outcomes from a randomised trial to compare integrated versus conventional care for asthma patients. The last column contains the 95 per cent confidence intervals for the ratio of population means for the treatment and control groups. You will see that *all* of the confidence intervals contain 1, indicating that the population mean number of bronchodilators used, the number of inhaled steroids prescribed and so on, was no larger (or smaller) in one population than in the other.

The *sample* ratio furthest away from 1 is 1.31, for the ratio of mean number of hospital admissions, i.e. the *sample* of integrated care group patients had 31 per cent more admissions than the conventionally treated control group patients. However, the 95 per cent confidence interval of (0.87 to 1.96) includes 1, which implies that this is generally *not* the case in the populations.

Confidence interval for a population risk ratio

Table 6.1 showed the contingency table for a cohort study into the risk of coronary heart disease (CHD) as an adult, among men who weighed 18 lbs or less at 12 months old (the risk factor). On p. 104 we derived a risk ratio of 1.93 from this sample cohort. In other words, men who weighed 18 lbs or less at one year, appear to have nearly twice the risk of CHD when an adult, as men who weighed more than 18 lbs at one year. But is this true in the *population* of such men, or no more than a *chance* departure from a population ratio of 1? You now know that you can answer this question by examining the 95 per cent confidence interval for this risk ratio.

The 95 per cent confidence interval for the CHD risk ratio turns out to be (0.793 to 4.697).[1] Since this interval contains 1, you can conclude, that despite a *sample* risk ratio of nearly 2, that

---

[1] The calculation of confidence intervals for risk ratios and odds ratios is a step too far for this book. Those interested in doing the calculation by hand can consult Altman (1991) who gives the necessary formulae.

weighing 18 lbs or less at one year is *not* a significant risk factor for coronary heart disease in adult life in the sampled *population*. Notice that, in general, the value of a sample risk or odds ratio, as in this example, does *not* lie in the centre of its confidence interval, but is usually closer to the lower value.

An example from practice

Table 11.1 is from a cohort study of 552 men surviving acute myocardial infarction, in which each subject was assessed for depression at the beginning of the study (Ladwig *et al.* 1994). 14.5 per cent were identified as severely depressed, 2.3 per cent as moderately depressed, and 63.2 per cent had low levels of depression. The subjects were followed up at 6 months, and a number of outcomes measured, including: suffering angina, returning to work, emotional stability and smoking. The researchers were interested in examining the role of moderate and of severe depression (compared to low depression), as risk factors for each of these outcomes.

The results show the crude and adjusted risk ratios (labelled 'relative risks' by the authors) for each outcome. The crude risk ratios are *not* adjusted for any confounding factors, whereas the adjusted risk ratios *are* adjusted for the factors listed in the table footnote (review the material on confounding and adjustment in Chapter 7 if necessary).

Let's interpret the 95 per cent risk ratios for 'return to work'. The *crude* risk ratios for a return to work indicate lower rates of return to work for men both moderately depressed (risk

Table 11.1 The crude and adjusted risk ratios (labelled relative risk by the authors), for a number of outcomes related to the risk factor of experiencing moderate and severe levels of depression compared to low depression. Reprinted courtesy of Elsevier (*The Lancet*, 1994, Vol No. **343**, page 20–3)

	Relative risk (95% CI)	
Depression level	Crude	Adjusted[*]
Angina pectoris		
Moderate	1.36 (0.83 to 2.23)	0.97 (0.55 to 1.70)
Severe	3.12 (1.58 to 6.16)	2.31 (1.11 to 4.80)
Return to work		
Moderate	0.41 (0.22 to 0.77)	0.58 (0.28 to 1.17)
Severe	0.39 (0.18 to 0.88)	0.54 (0.22 to 1.31)
Emotional Instability		
Moderate	2.21 (1.33 to 3.69)	1.87 (1.07 to 3.27)
Severe	5.55 (2.87 to 10.71)	4.61 (2.32 to 9.18)
Smoking		
Moderate	1.39 (0.71 to 2.73)	1.19 (0.56 to 2.51)
Severe	2.63 (1.23 to 5.60)	2.84 (1.22 to 6.63)
Late potentials		
Moderate	1.30 (0.76 to 2.22)	1.54 (0.86 to 2.74)
Severe	0.70 (0.33 to 1.47)	0.75 (0.35 to 2.17)

[*]Adjusted for age, social class, recurrent infarction, rehabilitation, cardiac events and helplessness

ratio = 0.41), and severely depressed (risk ratio = 0.39), compared to men with low levels of depression. Neither of the confidence intervals, (0.22 to 0.77) and (0.18 to 0.88), includes 1, indicating statistical significance. However, after adjusting for possible confounding variables, the *adjusted* risk ratios are 0.58 and 0.54, and are no longer statistically significant, because the confidence intervals for both risk ratios, for moderate depression (0.28 to 1.17), and severe depression (0.22 to 1.31), now include 1.

Exercise 11.1   Table 11.2 is from the same cohort study referred to in Exercise 8.9, to investigate dental disease, and risk of coronary heart disease (CHD) and mortality, involving over 20 000 men and women aged 25–74, who were followed up between 1971– 4 and 1986–7 (DeStefano *et al.* 1993).

The results give the risk ratios (called relative risks here) for CHD and mortality in those with a number of dental diseases compared to those without (the referent group), adjusted for a number of possible confounding variables (see table footnote for a list of the variables adjusted for).

Briefly summarise what the results show about dental disease as a risk factor for CHD and mortality. Note: the periodontal index (range from 0-8, higher is worse) measures the average degree of periodontal disease in all teeth present, and the oral hygiene index (range 0-6, higher is worse) measures the average degree of debris and calculus on the surfaces of six selected teeth.

Confidence intervals for a population odds ratio

Table 6.2 showed the data for the case-control study into exercise between the ages of 15 and 25, and stroke later in life. The risk factor was 'not exercising', and you calculated the *sample crude odds ratio* of 0.411 for a stroke, in those who hadn't exercised compared to those who

Table 11.2 Adjusted risk ratios for CHD and mortality among those with dental disease compared to those without dental disease*. Reproduced by permission of BMJ Publishing Group. (*BMJ*, 1993, Vol. **306**, pages 688–691)

Indicator	No of subjects[†]	Coronary heart disease	Total mortality
Periodontal class:			
No disease	673	1.00	1.00
Gingivitis	529	0.98 (0.63 to 1.54)	1.42 (0.84 to 2.42)
Periodontitis	300	1.72 (1.10 to 2.68)	2.12 (1.24 to 3.62)
No teeth	92	1.71 (0.93 to 3.15)	2.60 (1.33 to 5.07)
Periodontal index (per unit)	1502	1.09 (1.00 to 1.19)	1.11 (1.01 to 1.22)
Oral hygiene index (per unit)	1436	1.11 (0.96 to 1.27)	1.23 (1.06 to 1.43)

*Adjusted for age, sex, race, education, poverty index, marital state, systolic blood pressure, total cholesterol concentration, diabetes, body mass index, physical activity, alcohol consumption, and cigarette smoking.
[†]Excluding those with missing data for any variable and, for periodontal index and hygiene index, those who had no teeth.

had (see p. 105). So the exercising group appear to have under half the odds for a stroke as the non-exercising group. However, you need to examine the confidence interval for this odds ratio to see if it contains 1 or not, before you can come to a conclusion about the statistical significance of the *population* odds ratio.

SPSS produces an odds ratio of 0.411, with a 95 per cent confidence interval of (0.260 to 0.650). This does not contain 1, so you can be 95 per cent confident that the odds ratio for a stroke in the *population* of those who did exercise compared to the population of those who didn't exercise is somewhere between 0.260 and 0.650. So early-life exercise does seem to reduce the odds for a stroke later on. Of course this is a crude, unadjusted odds ratio, which takes no account of the contribution, positive or negative, of any other relevant variables.

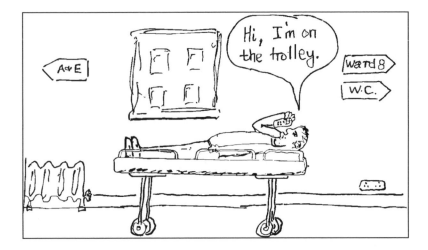

An example from practice

Table 11.3 shows the results from this same exercise/stroke study, where the authors provide both crude odds ratios and ratios *adjusted* for a number of different variables (Shinton and Sagar 1993).

We have been looking at exercise between the ages of 15 and 25, the first row of the table. Compared to the *crude* odds ratio calculated above of 0.411, the authors report an odds ratio for stroke, *adjusted* for age and sex, among those who exercised compared to those who didn't exercise, as 0.33, with a 95 per cent confidence interval of (0.20 to 0.60). So even after the effects of any differences in age and sex between the two groups has been adjusted for, exercising remains a statistically significant 'risk' factor for stroke (although *beneficial* in this case). Adjustment for possible confounders is crucial if your results are to be of any use, and I will return to adjustment and how it can be achieved in Chapter 18.

Table 11.3 Odds ratios for stroke*, according to whether, and at what age, exercise was undertaken by patients, compared to controls without stroke. Reproduced by permission of BMJ Publishing Group. (*BMJ*, 1993, Vol. **307**, pages 231–234)

	Exercise not undertaken		Exercise undertaken	
	Odds ratio	No of cases: no of controls	Odds ratio (95% confidence interval)	No of cases: no of controls
Age when exercise undertaken (years):				
15–25	1.0	70:68	0.33 (0.2 to 0.6)	55:130
25–40	1.0	103:136	0.43 (0.2 to 0.8)	21:57
40–55	1.0	101:139	0.63 (0.3 to 1.5)	10:22

*Adjusted for age and sex

Exercise 11.2. (a) Explain briefly why, in Table 11.3, age and sex differences between the groups have to be adjusted for. (b) What do the results indicate about exercise as a risk factor for stroke among the 25–40 years and 40–55 years groups?

Exercise 11.3. Refer back to Table 1.7, the results from a cross-section study into thrombotic risk during pregnancy. Identify and interpret any statistically significant odds ratios.

VI

Putting it to the Test

12

Testing hypotheses about the *difference* between two population parameters

Medical Statistics from Scratch, Second Edition   David Bowers
© 2008 John Wiley & Sons, Ltd

- Explain the power of a test and how it is calculated.

- Explain the connection between power and sample size.

- Calculate sample size required in some common situations.

The research question and the hypothesis test

The procedures discussed in the preceding three chapters have one primary aim: to use confidence intervals to estimate population parameter values, and their differences and ratios. We were able to make statements like, 'We are 95 per cent confident that the range of values defined by the confidence interval will include the value of the population parameter,' or, 'The confidence interval represents a plausible range of values for the population parameter.'

There is, however, an alternative approach called *hypothesis testing*, which uses exactly the same sample data as the confidence interval approach, but focuses not on *estimating* a parameter value, but on *testing* whether its value is the same as a previously specified or *hypothesised* value. In recent years, the estimation approach has become more generally favoured, primarily because the results from a confidence interval provides *more information* than the results of a hypothesis test (as you will see a bit later). However, hypothesis testing is still very common in research publications, and so I will describe a few of the more common tests.[1] Let's first establish some basic concepts.

The null hypothesis

As we have seen, almost all clinical research begins with a question. For example, is Malathion a more effective drug for treating head lice than *d*-phenothrin? Is stress a risk factor for breast cancer? To answer questions like this you have to transform the *research question* into a *testable hypothesis* called the *null hypothesis*, conventionally labelled H_0. This usually takes the following form:

H_0: Malathion is *NOT* a more effective drug for treating head lice than *d*-phenothrin.

H_0: Stress is *NOT* a risk factor for breast cancer.

Notice that both of these null hypotheses reflect the conservative position of *no* difference, *no* risk, *no* effect, etc., hence the name, '*null*' hypothesis. To *test* this null hypothesis, researchers will take samples and measure outcomes, and decide whether the data from the sample provides strong enough evidence to be able to refute or *reject* the null hypothesis or not. If evidence against the null hypothesis is strong enough for us to be able to reject it, then we are implicitly accepting that some specified alternative hypothesis, usually labelled H_1, is probably true.

---

[1] And there are some situations where there is no reasonable alternative to a hypothesis test.

The hypothesis testing process

The hypothesis testing process can be summarised thus:

- Select a suitable outcome variable.

- Use your research question to define an appropriate and testable null hypothesis involving this outcome variable.

- Collect the appropriate sample data and determine the relevant sample statistic, e.g. sample mean, sample proportion, sample median, (or their difference or ratio), etc.

- Use a decision rule that will enable you to judge whether the sample evidence supports or does not support your null hypothesis.

- Thus, on the strength of this evidence, either reject or do not reject your null hypothesis.

Let's take a simple example. Suppose you want to test whether a coin is fair, i.e. not weighted to produce more heads or more tails than it should. Your null hypothesis is that the coin is fair, i.e. will produce as many heads as tails, so that the population proportion π, equals 0.5. Your outcome variable is the sample proportion of heads, p. You toss the coin 100 times, and get 42 heads, so $p = 0.42$. Is this outcome compatible with your hypothesised value of 0.5? Is the difference between 0.5 and 0.42 statistically significant or could it be due to chance?

You can probably see the problem. How do we decide *what* proportion of heads we might expect to get if the coin is fair? As it happens, there is a generally accepted rule, which involves something known as the *p-value*.

The p-value and the decision rule

The hypothesis test decision rule is: *If the probability of getting the number of heads you get (or even fewer) is less than 0.05,*[2] *when the null hypothesis is true, then this is strong enough evidence against the null hypothesis and it can be rejected.* The beauty of this rule is that you can apply it to any situation where the probability of an outcome can be calculated, not just to coin tossing.

As a matter of interest, the probability of getting say 42 *or fewer* heads if the coin is fair is 0.0666, which is *not* less than 0.05. This is *not* strong enough evidence against the null hypothesis. However, if you had got 41 heads or fewer, the probability of which is 0.0443, this *is* less than 0.05, now the evidence against H$_0$ *is* strong enough and it can be rejected. The coin is not fair. This crucial threshold outcome probability (0.0443 in this example), is called the p-*value*, and defined thus:

A *p*-value is the probability of getting the outcome observed (or one more extreme), assuming the null hypothesis to be true.

---

[2] Or 0.01. There is nothing magical about these values, they are quite arbitrary.

So, in the end, the decision rule is simple:

- Determine the p-*value* for the output you have obtained (using a computer).

- Compare it with the *critical value*, usually 0.05.

- If the *p*-value is *less* than the critical value, reject the null hypothesis; otherwise do not reject it.

When you reject a null hypothesis, it's worth remembering that although there is a probability of 0.95 that you are making the correct decision, there is a corresponding probability of 0.05 that your decision is incorrect. In fact, you *never* know whether your decision is correct or not,[3] but there are 95 chances in 100 that it is. Compare this with the conclusion from a confidence interval where you can be 95 per cent confident that a confidence interval will include the population parameter, but there's still a 5 per cent chance that it will not.

It's important to stress that the *p*-value is *not* the probability that the null hypothesis is true (or not true). It's a measure of the *strength of the evidence against* the null hypothesis. The smaller the *p*-value, the stronger the evidence (the less likely it is that the outcome you got occurred by chance). Note that the critical value, usually 0.05 or 0.01, is called the *significance level* of the hypothesis test and denoted α (alpha). We'll return to alpha again shortly.

Exercise 12.1   Suppose you want to check your belief that as many males as females use your genito-urinary clinic. (a) Frame your belief as a research question. (b) Write down an appropriate null hypothesis. (c) You take a sample of 100 patients on Monday and find that 40 are male. The *p*-value for 40 or fewer males from a sample of 100 individuals is 0.028. Do you reject the null hypothesis? (d) Your colleague takes a sample of 100 patients on the following Friday and gets 43 males, the *p*-value for which is 0.097. Does your colleague come to the same decision as you did? Explain your answer.

A brief summary of a few of the commonest tests

Some hypothesis tests are suitable only for metric data, some for metric and ordinal data, and some for ordinal and nominal data. Some require data to have a particular distribution (often Normal); these are *parametric* tests. Some have no or less strict distributional requirements; the *non-parametric* tests. Before I discuss a few tests in any detail, I have listed in Table 12.1 a brief summary of the more commonly used tests, along with their data and distributional requirements, if any. I am ignoring tests of single population parameters since these are not required often enough to justify any discussion.

---

[3] Because you'll never know what the value of any population parameter is.

Table 12.1 Some of the more common hypothesis tests

Two-sample *t* test. Used to test whether or not the difference between two *independent* population means is zero (i.e. the two means are equal). The null assumption is that it is. Both variables must be metric and Normally distributed (this is a parametric test). In addition the two population standard deviations should be similar (but for larger sample sizes this becomes less important).

Matched-pairs *t* test. Used to test whether or not the difference between two *paired* population means is zero. The null assumption is that it is, i.e. the two means are equal. Both variables must be metric, and the *differences* between the two must be Normally distributed (this is a parametric test).

Mann-Whitney test. Used to test whether or not the difference between two *independent* population medians is zero. The null assumption is that it is, i.e. the two medians are equal. Variables can be either metric or ordinal. No requirement as to shape of the distributions, but they need to be similar. This is the non-parametric equivalent of the two-sample *t* test.

Kruskal-Wallis test. Used to test whether the medians of three of more *independent* groups are the same. Variables can be either ordinal or metric. Distributions any shape, but all need to be similar. This non-parametric test is an extension of the Mann-Whitney test.

Wilcoxon test. Used to test whether or not the difference between two *paired* population medians is zero. The null assumption is that it is, i.e. the two medians are equal. Variables can be either metric or ordinal. Distributions any shape, but the *differences* should be distributed symmetrically. This is the non-parametric equivalent of the matched-pairs *t* test.

Chi-squared test. (χ^2). Used to test whether the proportions across a number of categories of two or more *independent* groups is the same. The null hypothesis is that they are. Variables must be categorical.[a] The chi-squared test is also a test of the independence of the two variables (and has a number of other applications). We will deal with the chi-squared test in Chapter 14.

Fisher's Exact test. Used to test whether the proportions in two categories of two *independent* groups is the same. The null hypothesis is that they are. Variables must be categorical. This test is an alternative to the 2×2 chi-squared test, when cell sizes are too small (I'll explain this later).

McNemar's test. Used to test whether the proportions in two categories of two *matched* groups is the same. The null hypothesis is that they are. Variables must be categorical.

---

[a]Categorical will normally be nominal or ordinal, but metric discrete or grouped metric continuous might be used provided the number of values or groups is small.

Interpreting computer hypothesis test results for the difference in two independent population means – the two-sample *t* test

Since the two-sample *t* test is one of the more commonly used hypothesis tests, it will be helpful to have a look at the computer output. For example, let's apply the two-sample *t* test to test the null hypothesis of no difference in the population mean birthweight of maternity-unit-born infants and the mean birthweight of home-born infants (data in Table 10.1). The null hypothesis is:

$$H_0: \mu_M = \mu_H$$

Where, μ_M = population mean birthweight of maternity-unit-born infants, and μ_H = the population mean birthweight of home-born infants.[4]

With SPSS

Look back at Figure 10.1, which shows the output from SPSS, which, in addition to the 95 per cent confidence interval, gives the result of the two-sample *t* test of the equality of the two population mean birthweights. The test results are given in columns five, six and seven. The column headed 'Sig. (2-tailed)' gives the *p*-value of 0.407. Since this is not less than 0.05, you cannot reject the null hypothesis. You thus conclude that there is no difference in the two population mean birthweights.

With Minitab

The Minitab output in Figure 10.2 gives the same *p*-value value as SPSS (0.407), confirming that the two population means are not significantly different.

Some examples of hypothesis tests from practice

Two independent means – the two-sample *t* test

Table 12.2 shows the baseline characteristics of two independent groups in a randomised controlled trial to compare conventional blood pressure measurement (CBP) and ambulatory blood pressure measurement (ABP) in the treatment of hypertension (Staessen *et al.* 1997). *p*-values for the differences in the basic characteristics of the two groups are shown in the last column.

The authors used a variety of tests to assess the difference between several parameters for these independent groups (although these are referred to in the text, this information should have been available somewhere in the table itself). To assess the difference in population mean age, and mean body mass index, they used a two-sample *t* test. For age, the *p*-valuc is 0.03, so you can reject the null hypothesis of equal mean ages and conclude that the difference is statistically significant. The *p*-value for the difference in mean body mass index is 0.39, so you can conclude that the mean body mass index in the two populations is the same.

Exercise 12.2   Comment on what the results in Table 12.2 indicate about the difference between the two populations in terms of their mean serum creatinine and serum total cholesterol levels.

Exercise 12.3   Refer back to Table 1.6, showing the basic characteristics of women in the breast cancer and stressful life events case-control study. Comment on what the *p*-values tell you about the equality or otherwise, between cases and controls, of the means of the seven metric variables (shown with an * – see table footnote).

---

[4] Note that *differences in independent percentages* can also be tested with the two-sample *t* test.

Table 12.2 Baseline characteristics of two *independent* groups, from a randomised controlled trial to compare conventional blood pressure measurement (CBP) and ambulatory blood pressure measurement (ABP) in the treatment of hypertension. Reproduced from *JAMA*, **278**, 1065–72, courtesy of the American Medical Association

Characteristics	CBP Group ($n = 206$)	ABP Group ($n = 213$)	P
Age, mean (SD), y	51.3 (11.9)	53.8 (10.8)	.03
Body mass index, mean (SD), kg/m²	28.5 (4.8)	28.2 (4.4)	.39
Women, No. (%)	102 (49.5)	124 (58.2)	.07
Receiving oral contraceptives, No. (%)*	14 (13.7)	10 (8.1)	.17
Receiving hormonal substitution, No. (%)*	19 (18.6)	19 (15.3)	.51
Previous antihypertensive treatment, No. (%)†	134 (65.0)	139 (65.3)	.95
Diuretics, No. (%)*	47 (35.1)	59 (42.4)	.26
β-Blockers, No. (%)*	65 (48.5)	80 (57.6)	.17
Calcium channel blockers, No. (%)*	45 (33.6)	38 (27.3)	.32
Angiotensin-converting enzyme inhibitors, No. (%)*	50 (37.3)	48 (34.5)	.72
Multiple-drug treatment, No. (%)*	62 (46.3)	65 (46.8)	.97
Smokers, No. (%)	42 (20.5)	35 (16.4)	.29
Alcohol use, No. (%)	115 (55.8)	102 (47.9)	.10
Serum creatinine, mean (SD), μmol/L‡	85.75 (15.91)	88.4 (16.80)	.25
Serum total cholesterol, mean (SD), mmol/L‡	6.00 (1.03)	6.10 (1.19)	.32

*Percentages and values of P computed considering only women receiving antihypertensive drug treatment before their enrollment.
†Defined as antihypertensive drug treatment within 6 months before the screening visit.
‡Divide creatinine by 88.4 and cholesterol by 0.02586 to convert milligrams per deciliter.

Two matched means – the matched-pairs *t* test

Table 10.3 provides an example from practice, and shows the *p*-values for the differences in population mean bone mineral densities between two individually matched groups of depressed and normal women (which we have already discussed in confidence interval terms). As you can see, only at the radius are the population mean bone mineral densities the same, indicated by a *p*-value of 0.25. All the other *p*-values are less than 0.05. Notice that this confirms the confidence interval results.[5]

Two independent medians – the Mann-Whitney test

With two independent groups, and when the data is ordinal or skewed metric, the median is the preferred measure of location. In these circumstances, the Mann-Whitney test can be used to test the null hypothesis that the two population medians are the same.

Recall that in Chapter 10, I introduced the Mann-Whitney procedure to calculate confidence intervals for the difference between two independent population median treatment times. These

---

[5] Note that differences in matched percentages can also be tested with the matched-pairs *t* test.

were from a study of the use of ketorolac versus morphine to treat limb injury pain. Table 10.4 contains both 95 per cent confidence intervals and *p*-values from this study. Only one confidence interval does not include zero, that for the time between receiving analgesia and leaving A&E (4.0 to 39.0). This outcome has a *p*-value of 0.02, less than 0.05, which confirms the fact that the difference in treatment time between the two population median times is statistically significant.

However there is a problem with the time for preparation of the analgesia. Table 10.4 shows this has a 95 per cent confidence interval of (0 to 5.0), which includes zero, implying no significant difference in treatment times. But the *p*-value is given as 0.0002, which suggests a highly significant difference in population medians. In the accompanying text the authors indicate that this difference is significant and quote the low *p*-value, so I can only assume a typographical error in the confidence interval.

Interpreting computer output for the Mann-Whitney test

In view of the widespread use of the Mann-Whitney test you might find it helpful to see the output for this procedure from both SPSS and Minitab.

With SPSS

With the Apgar scores in Table 10.1, you can use the Mann-Whitney test to check if the population median Apgar scores for infants born in a maternity unit and those born at home are the same and differ in the sample only by chance. The null hypothesis is that these medians are equal. The output from SPSS is shown in Figure 12.1. The *p*-value of 0.061 is labelled 'Asymp. Sig. (2-tailed)'. Since this is not less than 0.05 you *cannot* reject the null hypothesis of no difference in population median Apgar scores between the two groups.

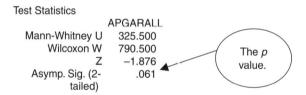

Test Statistics

	APGARALL
Mann-Whitney U	325.500
Wilcoxon W	790.500
Z	−1.876
Asymp. Sig. (2-tailed)	.061

The *p* value.

Figure 12.1   Output from SPSS for the Mann-Whitney test of the difference between population medians of the two independent Apgar scores (raw data in Table 10.1)

With Minitab

If you refer back to Figure 10.3, you will see the results of Minitab's Mann-Whitney test three rows from the bottom.[6] The *p*-value is given in the second row up as 0.0616 and since this is

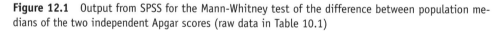

---

[6] 'ETA' is Minitab's word for the population median.

not less than 0.05 you *cannot* reject the null hypothesis. This is confirmed in the bottom row of the table, and enables you to conclude that the population median Apgar scores are the same in both groups of infants.

Two matched medians – the Wilcoxon test

In the same circumstances as for the Mann-Whitney test described above, but with *matched* populations, the Wilcoxon test is appropriate. Look back at Table 10.5, which was from a matched case-control study into the dietary intake of schizophrenic patients living in the community in Scotland. Here the authors have used the Wilcoxon matched-pairs test to test for differences in the population median daily intakes of a number of substances between 'All Patients' and 'All Controls'. The *p*-values are in the column headed 'P'. As you can see, the only *p* value *not* less than 0.05 is that for protein (*p*-value = 0.07), so this is the only substance whose median daily intake does *not* differ between the two populations. Once again this confirms the confidence interval results.

Confidence intervals versus hypothesis testing

I said at the beginning of this chapter that where possible, confidence intervals are preferred to hypothesis tests because the confidence intervals are more informative. How so? Have another look at Table 10.4, from the study comparing ketorolac and morphine for limb injury pain. The authors give both 95 per cent confidence intervals and *p*-values for differences in a number of different treatment times, between two groups of limb injury patients. Let's take the last of these. For the 'interval between receiving analgesia and leaving A&E', the *p*-value of 0.02 enables us to reject the null hypothesis, and you would conclude that the difference between the two population median treatment times is statistically significant.

The 95 per cent confidence interval of (4.0 to 39.0) minutes, tells us, *not only* that the difference between the population medians is statistically significant – because the confidence interval does not contain zero – but in *addition*, that the value of this difference in population medians is likely to be somewhere between 4.0 minutes and 39 minutes. So the confidence interval does everything that the hypothesis test does – it tells us if the medians are equal or not, but it *also* gives us extra information – on the likely range of values for this difference. Moreover, unlike a *p*-value, the confidence interval is in *clinically meaningful* units, which helps with the interpretation. So whenever possible, it is good practice to use confidence intervals in preference to *p*-values.

Nobody's perfect – types of error

Suppose you are investigating a new drug for the treatment of hypertension. Your null hypothesis is that the drug has no effect. Let's suppose that the drug *does* actually reduce mean systolic blood pressure, but, on average, by only 5 mmHg. However, the hypothesis test you use can only detect a change of 10 mmHg or more. As a consequence, you will not find strong enough evidence to reject the null hypothesis, and you'll conclude, mistakenly, that the new drug is *not* effective. But the effect is there, it's just that your test does not have enough *power* to detect it.

There are three questions here. First, what exactly is the power of a test and how can we measure it? Second, how can we increase the power of the test we are using? Third, is there a more powerful test that we can use instead? Before I address these questions, a few words on *types of error*.

Whenever you decide either to reject or not reject a null hypothesis, you could be making a mistake. After all, you are basing your decision on *sample* evidence. Even if you have done everything right, your sample could still, by chance, not be very representative of the population. Moreover, your test might not be powerful enough to detect an effect if there is one. There are two possible errors:

Type I error. Rejecting a null hypothesis when it is true. Also known as a *false positive*. In other words, concluding there *is* an effect when there isn't. The probability of committing a type I error is denoted α (alpha), and is the *same* alpha as the significance level of a test.

Type II error: Not rejecting a null hypothesis when it is false. Also known as a *false negative*. That is, concluding there is *no* effect when there is. The probability of committing a type II error is denoted β (beta).

Ideally, you would like a test procedure which minimised the probability of a type I error, because in many clinical situations such an error is potentially serious – judging some procedure to be effective when it is not. When you set the significance level of a test to $\alpha = 0.05$, it's because you want the probability of a type I error to be no more than 0.05. Nonetheless, if there *is* a real effect you would certainly like to detect it, so you also want to minimise the probability of β, a type II error, or put another way, you want to make $(1 - \beta)$ as large as possible.

Exercise 12.4   Explain, with examples, what is meant in hypothesis testing by: (a) a false positive; (b) a false negative.

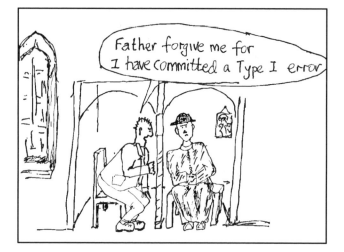

The power of a test

We can now come back to the three questions above. To answer the first question – the *power* of a test is defined to be $(1 - \beta)$; it is a measure of its capacity to reject the null hypothesis when it is false. In other words, to detect an effect if one is present. In practice, β is typically set at 0.2 or 0.1. This provides power values of 0.80 (or 80 per cent), and 0.90 (or 90 per cent) respectively. So if there *is* an effect, then the probability of the test detecting it is 0.80 or 0.90.

The *power* of a test is a measure of its capacity to reject the null hypothesis when it is false. In other words, its capacity to detect an effect if one is present.

Although you would like to minimise both α and β, unfortunately they are, for a given sample size, linked. You can't make β smaller without making α larger, and vice versa. Thus when you decide a value for α, you are also inevitably fixing the value of β. To answer the second question – the only way to reduce both simultaneously (and increase the power of a test) is to increase the sample size.

To answer the third question, is there a more powerful test? Briefly, parametric tests are more powerful than non-parametric tests (see p. 127 on the meaning of these terms). For example, a Mann-Whitney test has 95 percent of the power of the two-sample t test.[7] The Wilcoxon matched-pairs test similarly has 95 per cent of the power of the matched-pairs t test. As for the chi-squared test, there is usually no obvious alternative when used for categorical data, so comparisons of power are less relevant, but it is known to be a powerful test. Generally you should of course use the most powerful test that the type of data, and its distributional shape, will allow.

An example from practice

The following is an extract from the RCT of epidural analgesic in the prevention of stump and phantom pain after amputation, referred to in Table 5.3. The authors of the study outline their thinking on power thus:

> The natural history of phantom pain after amputation shows rates of about 70%, and in most patients the pain is not severe. Since epidural treatment is an invasive procedure, we decided that a clinically relevant treatment should reduce the incidence of phantom pain to less than 30% at week 1 and then at 3, 6, and 12 months after amputation. Before the start of the study, we estimated that a sample size of 27 patients per group would be required to detect a between-group difference of 40% in the rate of phantom pain (type I error rate 0.05; type II error rate 0.2; power = 0.8).

---

[7] In view of the restrictions associated with the two-sample t test, the Mann-Whitney test seems an excellent alternative!

> **Exercise 12.5**   a) Explain, with the help of a few clinical examples, why you would normally want to minimise α, when testing a hypothesis. (b) α is conventionally set to 0.05, or 0.01. Why, if you want to minimise it, don't you set it at 0.001 or 0.000001, or even 0?

Maximising power – calculating sample size

Generally, the bigger the sample, the more powerful the test.[8] The minimum size of a sample for a given power is determined both by the chosen level of alpha, as well as the power required. The sample size calculation can be summarised thus:

- Decide on the minimum size of the *effect* that would be clinically useful (or otherwise of interest).

- Decide the significance level α, usually 0.05.

- Decide the power required, usually 80 per cent.

- Do the sample size calculation, using some appropriate software, or the rule of thumb described below.

Minitab has an easy to use sample size calculator for the most commonly used tests. Machin, *et al.* (1987) is a comprehensive collection of sample size calculations for a large number of different test situations.

Rules of thumb[9]

Comparing the means of two independent populations (metric data)

The required sample size n is given by the following expression:

$$n = \frac{2 \times \text{s.d.}^2}{E^2} \times k$$

Where s.d. is the population standard deviation (assumed equal in both populations). This can be estimated using the sample standard deviations, if they are available from a pilot study, say. Otherwise the s.d. will have to be guessed using whatever information is available. E is the minimum change in the mean that would be clinically useful or otherwise interesting. k is a magic number which depends on the power and significance levels required, and is obtained from Table 12.3.

---

[8] These sample size calculations also apply if you are calculating confidence intervals. Samples that are too small produce wide confidence intervals, sometimes too wide to enable a real effect to be identified.
[9] I am indebted to Andy Vail for this material.

Table 12.3 Table of magic numbers for sample size calculations

		Power, $(1 - \beta)$			
		70 %	80 %	90 %	95 %
Significance level, α	0.05	6.2	7.8	10.5	13.0
	0.01	9.6	11.7	14.9	17.8

For example, suppose you propose to use a case-control study to examine the efficacy of a program of regular exercise, as an alternative to your current drug of choice, in treating moderately hypertensive patients. The minimal difference in mean systolic blood pressures between the cases (given the exercise program), and the controls (given the existing drug), that you think clinically worthwhile is 10 mmHg. You will have to make an intelligent guess as to the standard deviation of systolic blood pressure (assumed the same in both groups – see above). Information on this, and many other measures, is likely to be available from reference sources, from the research literature, from colleagues, etc. Let's assume systolic blood pressure s.d. = 12 mmHg. If power required is 80 per cent, with a significance level of 0.05, then from Table 12.3, $k = 7.8$, and the sample size required per group is:

$$ n = \frac{2 \times 12^2}{10^2} \times 7.8 = 22.5 $$

So you will need at least 23 subjects in each of the two groups (always round up to next highest integer) to detect a difference between the means of 10 mmHg. Note that these sample sizes will also be large enough for two matched populations since these require smaller sample sizes for the same power.

Comparing the proportions in two independent populations (binary data)

The required sample size, n, is given by:

$$ n = \frac{[P_a \times (1 - P_a)] + [P_b \times (1 - P_b)]}{(P_a - P_b)^2} \times k $$

Where P_a is the proportion with treatment a, P_b is proportion with treatment b, so $(P_a - P_b)$ is the effect size; and k is the magic number from Table 12.3.

For example, suppose the percentage of elderly patients in a large district hospital with pressure sores is currently around 40 per cent, or 0.40. You want to test a new pressure-sore-reducing mattress, and you would like the percentage with pressure sores to decrease to at least 20 per cent, or 0.20. So $P_a = 0.40$, and $(1 - P_a) = 0.60$; $P_b = 0.20$, and $(1 - P_b) = 0.80$; therefore $(P_a - P_b) = (0.40 - 0.20) = 0.20$. If power required is 80 per cent and significance level $\alpha = 0.05$, then required sample size per group is:

$$n = \frac{(0.40 \times 0.60) + (0.20 \times 0.80)}{0.20^2} \times 7.8 = 78.0$$

Thus you would need at least 78 subjects in each group, which would also be big enough for matched proportions.

Exercise 12.6   In the above examples for: (a) hypertension and (b) the pressure sore example; what sample sizes would be required if power and significance levels were respectively: (i) 90 per cent and 0.05; (ii) 90 per cent and 0.01; (iii) 80 per cent and 0.01?

Exercise 12.7   Suppose you are proposing to use a randomised controlled trial to study the effectiveness of St John's Wort, as an alternative to an existing drug for the treatment of mild to moderate depression. The percentage of patients reporting an improvement in mood three months after existing drug treatment is 70 per cent. You would be satisfied if the percentage reporting mood improvement after three months of St John's Wort was 80 per cent. How big a sample would you require to detect this improvement if you wanted your test to have, (a) 80 per cent power and an α of 0.05; (b) 90 per cent power and an α of 0.01?

13

Testing hypotheses about the *ratio* of two population parameters

---

Learning objectives

When you have finished this chapter you should be able to:

- Describe the usual form of the null hypothesis in the context of testing the ratio of two population parameters

- Outline the differences between tests of ratios and tests of differences.

- Interpret published results on tests of risk and odds ratios.

Testing the risk ratio

In Chapter 11 you saw that if the confidence interval for a sample risk ratio contains 1, then the population risk ratio is most probably not statistically significant, i.e. not significantly different from 1. This in turn means that the risk factor in question is *not* a statistically significant risk. You can also use the *hypothesis* test approach to find out whether any departure in the sample risk ratio from 1 is statistically significant, or is more likely due to chance. The null hypothesis

---

Medical Statistics from Scratch, Second Edition   David Bowers
© 2008 John Wiley & Sons, Ltd

is that the population risk ratio equals 1, the alternate hypothesis is that it isn't equal to 1. That is:

$$H_0: \quad \text{population risk ratio} = 1$$

$$H_1: \quad \text{population risk ratio} \neq 1$$

In other words, if H_0 is true, the risk factor in question does not significantly increase or decrease the risk for the condition or disease. If the associated p value is less than 0.05 (or 0.01), you can reject the null hypothesis H_0, and conclude that the population risk ratio in question is statistically significant, and the risk factor in question is a *statistically significant* risk.

An example from practice

Table 13.1 is from a randomised trial into the efficacy of long-term treatment with subcutaneous heparin in unstable coronary-artery disease (FRISC II Investigators 1999), and shows the risk ratios, 95 per cent confidence intervals and p values for a number of clinical outcomes, in two independent groups, one group given heparin, the other a placebo.

As you can see from the p values in the last column, three out of the six risk ratios were statistically significant: death, myocardial infarction or both, at one month (p value = 0.048); death, myocardial infarction or revascularisation, at one month (p value = 0.001); and death, myocardial infarction or revascularisation, at three months (p value = 0.031). All three of these p values are less than 0.05, the remaining three are all greater than 0.05. Notice that these results are confirmed by the corresponding 95 per cent confidence intervals.

Table 13.1 Risk ratios, 95 per cent confidence intervals, and p-values, for a number of clinical outcomes, at 1 month, 3 months and 6 months, in two independent groups, one group given heparin and the other group a placebo. Reprinted courtesy of Elsevier (*The Lancet*, 1999, Vol No. **354**, page 701–7)

Variable	Dalteparin ($n = 1129$)	Placebo ($n = 1121$)	Risk ratio (95% CI)	p
1 month				
Death, MI, or both	70 (6.2%)	95 (8.4%)	0.73 (0.54–0.99)	0.048
Death, MI, or revascularisation	220 (19.5%)	288 (25.7%)	0.76 (0.65–0.89)	0.001
3 months				
Death, MI, or both	113 (10.0%)	126 (11.2%)	0.89 (0.70–1.13)	0.34
Death, MI, or revascularisation	328 (29.1%)	374 (33.4%)	0.87 (0.77–0.99)	0.031
6 months*				
Death, MI, or both	148 (13.3%)	145 (13.1%)	1.01 (0.82–1.25)	0.93
Death, MI, or revascularisation	428 (38.4%)	440 (39.9%)	0.96 (0.87–1.07)	0.50

MI = myocardial infarction.
*Dalteparin ($n = 1115$), placebo ($n = 1103$).

Table 13.2 Relative risk for a number of non-cerebral bleeding complications in patients receiving tenecteplase compared to those receiving alteplase, in the treatment of acute myocardial infarction. Reprinted courtesy of Elsevier (*The Lancet*, 1999, Vol No. **354**, page 716–21)

Complication	Frequency (%) Tenecteplase ($n = 8461$)	Alteplase ($n = 8488$)	Relative risk (95% CI)	p
Reinfarction	4.1	3.8	1.078 (0.929–1.250)	0.325
Recurrent angina	19.4	19.5	0.995 (0.935–1.058)	0.877
Sustained hypotension	15.9	16.1	0.988 (0.921–1.058)	0.737
Cardiogenic shock	3.9	4.0	0.965 (0.832–1.119)	0.664
Major arrhythmias	20.5	21.2	0.968 (0.913–1.027)	0.281
Pericarditis	3.0	2.6	1.124 (0.941–1.343)	0.209
Invasive cardiac procedures				
PTCA	24.0	23.9	1.006 (0.953–1.061)	0.843
Stent placement	19.0	19.7	0.968 (0.910–1.029)	0.302
CABG	5.5	6.2	0.884 (0.783–0.999)	0.049
IABP	2.6	2.7	0.968 (0.805–1.163)	0.736
Killip class $>$I	6.1	7.0	0.991 (0.982–0.999)	0.026
Tamponade or cardiac rupture	0.6	0.7	0.816 (0.558–1.193)	0.332
Acute mitral regurgitation	0.6	0.7	0.886 (0.613–1.281)	0.571
Ventricular septum defect	0.3	0.3	0.817 (0.466–1.434)	0.568
Anaphylaxis	0.1	0.2	0.376 (0.147–0.961)	0.052
Pulmonary embolism	0.09	0.04	2.675 (0.710–10.080)	0.145

PTCA = Percutaneous transluminal coronary angioplasty; CABG = coronary-artery bypass graft; IABP = Intra-aortic balloon pump.

Exercise 13.1 Table 13.2 is from a double blind RCT to assess the efficacy of tenecteplase as a possible alternative to alteplase in the treatment of acute myocardial infarction (ASSENT-2 Investigators 1999). The table contains the risk ratios (relative risks) for a number of in-hospital cardiac events and procedures, for patients receiving tenecteplase, compared to those receiving alteplase.[1]

Identify and comment on those cardiac events and procedures for which patients on alteplase had a significant higher risk of experiencing than those on tenecteplase. Note: the key to the cardiac procedures is given in the table footnote. The Killip scale is a classification system for heart failure in patients with acute myocardial infarction, and varies from I (least serious, no heart failure, 5 per cent expected mortality), to IV (most serious, cardiogenic shock, 90 per cent expected mortality).

[1] As a background note: rapid infusion of alteplase, with aspirin and heparin, is the current gold standard for pharmacological reperfusion in acute myocardial infarction. Tenecteplase is a mutant of alteplase with fewer of the limitations of alteplase.

Testing the odds ratio

Here the null hypothesis is that the population odds ratio is not significantly different from 1. That is:

$$H_0: \quad \text{population odds ratio} = 1$$

$$H_1: \quad \text{population odds ratio} \neq 1$$

In other words, in the population, if H_0 is true the risk factor in question does not significantly increase or decrease the odds for the condition or disease. Only if the p value for the sample odds ratio is less than 0.05, can you reject the null hypothesis, and conclude that the risk factor is statistically significant.

An example from practice

Table 13.3 is from an unmatched case-control study into the effect of passive smoking as a risk factor for coronary heart disease (CHD), in Chinese women who had never smoked (He *et al.* 1994). The cases were patients with CHD, the controls women without CHD. The study looked at both passive smoking at home from husbands who smoked, and at work from smoking co-workers. The null hypotheses were that the population odds ratio was equal to 1, both at home and at work, i.e. passive smoking has no effect on the odds for CHD. The

Table 13.3 Odds ratios, 95 per cent confidence intervals and p values, from an unmatched case-control study into the effect of passive smoking as a risk factor for coronary heart disease. The cases were patients with coronary heart disease, the controls individuals without coronary heart disease. Reproduced from *BMJ*, **308**, 380–4, courtesy of BMJ Publishing Group

	Adjusted odds ratio (95% confidence interval)*	P value
Final model (factors 1 to 7):		
1 Age (years)	1.13 (1.04 to 1.22)	0.003
2 History of hypertension	2.47 (1.14 to 5.36)	0.022
3 Type A personality	2.83 (1.31 to 6.37)	0.008
4 Total cholesterol (mg/dl)	1.02 (1.01 to 1.03)	0.0006
5 High density lipoprotein cholesterol (mg/dl)	0.94 (0.90 to 0.98)	0.003
6 Passive smoking from husband	1.24 (0.56 to 2.72)	0.60
7 Passive smoking at work	1.85 (0.86 to 4.00)	0.12
Other model (factors 1 to 5 and passive smoking at work)	1.95 (0.90 to 4.10)[†]	0.087
Other model (factors 1 to 5 and passive smoking from husband or at work, or both)	2.36 (1.01 to 5.55)[†]	0.049

*Adjusted for the other variables in the final model.
[†]Adjusted for the first five varibles above; odds ratios for these variables in the other models were essentially the same as those shown above and are not shown.

table contains the adjusted odds ratios for CHD for a number of risk factors, with 95 per cent confidence intervals and p values.

As you can see, the adjusted odds ratio for CHD because of passive smoking from the husband was 1.24, with a p value of 0.60, so you *cannot* reject the null hypothesis. You conclude that passive smoking from husbands is not a statistically significant risk factor for CHD in wives. The same conclusions can be drawn for the odds ratio of 1.85 for passive smoking at work, p value equals 0.12.

Exercise 13.2 In Table 13.3, identify those risk factors which are statistically significant for CHD in the population from whom this sample of women was drawn.

14

Testing hypotheses about the equality of population proportions: the chi-squared test

Learning objectives

When you have finished this chapter you should be able to:

- Describe the rationale underlying the chi-squared hypothesis test.

- Explain the difference between observed and expected values.

- Calculate expected values and the test statistic.

- Outline the procedure for the chi-squared test for the independence of two variables in a population.

- Outline the procedure for the chi-squared test for the equality of two population proportions, and show this is equivalent to the test of the independence of two variables.

- Perform a chi-squared test in 2×2, 2×3, 2×4 and 3×4 cases.

- Interpret SPSS and Minitab chi-squared test results.

- Interpret published results of chi-squared tests.

- Outline the procedure for the chi-squared test for trend.

Medical Statistics from Scratch, Second Edition   David Bowers
© 2008 John Wiley & Sons, Ltd

Table 14.1 Observed values in the sample of mothers giving birth in maternity units and at home, and whether they smoked during their pregnancy (raw data in Table 10.1)

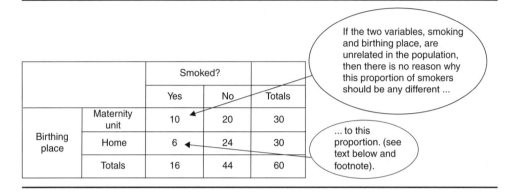

		Smoked?		
		Yes	No	Totals
Birthing place	Maternity unit	10	20	30
	Home	6	24	30
	Totals	16	44	60

If the two variables, smoking and birthing place, are unrelated in the population, then there is no reason why this proportion of smokers should be any different ...

... to this proportion. (see text below and footnote).

Of all the tests in all the world . . . the chi-squared (χ^2) test

Two hypothesis tests are prominent in general clinical research. One is the two-sample t test, (see Chapter 12), which, as you have seen, is used with metric data to test the equality of two independent population means. The second is the *chi-squared test*[1] (denoted χ^2).[2] This has two common applications: first as a test of whether two *categorical* variables are independent or not; second, as a test of whether two proportions are equal or not. As you will see, these tests are in fact equivalent.

The chi-squared test is applied to frequency data[3] in the form of a contingency table (i.e. a table of cross-tabulations), with the rows representing categories of one variable and the columns categories of a second variable. The null hypothesis is that the two variables are unrelated.

To explain the idea of the chi-squared test, let's refer back to the birthweight data in Table 10.1, and ask the question, 'Is there a relationship between the variables "birthing place" and "whether the mother smoked during pregnancy"?' The relevant data is summarised in the 2×2 table, Table 14.1. The columns of this table represent the two groups 'smokers' and 'non-smokers'. These two groups are *independent* - this is an essential requirement of the chi-squared test.[4] The rows of the table represent the variable *birthing place* (either maternity unit, or home birth), again independent.

---

[1] The test is called the chi-squared test because it uses the *chi-squared,* or χ^2, distribution. If a variable X is Normally distributed, then the variable X^2 has a χ^2 distribution. The χ^2 distribution is very skewed in small samples but becomes more similar in shape to the Normal distribution when samples are large.

[2] And pronounced as in *Ky*lie Minogue

[3] The method does not work for tables of percentages, proportions, or measurements.

[4] If the two groups are matched, then *McNemar's test* is appropriate (see Table 12.1).

If we want to know whether the variables 'birthing place' and 'smoking' are related, the competing hypotheses will be:

H_0 : Birthing place and smoking status are *not* related in the population, i.e. the two variables are *independent*.

H_1 : Birthing place and smoking status *are* related in the population. The two variables are *dependent*.

Now, if the two variables are unrelated, then there is no reason why the proportion of smokers among mothers giving birth in a maternity unit, should be any different to the proportion of smokers among home-birth mothers.[5] In other words, these two proportions should be the same. But we have already discussed a method for deciding whether two proportions are the same – by calculating a confidence interval for the difference in two population proportions – see p. 126 in Chapter 10. In fact, the two methods – asking if two variables are independent or if two proportions are the same - are equivalent whenever one of the variables *has only two* categories. However, although we can calculate a confidence interval in the two proportions approach as we saw in Chapter 10, we can't with the chi-squared approach.

You can see that 10 out of the sample of 30 maternity-unit mothers smoked (a proportion of 0.333), and six out of 30 home-birth mothers smoked (a proportion of 0.2000). These sample proportions are definitely *not* the same, but this could be due to chance.

The crucial question is this, 'What proportions would we *expect* to find if the null hypothesis of unrelated variables was true?' The answer is, since we've got 16 smokers in a total of 60 women, a proportion of 16/60 = 0.2667, we would expect to find 0.2667 or 26.67 per cent of the 30 in each category, which is 0.2667 × 30 = 8. So you'd expect about eight smokers in each group, rather than the observed values of 10 and six. An easier way to calculate *expected* frequencies is to use the expression:

$$\text{Expected cell frequency} = \frac{\text{Total of row cell is in} \times \text{total of column cell is in}}{\text{overall total frequency}}$$

For example, for the top left-hand cell, the row total is 30, the column total is 16 and the overall total is 60, so the expected value is (30×16)/60 = 8. Since in this example the row totals are both 30, this means that the other two cells must each have an expected value of 22. In other words, the two-by-two table you would *expect* to see if the null hypothesis was true is that shown in Table 14.2.

Exercise 14.1   Calculate the expected values for the contingency table of 'mother smoked' and 'Apgar score < 7', shown in Table 2.11.

---

[5] If there *was* a relationship, for example, maternity unit mothers tended to smoke more on average than home-birth mothers, then we would expect to find that the proportion of smokers among these mothers was consistently larger than among home-birth mothers. If there is *no* relationship, i.e. if the two variables are independent, then there is no reason to expect one proportion generally to be any larger or any smaller than the other.

Table 14.2   *Expected* cell values if the null hypothesis of unrelated variables (or equal proportions) is true

		Smoked?		
		Group 1: Yes	Group 2: No	Totals
Place of birth	Maternity unit	8	22	30
	Home	8	22	30
	Totals	16	44	60

Are the observed and expected values close enough?

As you've seen, even if the null hypothesis is true, you wouldn't expect the difference between the observed and expected values to be *exactly* zero. But how far away from zero does this difference have to be, before you accept that the sample results are indicative of a true difference in the proportions in the population, rather than chance?

You can use the *chi-squared test* to answer this question: if the *p*-value associated with the chi-squared test is less than 0.05 (or 0.01), you can reject the null hypothesis and conclude that the two variables are not independent or, put another way, there is a statistically significant difference in the proportions.

The chi-squared test can be used with more than two categories in each variable, but with small sample sizes the maximum number of either is limited by the proviso that none of the *expected* values should be less than 1, and that 80 per cent of expected values should be greater than 5.[6] There are two ways round the problem of low expected values. First, increase the sample size – usually impractical. Second, amalgamate two or more rows or columns, if this can be done and still make sense.

Calculation of a chi-squared test is not difficult to do by hand if the number of categories is small, but you would have to have available, and know how to use, a table of chi-squared values (I'm assuming here that calculation of the *p*-value is too difficult by hand, so this is a practical alternative). The procedure is as follows:

- Calculate the expected value *E*, for each cell in the table.

- For each cell calculate the value of $(O - E)$, where *O* is the observed value.

- Square each $(O - E)$ value.

- Divide each $(O - E)^2$ value by the *E* value for that cell.

- Sum all of the values in the previous step.

- This result is called the *test statistic*.[7]

---

[6] There is some dispute among statisticians about the validity of this condition – some suggest that the chi-squared test still works well even with low expected frequencies.

[7] For the mathematically minded, the test statistic $= \sum \left\{ \frac{(O - E)^2}{E} \right\}$.

Table 14.3 Table of critical values for χ^2 test with statistical significance of 0.05. To reject the null hypothesis of unrelated, i.e. independent variables, or of equal proportions, the value of the test statistic must exceed the value in column two for the given table sizes in column one

(No. rows $-$ 1) $\times$ (No. cols $-$ 1)	Value to be exceeded to reject null hypothesis of unrelated variables, or of equal proportions
1	3.84
2	5.99
4	9.49
6	12.59
9	16.92

To reject the null hypothesis of equal proportions, i.e. of independent variables, the value of the test statistic must exceed the critical chi-squared value obtained from a chi-squared table. Some of these values are shown in Table 14.3, for a level of significance of 0.05. For example, the test statistic must *exceed* 3.84 for a 2 × 2 table. In practice, you will, no doubt, use a computer program to supply the *p*-value for the chi-squared test, and thus to reject or not reject the null hypothesis that the two variables are independent, i.e. that the proportions are equal across categories.

> **Exercise 14.2**   Calculate the value of the test statistic using the expected values you calculated in Exercise 14.1. With the help of Table 14.3, can you reject the null hypothesis that 'smoking during pregnancy' and 'Apgar scores < 7', are independent? Explain.

An example from practice

Table 14.4 is from the randomised controlled trial into ketorolac versus morphine for the treatment of limb pain (first referred to in Table 10.4) and shows the basic characteristics of the patients participating in the trial. The chi-squared test has been used four times to test whether the proportions (expressed here as percentages) in the ketorolac group and the morphine group are the same. First for 'the proportion of men' (categories 'men' and 'not men'); then for 'fracture site'; then for 'referred for orthopaedic treatment'; and finally for 'admitted to hospital'.

As you can see, the chi-squared test applied to the fracture sites data, for example, tests whether the proportions between the two groups is the same for all six sites, and gives rise to a 2 × 6 table. The *p*-value is 0.91, which is not less than 0.05, so you can conclude that the null hypothesis of equal proportions cannot be rejected. In fact, the *p*-value for the chi-squared test on each of the other three items are also all considerably greater than 0.05 indicating no difference between the two groups in any of them.

Table 14.4 Basic characteristics of the patients participating in a randomised controlled trial of ketorolac versus morphine for the treatment of blunt injury limb pain (see Table 10.5). The chi-squared test has been used four times to test whether the proportions in the ketorolac and morphine groups are the same for a number of items. Values are numbers (percentage*) unless stated otherwise. Reproduced from *BMJ*, **321**, 1247–51, by permission of BMJ

Variable	Ketorolac group (n = 75)	Morphine group (n = 73)	P value
Mean (SD) age (years)	53.9 (21.7)	53.2 (21.8)	0.85‡
No (%) of men	38 (51)	33 (45)	0.51§
Mean (SD) body mass index (kg/m^2)	22.8 (3.2)	23.0 (3.7)	0.77‡
Mean (interquartile range) time between injury and arrival at hospital (minutes)	95 (30–630)	82 (33–921)	0.75
Cause of injury:			
Motor vehicle crash	6 (8)	4 (5)	0.58¶
Falls	46 (61)	51 (70)	
Crush	20 (27)	14 (19)	
Other	3 (4)	4 (5)	
Fractures:	50 (67)	48 (66)	0.91§
Clavicle, humerus, elbow	5 (7)	8 (11)	
Radius, ulnar	8 (11)	11 (15)	
Hand	15 (20)	13 (18)	
Femur, patella	14 (19)	12 (16)	
Tibia, fibula	5 (7)	3 (4)	
Foot	2 (3)	1 (1)	
Non-fractures:			
Dislocation, upper limb	2 (3)	1 (1)	
Soft tissue injury, upper limb	10 (13)	10 (14)	
Soft tissue injury, lower limb	14 (19)	14 (19)	
Initial mean (SD) pain score:			
At rest	3.8 (1.1)	3.9 (1.1)	0.65‡
With activity	8.1 (1.2)	8.1 (1.2)	0.85‡
Referred for orthopaedic assessment	41 (55)	36 (49)	0.52§
Admitted to hospital†	38 (51)	29 (40)	0.18§
Admitted with adverse effects	0	3 (4)	

*Percentages may not sum to 100 because of rounding.
†Patient's admitted to hospital (to orthopaedic or emergency observation ward).
‡*t* test for unpaired means comparison.
$^§\chi^2$ test.
¶Fisher's exact test.

Notice that the authors have used *Fisher's Exact* test (see Table 12.1 for a brief description) to compare the equality of the proportions between the two groups for 'cause of injury'. This is almost certainly because of low expected values in some cells.

The chi-squared test for trend

The *chi-squared trend test* is another useful application of the chi-squared distribution, and is appropriate if either variable has categories that *can be ordered*. I can best explain with a real example.

Table 14.5 Numbers of subjects by social class in cases and controls, in a study of stressful life events as a possible risk factor for breast cancer in women

Social class	Malignant diagnosis (cases) group	Benign diagnosis (control) group
I	10	20
II	38	82
III non-manual	28	72
III manual	13	24
IV	11	21
V	3	2
VI	3	4
Totals	106	226

An example from practice

Table 14.5 shows the social class categories (ordinal data) of the cases and controls in the unmatched case-control study of breast cancer in women (refer to Table 1.6). Recall that the subjects were women who attended with a breast lump. The cases were those women who received a malignant diagnosis, the controls those who received a benign diagnosis. These two groups are independent.

With two groups and seven ordered categories of 'social class', we have a 2 × 7 table. If you apply the chi-squared test here, you are testing whether the proportion of breast cancer cases is the same in each social class category, and simultaneously whether the two variables, diagnosis and social class, are independent. If the proportions are not the same you conclude that the variables are associated in some way.[8]

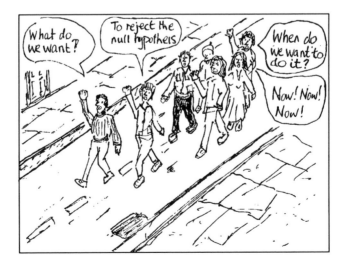

---

[8] Note that to perform the chi-squared test for trend we have to number the categories.

The problem is that if social class *is* associated with diagnosis, then you would *expect* the proportion getting a benign diagnosis to vary systematically, either increasing or decreasing, as social class increased.[9] In other words, the variability in the proportions may be due largely to this trend, rather than that the variables are associated.

In the chi-squared test for trend, the null hypothesis is that there is *no* trend, and the p-value is used in the usual way. Note that the test statistic for the trend test will always be less than that for the overall test described earlier. However, the trend test may produce a statistically significant result even when the overall test does not. This is because the test for trend is a *more powerful test*. The net result of all this is that if one or both of your variables has ordinal categories, you should use the chi-squared test for trend rather than the overall chi-squared test.

As a matter of interest, the overall chi-squared test for the data in Table 14.5 gives a *p*-value of 0.784, while the chi-squared trend test gives a *p*-value of 0.094. As it happens, neither of these is statistically significant, but is an illustration of how different the results from the two tests can be.

Exercise 14.3   Refer back to Table 1.6, the breast cancer and stress case-control study. The table footnote indicates four chi-squared trend tests. Comment on what each *p*-value reveals about the existence of a trend in the categories of each of the variable concerned.

The chi-squared test has a large number of other applications, one of which we'll meet in Chapter 19.

---

[9] The direction of change would depend on whether stressful life events were more, or less, common in higher social class groups.

VII

Getting up Close

15

Measuring the association between two variables

Association

When we say that two ordinal or metric variables are *associated*, we mean that they behave in a way that makes them appear 'connected' - changes in either variable seem to coincide with changes in the other variable. It's important to note (at this point anyway), that we are not suggesting that change in either variable is *causing* the change in the other variable, simply that they exhibit this commonality. As you will see, association, if it exists, may be *positive* (low values of one variable coincide with low values of the other variable, and high values with high values) or *negative* (low values with high values and vice versa).

In this chapter, I want to discuss two alternative methods of detecting an association. The first method relies on a plot of the sample data, called a *scatterplot*, in which values of one variable are plotted on the vertical axis and values of the other on the horizontal axis. The second approach is numeric, making both comparison and inference possible.

The scatterplot

A scatterplot will enable you to see if there is an association between the variables, and if there is, its strength and direction. But the scatterplot will only provide a *qualitative* assessment, and thus has obvious limitations. First, it's not always easy to say which of two sample scatterplots indicates the stronger association and second, it doesn't allow us to make *inferences* about possible associations in the population.

An example from practice

As part of a study of the possible association between Crohn's disease (CD) and ulcerative colitis (UC), researchers in Canada (Blanchard *et al.* 2001) produced the scatterplot shown in Figure 15.1. It doesn't matter which variable is plotted on which axis for the scatterplot itself, but in the study of causal *relationships* between variables (which I will discuss in Chapter 17), the choice of axis becomes more important.

Looking at the scatterplot it's not difficult to see that something is going on here. The scatter is not just a random cloud of points, but appears to display a pattern – low CD levels seem to be associated with low UC levels, and higher CD levels with high UC levels. You could justly claim that the two variables appear to be *positively associated*.

As a second example, Figure 15.2 shows a scatterplot taken from a study into the possible relationship between percentage mortality from aortic aneurysm, and the number of aortic aneurysm episodes dealt with per year, in each of 22 hospitals (McKee and Hunter 1995). This scatterplot displays a *negative association* between the two variables, low values for number of episodes seem to be associated with high values for percentage mortality, and vice versa.

As a final example from practice, Figure 15.3 shows a scatterplot taken from the cross-section study into the possible contribution of channel blockers (prescribed for depression), to the suicide rate in 284 Swedish municipalities (Lindberg *et al.* 1998), first referred to in Figure 3.10. The scatterplot here is very much more fuzzy than the two previous plots, and it would be hard to claim, merely from eyeballing it, that there is any notable association between the two variables (although admittedly there is some evidence of a rather weak positive association).

When you set out to investigate a possible association between two variables, a scatterplot is almost always worthwhile, and will often produce an insight into the way the two variables co-behave. In particular, it may reveal whether an association between them is *linear*. The

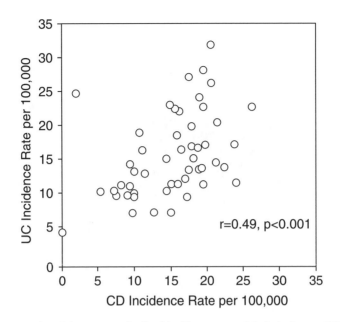

Figure 15.1 Scatterplot of the age-standardised incidence rates of Crohn's disease (CD) and ulcerative colitis (UC) by Manitoba postal area, Canada, 1987–1996. The scatterplot suggests a positive association between the two variables. Reproduced from *Americal Jnl of Epidemiology* 2001, **154**: 328–33, Fig. 3 p. 331, by permission of OUP

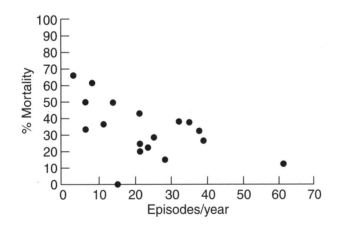

Figure 15.2 A scatterplot of percentage mortality from aortic aneurysm, and number of aortic aneurysm episodes dealt with per year, in 22 hospitals. The plot suggests a negative association between the two variables. Reproduced from *Quality in Health Care*, **4**, 5–12, courtesy of BMJ Publishing Group

property of linearity is important in some branches of statistics and we'll meet it again ourselves in Chapter 17. Put simply, a linear association is one in which the points in the scatterplot seem to cluster around a straight line. The two scatterplots in Figure 15.4 illustrate the difference between a linear and a non-linear association. The scatter in Figure 15.4a seems to be linear; but in Figure 15.4b it shows some curviness.

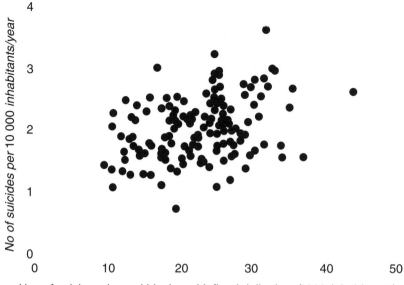

Figure 15.3   A scatterplot taken from a cross-section study into the possible contribution of channel blockers (prescribed for depression) to the suicide rate, in 284 Swedish municipalities. The plot suggests a weak, if any, relationship between the variables. Reproduced courtesy of BMJ Publishing Group

Exercise 15.1   Draw a scatterplot of Apgar score against birthweight for the 30 maternity-unit born infants using the data in Table 2.5, and comment on what it shows about any association between the two variables.

Exercise 15.2   The scatterplot in Figure 15.5 is from a study into the effect of passive smoking on respiratory symptoms (Janson *et al.* 2001). In addition, the 'best' straight line has been drawn through the points.[1] Comment on what the scatterplot suggests about the nature and strength of any association between the two variables.

Exercise 15.3   The scatterplot of percentage body fat against body mass index (bmi) in Figure 15.6 is from a cross-section study into the relationship between body mass index and body fat, in black populations in Nigeria, Jamaica and the USA (Luke *et al.* 1997). The aim of the study was to investigate whether per cent body fat rather than bmi could be used as a measure of obesity. What does the scatterplot tell you about the nature and strength of any association between these two variables?

---

[1] I'll have more to say about what constitutes the *best* straight line in Chapter 17, but loosely speaking, it's the line which passes as close as possible to all the points.

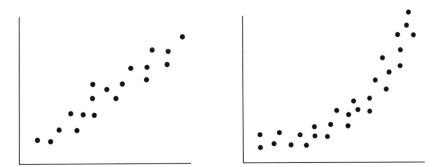

Figure 15.4   (a) A linear association (b) A non-linear association

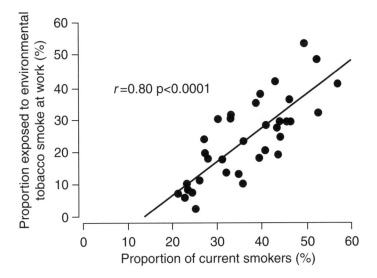

Figure 15.5   Scatterplot from a study into the effect of passive smoking on respiratory symptoms. Reprinted courtesy of Elsevier (*The Lancet* 2001, **358**, 2103–9, Fig. 1, p. 2105)

The correlation coefficient

The principal limitation of the scatterplot in assessing association is that it does not provide us with a *numeric* measure of the strength of the association; for this we have to turn to the *correlation coefficient*. Two correlation coefficients are widely used: *Pearson's* and *Spearman's*.

Pearson's correlation coefficient

Pearson's product-moment correlation coefficient, denoted ρ (Greek rho), in the population, and r in the sample, measures the strength of the *linear* association between two variables. Loosely speaking, the correlation coefficient is a measure of the average distance of all of the points from an imaginary straight line drawn through the scatter of points (analogous to the standard deviation measuring the average distance of each value from the mean).

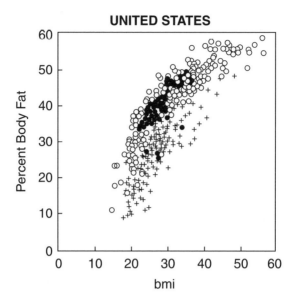

Figure 15.6 Scatterplot of per cent body fat against body mass index from a cross-section study into the relationship between bmi and body fat, in black population samples from Nigeria, Jamaica and the USA. Reproduced from *Amer. J. Epid.*, **145**, 620–8, courtesy of Oxford University Press

For Pearson's correlation coefficient to be appropriately used, both variables must be *metric continuous* and, if a confidence interval is to be determined, also approximately *Normally* distributed. The value of Pearson's correlation coefficient can vary as follows: from −1, indicating a perfect negative association (all the points lie exactly on a straight line); through 0, indicating no association; to +1, indicating perfect positive association (all points exactly on a line). In practice, with real sample data, you will never see values of –1, 0 or +1. Calculation of r by hand is very tedious and prone to error, so we will avoid it here. But it can be done in a flash with a computer statistics program, such as SPSS or Minitab.

Is the correlation coefficient statistically significant in the population?

To assess the statistical significance of a *population* correlation coefficient and hence decide whether there is a statistically significant association between the two variables, you can either perform a hypothesis test (is the *p*-value less than 0.05?), or calculate a confidence interval (does it include zero?). For the hypothesis test, the hypotheses are:

$$H_0: \rho = 0$$

$$H_1: \rho \neq 0$$

For example, for the data shown in the scatterplot in Figure 15.1, the sample $r = 0.49$, with a *p*-value < 0.001. This indicates a statistically significant positive association in the population between incidence rate of Crohn's disease and ulcerative colitis.

A useful rule of thumb if you have a value for r but no confidence interval or p-value, is that to be statistically significant, r must be greater than $2/\sqrt{n}$, where n is the sample size. For example, if $n = 100$, then r has to be greater than $2/10 = 0.200$ to be statistically significant.

An example from practice

Table 15.1 is taken from the same cross-section study as Exercise 15.3, and shows the sample Pearson's correlation coefficient for the association between bmi and per cent body fat, with blood pressure, and waist and hip measurements, along with an indication of the statistical significance or otherwise of the p-value.

Unfortunately, the authors have not given the actual p-values, but only indicated whether they were less than 0.05 or less than 0.01. This is not good practice; the actual p-values should always be provided. As you can see, the population correlation coefficient between both bmi and per cent body fat, with waist and hip circumference, is positive and statistically significant in every case. However, bmi is more *closely* associated (higher r values) than body fat, except in Jamaican men. Apart from the association with systolic blood pressure in US males, there is no statistically significant association with either of the blood pressure measurements.

> **Exercise 15.4** Table 15.2 is from a case-control study of medical record validation (Olson *et al.* 1997), and shows the value of Pearson's r, and the 98 per cent confidence intervals, for the correlation between gestational age, as estimated by the mother, and as determined from medical records, for a number of demographic sub-groups (ignore the last column). The cases were the mothers of child leukaemia patients, the matched controls were randomly selected by random telephone calling. Identify: (a) any correlation coefficients not statistically significant; (b) the strongest correlation; (c) the weakest correlation.

Spearman's rank correlation coefficient

If *either* (or both) of the variables is ordinal, then *Spearman's rank correlation coefficient* (usually denoted ρ_s in the population and r_s in the sample) is appropriate. This is a non-parametric measure. As with Pearson's correlation coefficient, Spearman's correlation coefficient varies from -1, through 0, to $+1$, and its statistical significance can again be assessed with a p-value or a confidence interval. The null hypothesis is that the population correlation coefficient $\rho_s = 0$. Spearman's r_s is not quite as bad to calculate by hand as Pearson's r but bad enough, and once again you would want to do it with the help of a computer program.

An example from practice

Table 15.3 is from the same cross-section study first referred to in Figure 4.3, into the use of the Ontario mammography services. The authors wanted to know whether the variation in

Table 15.1 Correlation coefficients from a cross-section study into the relationship between body mass index (bmi) and body fat, in black population samples from Nigeria, Jamaica, and the USA. The aim of the study was to investigate whether body fat rather than bmi could be used as a measure of obesity.[‡,§] Reproduced from *Amer. J. Epid.*, **145**, 620–8, courtesy of Oxford University Press

	Women						Men					
	Nigeria		Jamaica		United States		Nigeria		Jamaica		United States	
Variable	BMI	% fat	BMI	% fat	BMI	% fat	BMI	% fat	BMI	% fat	BMI	% fat
Waist circumference	0.90**	0.77**	0.87**	0.77**	0.91**	0.85**	0.89**	0.79**	0.69**	0.76**	0.93**	0.83**
Hip circumference	0.93**	0.81**	0.91**	0.82**	0.93**	0.87**	0.89**	0.76**	0.64**	0.72**	0.93**	0.82**
Systolic blood pressure	0.24	0.24	0.16	0.15	0.21	0.21	0.09	0.09	0.24	0.24	0.24*	0.23*
Diastolic blood pressure	0.16	0.14	0.20	0.16	0.07	0.10	0.31	0.24	0.16	0.11	0.22	0.20

* $p < 0.05$; ** $p < 0.01$.
† Weight (kg)/height (m)².
‡Data were adjusted for age.
§No significant difference was found between correlation coefficients for body mass index and percentage of body fat.

the ranked utilisation rates (number of visits per 1000 women) was similar across the age groups. They did this by measuring the strength of the association between the ranked rates for each pair of different age groups. When the association was strong and significant, they concluded that the variation in the usage rate was similar.

The results show that the r_s for the association between the ranked usage rates for 30–39 year-olds, and the 40–49 year-olds, across the 33 districts was 0.6496 (first row of table), with a p-value of 0.0005. So this association is positive and statistically significant in these two age group populations. Indeed, the correlation coefficients between all pairs of age groups are statistically significant, with all p-values < 0.05. The authors thus concluded that variation in

Table 15.2 Pearson's r and 98 per cent confidence intervals for the association between gestational age, as estimated by the mother and from medical records, for a number of demographic sub-groups. Reproduced from *Amer. J. Epid.*, **145**, 58–67, courtesy of Oxford University Press

	Correlation of gestational age	98% CI[*]	Kappa statistic[†]
All gestational ages	0.839	0.817–0.859	0.62
Case/control status			
Cases	0.849	0.813–0.878	0.63
Controls	0.835	0.805–0.861	0.61
Education			
<High school	0.694	0.553–0.797	0.51
High school	0.833	0.790–0.868	0.63
>High school	0.835	0.804–0.861	0.62
Household income			
<$22,000	0.791	0.734–0.837	0.59
$22,000–$ 34,999	0.882	0.849–0.908	0.62
≥$35,000	0.843	0.800–0.877	0.65
Unknown	0.745	0.641–0.823	0.60
Time (years) from delivery to interview			
<2	0.896	0.862–0.921	0.64
2–3.9	0.821	0.784–0.852	0.63
4–5.9	0.828	0.775–0.869	0.61
6–8	0.852	0.734–0.920	0.42
Maternal age (years)			
<25	0.822	0.773–0.861	0.64
25–29	0.889	0.862–0.912	0.63
30–34	0.760	0.694–0.813	0.57
≥35	0.888	0.824–0.930	0.64
Birth order			
First born	0.880	0.853–0.903	0.67
Second born	0.815	0.778–0.846	0.57
≥Third born	0.632	0.416–0.781	0.52
Maternal race			
White	0.846	0.822–0.866	0.64
Other	0.782	0.680–0.855	0.42

[*]CI, confidence Interval.
[†] Three categories, <38, 38–41, ≥42 weeks.

Table 15.3 Spearman correlation coefficients from a cross-section study of the use of the Ontario mammography services in relation to age. Each correlation coefficient measures the strength of the association in the variation between the ranked usage rate across the 33 heath districts for each pair of age groups. Reproduced from *J. Epid. Comm. Health*, **51**, 378–82, courtesy of BMJ Publishing Group

Age group (y)	30–39y	40–49y	50–69y	70+y
30–39	1.0000	0.6496 (p < 0.0001)	0.5949 (p = 0.0005)	0.5488 (p = 0.0014)
40–49		1.0000	0.9021 (p < 0.0001)	0.8985 (p < 0.0001)
50–69			1.0000	0.9513 (p < 0.0001)
70+				1.0000

usage rate was similar for the four age groups across the 33 health districts. However, whether association is the correct way to measure similarity in two sets of values is a question I will return to in the next chapter.

Two other correlation coefficients can only be mentioned briefly. Kendal's rank-order correlation coefficient, denoted τ (tau), is appropriate in the same circumstances as Spearman's r_s, i.e. with ranked data (which may be ordinal or continuous). Tau is available in SPSS, but not in Minitab. The *point-biserial* correlation coefficient is appropriate if one variable is metric continuous and the other is truly dichotomous (which means that the variable can take only two values; alive or dead, male or female, etc.). Unfortunately, this latter measure of association is not available in either SPSS or Minitab.

If you plan to use a correlation coefficient you should ensure that the assumptions referred to above are satisfied, in particular that the association is linear - which can be checked by a scatterplot. Moreover, with Pearson's correlation coefficient you should interpret any results with suspicion if there are outliers present in either data set, since these can distort the results.

Finally it is worth noting again that just because two variables are significantly associated, does *not* mean that there is a cause–effect *relationship* between them.

16

Measuring agreement

Learning objectives

When you have finished this chapter you should be able to:

- Explain the difference between association and agreement.

- Describe Cohen's kappa, calculate its value and assess the level of agreement.

- Interpret published values for kappa.

- Describe the idea behind ordinal kappa.

- Outline the Bland–Altman approach to measuring agreement between metric variables.

To agree or not agree: that is the question

Association is a measure of the inter-connectedness of two variables; the degree to which they tend to change together, either positively or negatively. *Agreement* is the degree to which the values in two sets of data actually *agree*. To illustrate this idea look at the hypothetical data in Table 16.1, which shows the decision by a psychiatrist and by a psychiatric social worker (PSW) whether to section (Y), or not section (N), each of 10 individuals with mental ill-health. We would say that the two variables were in perfect *agreement* if every pair of values were the same.

Medical Statistics from Scratch, Second Edition   David Bowers
© 2008 John Wiley & Sons, Ltd

Table 16.1 Decision by a psychiatrist and a psychiatric social worker whether or not to section 10 individuals suffering mental ill-health

Patient	1	2	3	4	5	6	7	8	9	10
Psychiatrist	Y	Y	N	Y	N	N	N	Y	Y	Y
PSW	Y	N	N	Y	N	N	Y	Y	Y	N

In practical situations this won't happen, and here you can see that only seven out of the 10 decisions are the same, so the *observed* level of *proportional agreement* is 0.70 (70 per cent).

Cohen's kappa

However, if you had asked each clinician simply to toss a coin to make the decision (heads – section, tails – don't section), some of their decisions would probably still have been the same – by *chance* alone. You need to adjust the observed level of agreement for the proportion you would have *expected* to occur by chance alone. This adjustment gives us the *chance-corrected proportional agreement statistic*, known as Cohen's *kappa, κ*:

$$\kappa = \frac{(\text{proportion of observed agreement} - \text{proportion of expected agreement})}{(1 - \text{proportion of expected agreement})}$$

We can calculate the *expected* values using a contingency table in exactly the same way as we did for chi-squared (row total × column total ÷ overall total – see Chapter 14). Table 16.2 shows the data in Table 16.1 expressed in the form of a contingency table, with the psychiatrist's scores in the rows, the PSW's scores in the columns, and with row and column totals added. The expected values are shown in brackets in each cell.

Table 16.2 Contingency table showing observed (and *expected*) decisions by a psychiatrist and a psychiatric social worker on whether to section 10 patients (data from Figure 16.1)

		Psychiatric Social Worker		Totals	Expected value: (5 × 6)/10 = 3
		Yes	No		
Psychiatrist	Yes	4 (3)	2 (3)	6	
	No	1 (2)	3 (2)	4	
	Totals	5	5	10	

We have seen that the *observed* agreement is 0.70, and we can calculate the expected agreement to be 5 out of 10 or 0.50.[1] Therefore:

$$\kappa = (0.70 - 0.50)/(1 - 0.50) = 0.20/0.50 = 0.40$$

---

[1] We can expect the two clinicians to agree on 'Yes' three times, and 'No' two times, making five agreements in total.

Table 16.3 How good is the agreement – assessing kappa

Kappa	Strength of agreement
≤0.20	Poor
0.21–0.40	Fair
0.41–0.60	Moderate
0.61–0.80	Good
0.81–1.00	Very good

So after allowing for chance agreements, agreement is reduced from 70 per cent to 40 per cent. Kappa can vary between zero (agreement no better than chance), and one (perfect agreement), and you can use Table 16.3 to asses the quality of agreement. It's possible to calculate a confidence interval for kappa, but these will usually be too narrow (except for quite small samples) to add much insight to your result.

An example from practice

Table 16.4 is from a study into the development of a new quality of life scale for patients with advanced cancer and their families – the Palliative Care Outcome scale (POS) (Hearn *et al.* 1998). It shows agreement between the patient and staff (who also completed the scale questionnaires) for a number of items on the POS scale. The table also contains values of Spearman's r_s, and the proportion of agreements within one point on the POS scale. The level of agreement between staff and patient is either fair or moderate for all items, and agreement within one point is either good or very good.

Table 16.4 From a palliative care outcome scale (POS) study showing levels of agreement between the patient and staff assessment for a number of items on the POS scale. Reproduced from *Quality in Health Care*, **8**, 219–27, courtesy of BMJ Publishing Group

Item	No of patients	Patient score (% severe)	Staff score (% severe)	K	Spearman correlation	Proportion agreement within 1 score
At first assessment: 145 matched assessments						
Pain	140	24.3	20.0	0.56	0.67	0.87
Other symptoms	140	27.2	26.4	0.43	0.60	0.86
Patient anxiety	140	23.6	30.0	0.37	0.56	0.83
Family anxiety	137	49.6	46.0	0.28	0.37	0.72
Information	135	12.6	13.4	0.39	0.36	0.79
Support	135	10.4	14.1	0.22	0.32	0.79
Life worthwhile	133	13.6	16.5	0.43	0.54	0.82
Self worth	132	15.9	23.5	0.37	0.53	0.82
Wasted time	135	5.9	6.7	0.33	0.32	0.95
Personal affairs	129	7.8	13.2	0.42	0.49	0.96

Table 16.5 Injury Severity Scale (ISS) scores given from case notes by two experienced trauma clinicians to 16 patients in a major trauma unit. Reproduced from *BMJ*, **307**, 906–9. by permission of BMJ Publishing Group

Observer no.	Case no.															
	1	2	3	4	5	6	7	8	9	10	11	12	13	14	15	16
1	9	14	29	17	34	17	38	13	29	4	29	25	4	16	25	45
2	9	13	29	17	22	14	45	10	29	4	25	34	9	25	8	50

Exercise 16.1 Do the highest and the lowest levels of agreement in Table 16.4 coincide with the highest and lowest levels of correlation? Will this always be the case?

Exercise 16.2 Table 16.5 is from a study in a major trauma unit into the variation between two experienced trauma clinicians in assessing the degree of injury of 16 patients from their case notes (Zoltie *et al.* 1993). The table shows the Injury Severity Scale (ISS) score awarded to each patient.[2] Categorise the scores into two groups: ISS scores of less than 16, and of 16 or more. Express the results in a contingency table, and calculate: (a) the observed and expected proportional agreement; (b) kappa. Comment on the level of agreement.

A limitation of kappa is that it is sensitive to the proportion of subjects in each category (i.e. to prevalence), so caution is needed when comparing kappa values from different studies – these are only helpful if prevalences are similar. Moreover, Cohen's kappa as described above is only appropriate for *nominal* data, as in the sectioning example above, although most data can be 'nominalised', like the ISS values above. In the next paragraph, however, I describe, briefly, a version of kappa which can handle ordinal data.

Measuring agreement with ordinal data – weighted kappa

The idea behind weighted kappa is best illustrated by referring back to the data in Table 16.5. The two clinician's ISS scores agree for only five patients. So the proportional observed agreement is only 5/16 = 0.3125 (31.25 per cent). However, in several cases the scores have a 'near miss'; patient 2, for example, with scores of 14 and 13. Other pairs of scores are further apart, patient 15 is given scores of 25 and 8! Weighted kappa gives credit for near misses, but its calculation is too complex for this book.

Measuring the agreement between two metric continuous variables

When it comes to measuring agreement between two metric continuous variables the obvious problem is the large number of possible values – it's quite possible that *none* of them will be

---

[2] The ISS is used for the assessment of severity of injury, with a range from 0 to 75. ISS scores of 16 or above indicate potentially life-threatening injury, and survival with ISS scores above 51 is considered unlikely.

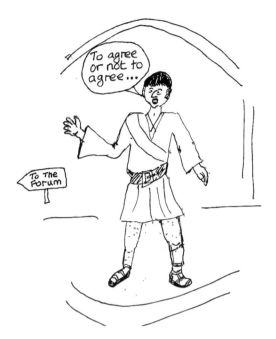

the same. One solution is to use a Bland-Altman chart (Bland and Altman 1986). This involves plotting, for each pair of measurements, the *differences* between the two scores (on the vertical axis) against the *mean* of the two scores (on the horizontal axis).

A pair of tramlines, called the 95 per cent *limits of agreement*, are drawn a distance of two s_d above and below the zero difference line (where s_d = standard deviations of the differences). If

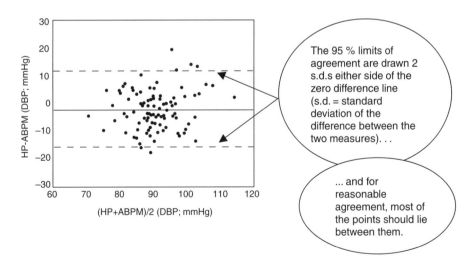

Figure 16.1 A Bland-Altman chart to measure agreement between two metric continuous variables; diastolic blood pressure as measured by patients at home with a cuff-measuring device (HP), and as measured by the same patients using an ambulatory device (ABPM). Reproduced from *Brit. J. General Practice*, **48**, 1585–9, courtesy of the Royal College of General Practitioners

all of the points on the graph fall between the tramlines, then agreement is 'acceptable', but the more points there are outside the tramlines, the less good the agreement. Moreover the spread of the points should be reasonably horizontal, indicating that differences are not increasing (or decreasing) as the values of the two variables increase.

An example from practice

The idea is illustrated in Figure 16.1, for agreement between two methods of measuring diastolic blood pressure (Brueren *et al.* 1998). In this example, there are only a few points outside the $\pm$ 2 standard deviation tramlines and the spread of points is broadly horizontal. We would assess this chart as suggesting reasonably good agreement between the two methods of blood pressure measurement.

The continuous horizontal line across the middle of the chart represents the mean of the differences between the two measures. Note that this is below the zero mark indicating some bias in the measures. It looks as if the ABPM values are greater on the whole than the HP values.

To sum up, two variables that are in reasonable agreement will be strongly associated, but the opposite is not necessarily true. The two measures are not equivalent; association does not measure agreement.

VIII

Getting into a Relationship

17

Straight line models:
linear regression

Medical Statistics from Scratch, Second Edition   David Bowers
© 2008 John Wiley & Sons, Ltd

- Interpret computer-generated linear regression results.

- Explain what goodness-of-fit is and how it is measured in the simple linear regression model.

- Explain the role of $\bar{R}^2$ in the context of multiple linear regression.

- Interpret published multiple linear regression results.

- Explain the adjustment properties of the regression model.

- Outline how the basic assumptions can be checked graphically.

Health warning!

Although the maths underlying the idea of linear regression is a little complicated, some explanation of the idea is necessary if you are to gain any understanding of the procedure and be able to interpret regression computer outputs sensibly. I have tried to keep the discussion as brief and as non-technical as possible, but if you have an aversion to maths you might want to skim the material in the next few pages.

Relationship and association

In Chapter 15, I emphasised the fact that an association between two variables does *not* mean that there is a cause-and-effect relationship between them. For example, body mass index and systolic blood pressure may appear to be closely associated, but this does *necessarily* mean that an increase in body mass index will *cause* a corresponding increase in systolic blood pressure (or indeed the other way round). In this chapter and the next, I am going to deal with the idea of a *causal* relationship between variables, such that changes in the value of one variable bring about or *cause* changes in the value of another variable. Or to put it another way, variation among a group of individuals in say their blood pressure is caused, or explained, by the variation among those same individuals in their body mass index.

In the clinical world demonstrating a cause–effect relationship is difficult, and requires a number of conditions to be satisfied; the relationship should be plausible, repeatable, predictable, with a proved mechanism, and so on. I will assume in the remainder of this chapter that a cause-effect relationship between the variables has been satisfactorily demonstrated, and that this relationship is *linear* (see pp. 172/3 for an explanation of linearity).

A causal relationship – explaining variation

Let's begin with a simple example. Suppose that systolic blood pressure (SBP), in mmHg, *is* effected by body mass index (bmi) in kg/m^2, and the two variables are related by the following expression:

SBP equals 110 plus ³⁄₄ of bmi

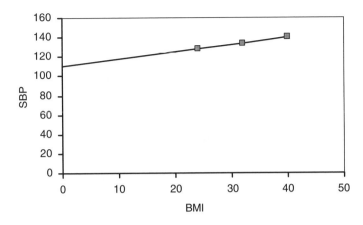

Figure 17.1 A plot of systolic blood pressure (SBP) against body mass index (bmi) produces a straight line, and shows that the relationship between the two variables is linear

So for example, when bmi = 40, SBP equals 110 plus 3/4 of 40, or 110 plus 30, which equals 140. This equation is a *linear* equation. If you plot it with pairs of values of bmi and SBP, you will see a straight line. For instance, when bmi = 24, SBP = 128, and when bmi = 32, SBP = 134. We already know that when bmi = 40, SBP = 140, and if we plot these three pairs of values, and draw a line through them, we get Figure 17.1. This is clearly a straight line.

We can write the above expression more mathematically as an equation:

$$SBP = 110 + 0.75 \times bmi$$

This equation explains the *variation* in systolic blood pressure from person to person, in terms of corresponding *variation* from person to person in body mass index. I have referred to this relationship as an equation, but I could also have described it as a *model*. We are *modelling* the variation in systolic blood pressure in terms of corresponding variation in body mass index. We can write this equation in a more general form in terms of two variables Y and X, thus:[1]

$$Y = b_0 + b_1 X$$

The term b_0 is known as the *constant coefficient*, or the coefficient of intersection – it's where the line cuts the Y axis (110 in our Figure 17.1). The term b_1 is known as the *slope coefficient*, (0.75 in our equation), and will be positive if the line slopes upwards from left to right (as in Figure 17.1), and negative if the line slopes down from left to right (as in Figure 15.2). Higher values of b_1 means more steeply sloped lines. One important point: the value of b_1 (+ 0.75 in the example) is the amount by which SBP would change if the value of bmi *increased* by 1 unit. I'll come back to this later.

---

[1] You may remember this from school as: $y = mx + c$, or some other variation.

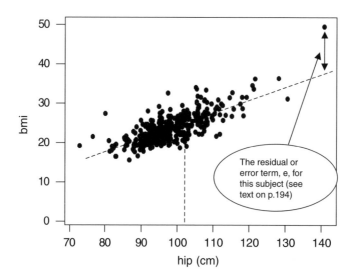

Figure 17.2 A scatterplot of body mass index against hip circumference, for a sample of 412 women in a diet and health cohort study. The scatter of values appears to be distributed around a straight line. That is, the relationship between these two variables appears to be broadly *linear*

Exercise 17.1 Plot the following values for the variables X and Y on a scatter plot and draw the straight line through the points. What is the equation of this line?

Y	5	4	2	1
X	2	4	8	10

The linear regression model

In Figure 17.1 all of the points lie *exactly* on the straight line. In practice this won't happen, and the scatterplot in Figure 17.2 is more typical of what you might see. Here we have body mass index, bmi, (in kg/m^2), and hip circumference, HIP (cm), for a sample of 412 British women from a study into the relationship between diet and health. Suppose we believe that there is a causal relationship between bmi and HIP – changes in hip measurement lead to changes in bmi. If we want to investigate the nature of this relationship then we need to do three things, which I'll deal with in turn:

- Make sure that the relationship is linear.[2]

- Find a way to determine the equation linking the variables, i.e. get the values of b_0 and b_1.

- See if the relationship is statistically significant, i.e. that it is present in the population.

---

[2] Because we are only dealing with linear relationships in this chapter.

Is the relationship linear?

One way of investigating the linearity of the relationship is to examine the scatterplot, such as that in Figure 17.2.

The points in the scatterplot do seem to cluster along a straight line (shown dotted), which I have drawn, 'by eye', through the scatter. This suggests a *linear* relationship between bmi and HIP. So far, so good. We can write the equation of this straight line as:

$$bmi = b_0 + b_1 \times HIP$$

This equation is known as *the sample regression equation*. The variable on the left-hand side of the equation, bmi, is known variously as the *outcome, response* or *dependent* variable. I'm going to refer to it as the dependent variable in this chapter. It must be *metric continuous*. It gives us the *mean* value of bmi for any specified HIP measurement. In other words, it would tell us (if we knew b_0 and b_1) what the mean body mass index would be for all those women with some particular hip measurement.

The variable on the right-hand side of the equation, HIP, is known variously as the *predictor, explanatory* or *independent* variable, or the covariate. I will use the term *independent variable* here. The independent variable can be of any type: nominal, ordinal or metric. This is the variable that's doing the 'causing'. It is changes in hip circumference that cause body mass index to change in response, but not the other way round.

Incidentally, my 'by eye' line has the equation:

$$bmi = -8.4 + 0.33 \times HIP$$

This means that the *mean* body mass index of *all* the women with, say, HIP = 100 cm in this sample is equal to 24.6 kg/m^2.

Clearly drawing a line by eye through a scatter is not satisfactory – ten people would get ten different lines. So the obvious question arises, 'What is the 'best' straight line that can be "drawn" through a scatter of sample values, and how do I find out what it is?'

Exercise 17.2 (a) Draw by eye the best straight line you can through the scatterplot in Figure 15.1, and write down the regression equation. By how much would the mean incidence rate of ulcerative colitis (UC) change if the rate of Crohn's disease (CD) changed by one unit? (b) Draw, by eye, the best straight line you can through the scatterplot in Figure 15.2, and write down the regression equation. What change in mean percentage mortality would you expect if the mean number of episodes per year increased by 1? (c) What is the equation of the regression line shown in Figure 15.5? What value of mean per cent exposed at work would you expect if per cent of current smokers in a workplace was 35 per cent?

Estimating b_0 and b_1 – the method of ordinary least squares (OLS)

The second problem is to find a method of getting the values of the sample coefficients b_0 and b_1, which will give us a line that fits the scatter of points better than any other line, and which will then enable us to write down the equation linking the variables. The most popular method used for this calculation is called *ordinary least squares*, or OLS. This gives us the values of b_0 and b_1, and the straight line that *best* fits the sample data. Roughly speaking, 'best' means the line that is, on average, closer to all of the points than any other line. How does it do this? Look back at Figure 17.2. The distance of each point in the scatter from the regression line is known as the *residual* or error, denoted e. I have shown the e for just one of the points. If all of these residuals are squared and then added together, to give the term Σe^2,[3] then the 'best' straight line is the one for which the sum, Σe^2, is smallest. Hence the name ordinary 'least squares'.

Now: the calculations involved with OLS are too tedious to do by hand, but you can use a suitable computer program to derive their values quite easily (both SPSS and Minitab will do this). It is important to note that the sample regression coefficients b_0 and b_1 are *estimates* of the population regression coefficients β_0 and β_1. In other words, we are using the sample regression equation:

$$Y = b_0 + b_1 X$$

to estimate the *population regression equation*:

$$Y = \beta_0 + \beta_1 X$$

Basic assumptions of the ordinary least squares procedure

The ordinary least squares procedure is only guaranteed to produce the line that best fits the data if the following assumptions are satisfied:

• The relationship between Y and X is linear.

• The dependent variable Y is metric continuous.

• The residual term, e, is Normally distributed, with a mean of zero, for each value of the independent variable, X.

• The spread of the residual terms should be the same, whatever the value of X. In other words, e shouldn't spread out more (or less) when X increases.

Let me explain the last two assumptions. Suppose you had, say, 50 women with a hip circumference of 100 cm. As the scatterplot in Figure 17.2 indicates, most of these women have a different body mass index. As you have seen, the difference between each individual woman's bmi and the regression line is the residual e. If you arranged these 50 residual values into a frequency distribution then the third assumption stipulates that this distribution should be Normal.

The fourth assumption demands that if you repeated the above exercise for each separate value of hip circumference, then the spreads (the standard deviations) of each distribution of

---

[3] Known as the sum of squares. Σ is the Greek 'sigma', which means sum all the values.

residual values should be the same, for all hip sizes. If the residual terms have this latter property then they are said to be *homoskedastic*.

These assumptions may seem complicated, but the consequences for the accuracy of the ordinary least squares estimators may be serious if they are violated. Needless to say, these assumptions need to be checked. I'll return to this later.

Back to the example – is the relationship statistically significant?

Having calculated b_1 and b_2, we now need to address the third question; is the relationship statistically significant in the population? We can use either confidence intervals for β_0 and β_1 or hypothesis tests, to judge statistical significance. We then ask: 'Does the confidence interval for β_1 include zero (or is its p value > 0.05)?' If the answer in either case is yes, then you *can't* reject the null hypothesis that β_1 *is* equal to zero; which means that the relationship is not statistically significant. Whatever the value of HIP, once multiplied by a b_1 equal to zero, it disappears from the regression equation and can have no effect on bmi.

SPSS and Minitab for example, will give you confidence intervals and/or p values. In practice we have very little interest in the constant coefficient β_0; it's only there to keep a mathematical equality between the left- and right-hand sides of the equation. Besides, in reality it often has no sensible interpretation. For example, in the current example, β_0 would equal the body mass index of individuals with a hip circumference equal to zero!

Thus the focus in linear regression analysis is to use b_1 to estimate β_1, and then examine its statistical significance. If β_1 *is* statistically significant, then the relationship is established (well at least with a confidence level of 95 per cent).

Using SPSS

If you use the SPSS linear regression program with the data on the 412 women in Figure 17.2, you will get the output shown in Figure 17.3. SPSS provides both a p value and a 95 per cent confidence interval.

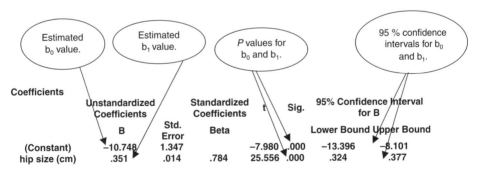

a Dependent Variable: Body Mass Index (weight/height^2) (kg/m2)
$R^2 = 0.614$; $R^2 = 0.613$[1].

---

[1] Values for R^2 amd R^{-2} appear in a separate table in the SPSS output. For convenience I have copied them to this table. See below for comment on R^2.

Figure 17.3 Output from SPSS for ordinary least squares regression applied to the body mass index/hip circumference example

Using Minitab

With Minitab you get the output shown in Figure 17.4. Minitab calculates only the p value, otherwise the results are the same as for SPSS.

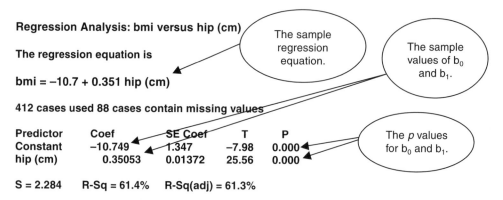

Regression Analysis: bmi versus hip (cm)

The regression equation is

bmi = −10.7 + 0.351 hip (cm)

412 cases used 88 cases contain missing values

Predictor	Coef	SE Coef	T	P
Constant	−10.749	1.347	−7.98	0.000
hip (cm)	0.35053	0.01372	25.56	0.000

S = 2.284   R-Sq = 61.4%   R-Sq(adj) = 61.3%

The sample regression equation.

The sample values of b_0 and b_1.

The p values for b_0 and b_1.

Figure 17.4 Output from Minitab for ordinary least squares regression applied to the body mass index/hip circumference example

Between them, Figure 17.3 and Figure 17.4 provide us with the estimates of b_0 and b_1, their 95 per cent confidence intervals and their p values, along with the value of R^2 (see below). Regression results are often summarised in a table such as that in Table 17.1.

Table 17.1 Summary of results from the regression of BMI on HIP

Dependent variable	Coefficient	Estimated value	(95 % CI)	(p-value)	R^2	$\bar{R}^2$
BMI	b_0	−10.748	(−13.396 to −8.101)	0.000		
	b_1	0.351	(0.324 to 0.377)	0.000	61.4%	61.3%

The 95 per cent confidence interval and the p value is shown alongside each sample coefficient. Both parameters β_0 and β_1 are statistically significant, since neither confidence interval includes zero, and both p values are less than 0.05. Thus the result of this analysis is that bmi and HIP are statistically significantly related through the linear regression equation:

$$bmi = -10.7 + 0.351 \times HIP^4$$

The value of +0.351 for b_1 means that for every unit (1 cm) increase in hip circumference, the mean bmi will increase by 0.351 kg/m^2. Knowing the equation, you can, if you wish, draw this best OLS estimated regression line onto the scatterplot.

The regression equation also enables us to *predict* the value of the mean bmi, for any value of hip circumference, *within* the range of the sample hip circumference values (71 cm to 140 cm). For example, for individuals with a hip circumference of 100 cm, you can substitute HIP = 100

---

[4] Compare with the by-eye line of: bmi = −8.4 + 0.33HIP.

into the sample regression equation and thus calculate a value for mean bmi of $24.4\,\text{kg/m}^2$. Prediction of bmi for hip circumference values *outside* the original sample data range requires a more complex procedure, and will not be discussed here.

> **Exercise 17.3**   What does the model predict for mean bmi for women with a hip circumference of 130 cm?

Goodness-of-fit – R^2

Figure 17.3, Figure 17.4, and Table 17.1, contain values for something called R^2, and $\bar{R}^2$ (SPSS calls the latter 'R-Sq(adj)'). What are these? Suppose you think that waist circumference, WST, might be used as a measure of obesity, so you repeat the above procedure, but use WST as your independent variable instead of HIP. Your results indicate that b_1 is again statistically significant. Now you have two models, in both of which the independent variable has a statistically significant linear relationship with bmi. But which model is best? The one with HIP or the one with WST?

In fact, the best model is the one that 'explains' the greatest proportion of the observed variation in bmi from subject to subject, that is, has the best *goodness-of-fit*. One such measure of this explanatory power is known as the *coefficient of determination*, and is denoted R^2.

As a matter of interest, $R^2 = 0.614$, or 61.4 per cent, for the hip circumference model, and $R^2 = 0.501$, or 50.1 per cent, for the waist circumference model. So variation in hip circumference explains 61 per cent of the observed variation in bmi, while variation in waist circumference explains only 50 per cent of the variation. So using hip circumference as your independent variable gives you a better fitting model.

Here's a thought. If only 61 per cent of the variation in bmi is explained by variation in hip circumference, what is the remaining 39 per cent explained by? One possibility is that the rest is due to chance, to random effects. A more likely possibility is that, as well as hip circumference, there are other variables that contribute something to the variation in bmi from subject to subject. It would be naïve to believe that variation in bmi, or any clinical variable, can be totally explained by only one variable. Which brings us neatly to the *multiple* linear regression model.

Multiple linear regression

A *simple* linear regression model is one with only one independent variable on the right-hand side. When you have *more* than one independent variable the regression model is called a *multiple linear regression model*. For example, having noticed that both hip and waist circumference are each significantly related to bmi, you might include them *both* as independent variables. This gives the following model, which now gives us *mean* bmi for the various possible combinations of sample values of both HIP and WST:

$$\text{bmi} = b_0 + b_1 \times \text{HIP} + b_2 \times \text{WST}$$

	Variable	Estimated coefficient	(95 % CI)	(p-value)	R^2	$\bar{R}^2$
Model (& dependent variable)	constant	$b_0 = -10.748$	$(-13.396$ to $-8.101)$	0.000		
1. BMI	HIP	$b_1 = 0.351$	$(0.324$ to $0.377)$	0.000	61.4%	61.3%
2. BMI	constant	$b_0 = -9.645$	$(-12.250$ to $-7.041)$	0.000		
	HIP	$b_1 = 0.261$	$(0.219$ to $0.303)$	0.000		
	WST	$b_2 = 0.105$	$(0.065$ to $0.144)$	0.000	63.7%	63.5%

Figure 17.5 Multiple linear regression output (last three rows) from SPSS for model with body mass index as the dependent variable and both hip and waist circumferences as independent variables

Note that when we move from the simple to the multiple linear regression model, we need to add a further basic assumption to the list on p. 194. That is, that there is no perfect association or *collinearity* between any of the independent variables. When this assumption is not met, we refer to the model as having *multicollinearity*. The consequence of this condition is wide and thus imprecise confidence intervals.

If you use SPPS to derive the OLS estimators of the above model containing both HIP and WST you get the output shown in Figure 17.5 (last three rows).

Using these results, we can write the estimated multiple linear regression model as:

$$\text{bmi} = -9.645 + 0.261 \times \text{HIP} + 0.105 \times \text{WST}$$

So for example, for all of those women in the sample for whom HIP = 100 and WST = 75, then the above equation estimates their *mean* bmi to be:

$$\text{bmi} = -9.645 + 0.261 \times 100 + 0.105 \times 75 = 24.330$$

The other information in Figure 17.5 tells us that parameters β_1 and β_2 are both statistically significant as neither confidence interval includes zero. Compared to the simple regression model containing only HIP as an independent variable, goodness of fit has improved marginally, with R^2 increasing from 61.4 per cent to 63.7 per cent. Note that in the multiple linear regression model, R^2 measures the explanatory power with *all* of the variables currently in the model acting together.

Exercise 17.4 If we add 'age' as a third independent variable to the bmi model, then Minitab produces the results shown in Figure 17.6. (a) Comment on the statistical significance of the three independent variables. (b) How does an increase in age effect mean body mass index values? (c) Has goodness of fit improved compared to the model with only HIP and WST included? (d) What is the mean body mass index of all of those women in the sample with a hip circumference of 100 cm, and a waist circumference of 75 cm, who are aged: (i) 30; (ii) 60?

Regression Analysis : BMI versus hip(cm), waist(cm), Age

```
The regression equation is

BMI = - 12.4 + 0.289 hip(cm) + 0.125 waist(cm) - 0.0249 Age

Predictor        Coef    SE Coef       T       P
Constant      -12.425      1.353   -9.18   0.000
Hip(cm)       0.28876    0.02041   14.15   0.000
Waist(cm)     0.12549    0.01762    7.12   0.000
Age          -0.02492    0.01104   -2.26   0.024

S = 2.24817    R-Sq = 64.0%   R-Sq(adj) = 63.8%
```

Figure 17.6 Output from Minitab for regression of bmi on HIP, WST and AGE

Dealing with nominal independent variables: design variables and coding

In linear regression, most of the independent variables are likely to be metric, or at least ordinal. However any independent variable that is *nominal* must be coded into a so-called *design* (or *dummy*) variable, before being entered into a model. There is only space for a brief description of the process here.

As an example, suppose in a study of hypertension, you have systolic blood pressure (SBP) as your dependent variable, and age (AGE) and smoking status (SMK), as your independent variables. SMK, is a nominal variable, having the categories: non-smoker, ex-smoker, and current smoker. This gives the model:

$$SBP = b_0 + b_1 AGE + b_2 SMK \qquad (1)$$

To enter SMK into your computer, you would have to score the three smoking categories in some way – but how? As 1, 2, 3, or as 0, 1, 2, etc. As you can imagine, the scores you attribute to each category will effect your results. The answer is to *code* these three categories into *two* design variables. Note that the number of design variables is always one *less* than the number of categories in the variable being coded. In this example, we set out the coding design as in Table 17.2.

So you replace smoking status (with its dodgy numbering), with two new design variables, D_1 and D_2, which take the values in Table 17.2, according to smoking status. The model now

Table 17.2 Coding design for a nominal variable with three categories

Smoking status	Design variable values	
	D_1	D_2
Non-smoker	0	0
Ex-smoker	0	1
Current smoker	1	0

becomes: $Y = b_0 + b_1 \text{Age} + b_2 D_1 + b_3 D_2$. For example, if the subject is a current smoker, $D_1 = 1$ and $D_2 = 0$; if an ex-smoker, $D_1 = 0$ and $D_2 = 1$; if a non-smoker, $D_1 = 0$ and $D_2 = 0$. Notice in the last situation that the smoking status variable effectively disappears from the model.

This coding scheme can be extended to deal with nominal variables with any reasonable number of categories, depending on the sample size.[5] The simplest situation is a nominal variable with only *two* categories, such as sex, which can be represented by one design variable with values 0 (if male) or 1 (if female).

Exercise 17.5   The first three subjects in the study of systolic blood pressure and its relationship with age and smoking status are, a 50-year-old smoker, a 55-year-old non-smoker and a 35-year-old ex-smoker, respectively. Fill in the first three rows of the data sheet shown in Table 17.3, as appropriate.

Table 17.3   Data sheet for systolic blood pressure relationship

Subject	Age	D_1	D_2
1			
2			
3			

Model building and variable selection

At the beginning of this chapter we chose body mass index as the variable to explain or model systolic blood pressure. In practice, researchers may or may not have an idea about which variables they think are relevant in explaining the variation in their dependent variable. Whether they do or they don't will influence their decision as to which variables to include in their model, i.e. their *variable selection procedure.*

There are two main approaches to the model-building process:

- First, *automated* variable selection – the computer does it for you. This approach is perhaps more appropriate if you have little idea about which variables are likely to be relevant in the relationship.

- Second, *manual* selection – *you* do it! This approach is more appropriate if you have a particular hypothesis to test, in which case you will have a pretty good idea which independent

---

[5] As a rule of thumb, you need at *the very least* 15 subjects for each independent variable in your model. If you've got, say, five ordinal and/or metric independent variables in your model, you would need a minimum of 75 subjects. If you want also to include a single nominal variable with five categories (i.e. four design variables), you would need another 60 subjects. In these circumstances, it might help to amalgamate some categories.

variable is likely to be the most relevant in explaining your dependent variable. However, you will almost certainly want to include other variables to control for confounding (see p. 81 for an account of confounding).

Both of these methods have a common starting procedure, as follows:[6]

- Identify a list of independent variables that you think might possibly have some role in explaining the variation in your dependent variable. Be as broad-minded as possible here.

- Draw a scatterplot of each of these candidate variables (if it is not a nominal variable), against the dependent variable. Examine for linearity. If any of the scatterplots show a strong, but not a linear relationship with the dependent variable, you will need to code them first before entering them into the computer data sheet. For example, you might find that the relationship between the dependent variable and 'age' is strong but not linear. One approach is to group the *age* values into four groups, using its three quartile values to define the group boundaries, and then code the groups with three design variables.

- Perform a series of univariate regressions, i.e. regress each candidate independent variable in turn against the dependent variable. Note the p-value in each case.

- At this stage, all variables that have a p-value of at least 0.2 should be considered for inclusion in the model. Using a p-value less than this may fail to identify variables that could subsequently turn out to be important in the final model.

  With this common starting procedure out of the way, we can briefly describe the two variable selection approaches, starting with automated methods.

Automated variable selection methods

- *Forwards selection*: The program starts with the variable that has the lowest p-value from the univariate regressions. It then adds the other variables one at a time, in lowest p-value order, regressing each time, retaining all variables with p-values < 0.05 in the model.

- *Backwards selection*: The reverse of forwards selection. The program starts with *all* of the candidate variables in the model, then the variable that has highest p-value > 0.05, is removed. Then the next highest p-value variable, and so on, until only those variables with a p-value < 0.05 are left in the model, and all other variables have been discarded.

- *Forwards or backwards stepwise selection*: After each variable is added (or removed), the variables which were already (or are left) in the model are re-checked for statistical significance; if no longer significant they are removed. The end result is a model where all variables have a p-value < 0.05.

---

[6] Note that the criteria used by the different computer regression programs to select and de-select variables differ.

These automated procedures have a number of disadvantages, although they may be useful when researchers have little idea about which variables are likely to be relevant. As an example of the automated approach, the authors of a study into the role of arginase in sickle cell disease, in which the outcome variable was $\log_{10}$ arginase activity (Morris *et al.* 2005), comment:

> This modelling used a stepwise procedure to add independent variables, beginning with the variables most strongly associated with $\log_{10}$ arginase with $P \leq 0.15$. Deletion of variables after initial inclusion in the model was allowed. The procedure continued until all independent variables in the final model had $P \leq 0.05$, adjusted for other independent variables, and no additional variables had $P \leq 0.05$.

Manual variable selection methods

Manual, DIY methods, are often more appropriate if the investigators know in advance which is likely to be their principal independent variable. They will include this variable in the model, together with any other variables that they think may be potential confounders. The identity of potential confounders will have been established by experience, a literature search, discussions with colleagues and patients and so on. There are two alternative manual selection procedures:

- *Backward elimination:* The main variable plus all of the potentially confounding variables are entered into the model at the start. The results will then reveal which variables are statistically significant (*p*-value < 0.05). Non-significant variables can then be dropped, one at a time in decreasing *p*-value order, from the model, regressing each time. However, if the coefficient of any of the remaining variables changes markedly[7] when a variable is dropped, the variable should be retained, since this may indicate that it is a confounder.

- *Forward elimination:* The main explanatory variable of interest is put in the model, and the other (confounding) variables are added one at a time in order of (lowest) *p*-value (from the univariate regressions). The regression repeated each time a variable is added. If the added variable is statistically significant it is retained, if not it is dropped, unless any of the coefficients of the existing variables change noticeably, suggesting that the new variable may be a confounder.

The end result of either of these manual approaches should be a model containing the same variables (although this model may differ from a model derived using one of the automated procedures). In any case, the overall objective is *parsimony*, i.e. having as few explanatory variables in the model as possible, while at the same time explaining the maximum amount of variation in the dependent variable. Parsimony is particularly important when sample size is on the small side. As a rule of thumb, researchers will need at least 15 observations for each independent variable to ensure mathematical stability, and at least 20 observations to obtain reasonable statistical reliability (e.g. narrow-ish confidence intervals).

As an example of the manual backwards selection approach, the authors of a study of birthweight and cord serum EPA concentration (Grandjean *et al.* 2000), knew that cord serum

---

[7] There is no rule about how big a change in a coefficient should be considered noteworthy. A value of 10 per cent has been suggested, but this seems on the small side.

EPA was their principal independent variable, and but wanted to include possible confounders in their model. They commented:

> Multiple regression analysis was used to determine the relevant importance of predictors of the outcome (variable). Potential confounders were identified on the basis of previous studies, and included maternal height and weight, smoking during pregnancy, diabetes, parity, gestational length, and sex of the child. Covariates[8] were kept in the final regression equation if statistically significant (p < 0.01) after backwards elimination.

Incidentally, the main independent variable, cord serum concentration, was found to be statistically significant (p-value = 0.037), as were all of the confounding variables.

Goodness-of-fit again: $\bar{R}^2$

When you add an *extra* variable to an existing model, and want to compare goodness-of-fit with the old model, you need to compare not R^2, but *adjusted* R^2, denoted $\bar{R}^2$. The reasons don't need to concern us here, but R^2 will increase when an extra independent variable is added to the model, without there necessarily being any increase in explanatory power. However, if $\bar{R}^2$ increases, then you know that the explanatory power (its ability to explain more of the variation in the dependent variable) of the model *has* increased. From Figure 17.3 or Figure 17.4, $\bar{R}^2 = 0.613$ in the *simple* regression model with only hip circumference as an independent variable. From Figure 17.5, with both hip and waist circumferences included, $\bar{R}^2$ increases to 0.635, so this multiple regression model does show a small but real improvement in goodness-of-fit, and would be preferred to either of the simple regression models. Of course, you might decide to explore the possibility that other independent variables might also have a significant role to play in explaining variation in body mass index; age is one obvious contender, as is sex, and should be included in the model.

Exercise 17.6 Table 17.4 contains the results of a multiple linear regression model from a cross-section study of disability, among 1971 adults aged 65 and over in 1986 (Kavanagh and Knapp 1998). The objective of the study was to examine the utilisation rates of general practitioners' time by elderly people resident in communal establishments. The dependent variable was the *natural log* of weekly utilisation (minutes) per resident.[9] There were 10 independent variables, as shown in the figure.
(a) Identify those independent variables whose relationship with the dependent variable is statistically significant. (b) What is the effect on the natural log of utilisation time, and what is this in actual minutes, if there is an increase of: (i) one person in the number in a

---

[8] i.e. independent variables.
[9] Probably because the researchers believed the utilisation rate to be skewed. See Figure 5.6 for an example of transformed data.

private residential home; (ii) one unit in the severity of disability score? (c) How much of the variation in general practitioners' utilisation time is explained by the variation in the independent variables?

Table 17.4   Sample regression coefficients from a linear regression model, where the dependent variable is the natural log of the utilisation time (minutes) of GPs, by elderly patients in residential care. The independent variables are as shown. Reproduced from *BMJ*, **317**, 322–7, courtesy of BMJ Publishing Group

Explanatory variable	β coefficient (SE)	P value
Constant	0.073 (0.353)	0.837
Age	<0.0005 (0.004)	0.923
Male sex	0.024 (0.060)	0.685
Severity of disability	0.043 (0.005)	<0.0001
Mental disorders	0.120 (0.061)	0.047
Nervous system disorders	0.116 (0.062)	0.063
Circulatory system disorders	0.122 (0.066)	0.063
Respiratory system disorders	0.336 (0.115)	0.003
Digestive system disorders	0.057 (0.070)	0.415
Type of accommodation:		
Local authority	—	—
Voluntary residential home	−0.084 (0.183)	0.649
Voluntary nursing home	0.562 (0.320)	0.079
Private residential home	−0.173 (0.157)	0.272
Private nursing home	0.443 (0.228)	0.053
Size of establishment (No of residents)		
Local authority	−0.004 (0.003)	0.170
Voluntary residential home	−0.004 (0.002)	0.069
Voluntary nursing home	−0.002 (0.002)	0.245
Private residential home	0.006 (0.002)	0.017
Private nursing home	−0.007 (0.007)	0.362

$R^2 = 0.1098$, $F_{(17,415)} = 9.71$, $P = $ <0.0001. Sample size = 1971 in 433 sampling units.

Adjustment and confounding

One of the most attractive features of the multiple regression model is its ability to *adjust* for the effects of possible association between the independent variables. It's quite possible that two or more of the independent variables will be associated. For example, hip (HIP) and waist (WST) circumference are significantly positively associated with $r = +0.783$ and p-value $= 0.000$. The consequence of such association is that increases in HIP are likely to be accompanied by increases in WST. The increase in HIP will cause bmi to increase both directly, but also indirectly via WST. In these circumstances it's difficult to tell how much of the increase in bmi is due *directly* to an increase in HIP, and how much to the *indirect* effect of an associated increase in WST.

    The beauty of the multiple regression model is that each regression coefficient measures only the *direct* effect of its independent variable on the dependent variable, and controls or adjusts for any possible interaction from any of the other variables in the model. In terms of the results in Figure 17.5, an increase in HIP of 1 cm will cause mean bmi to increase by 0.261 kg/m² (the value of b_1), and *all* of this increase is caused by the change in hip circumference (plus the inevitable random error). Any effect that a concomitant change in waist circumference might have is discounted. The same applies to the value of -0.0249 for b_3 on the 'age' variable in Figure 17.6.

We can use the adjustment property to deal with confounders in just the same way. You will recall that a confounding variable has to be associated with *both* one of the independent variables *and* the dependent variable (see the discussion in Chapter 6). Notice that the coefficient b_1, which was 0.351 in the simple regression model with HIP the only independent variable, decreases to 0.261 with two independent variables. A marked change like this in the coefficient of a variable already in the model when a new variable is added, is an indication that one of the variables is possibly a confounder. As you have already seen in the model-building section above, in these circumstances both variables should be retained in the model.

An example from practice

Table 17.5 is from a cross-section study into the relationship between bone lead and blood lead levels, and the development of hypertension in 512 individuals selected from a cohort study (Cheng *et al.* 2001). The table shows the outcome from three multiple linear regression models with systolic blood pressure as the dependent variable. The first model includes blood lead as an independent variable, along with six possible *confounding* variables.[10] The second and third models were the same as the first model, except tibia and patella lead, respectively, were substituted for blood lead. The results include 95 per cent confidence intervals and the R^2 for each model.

As the table shows, the tibia lead model has the best goodness-of-fit ($R^2 = 0.1015$), but even this model only explains 10 per cent of the observed variation in systolic blood pressure. However, this is the only model that supports the relationship between hypertension and lead levels; the 95 per cent confidence interval for tibia lead (0.02 to 2.73) does not include zero. The only confounders statistically significant in all three models are age, family history of hypertension and calcium intake.

Exercise 17.7   From the results in Table 17.5: (a) which independent variables are statistically significant in all three models? (b) Explain the 95 per cent confidence interval of (0.28 to 0.64) for *age* in the blood lead model. (c) In which model does a unit (1 year) increase in age change systolic blood pressure the most?

Diagnostics – checking the basic assumptions of the multiple linear regression model

The ordinary least squares method of coefficient estimation will only produce the best estimators if the basic assumptions of the model are satisfied. That is: a metric continuous

---

[10] The inclusion of Age^2 in the model is probably an attempt to establish the linearity of the relationship between systolic blood pressure and age. If the coefficient for Age^2 is not statistically significant then the relationship is probably linear.

Table 17.5 Multiple regression results from a cross-section study into the relationship between bone lead and blood lead levels and the development of hypertension in 512 individuals selected from a cohort study. The figure show the outcome from three multiple linear regression models, with systolic blood pressure as the dependent variable. Reproduced from *Amer. J. Epid.*, **153**, 164–71, courtesy of Oxford University Press

Variable	Baseline model + blood lead		Baseline model + tibia lead		Baseline model + patella lead	
	Parameter estimate	95% CI	Parameter estimate	95% CI	Parameter estimate	95% CI
Intercept	128.34		125.90		127.23	
Age (years)	0.46*	0.28, 0.64	0.39*	0.20, 0.58	0.44*	0.26, 0.63
Age squared (years²)	−0.02*	−0.04, −0.00	−0.02*	−0.04, −0.00	−0.02*	−0.04, −0.00
Body mass index (km/m²)	0.36*	0.01, 0.72	0.33	−0.02, 0.69	0.35	−0.00, 0.71
Family history of hypertension (yes/no)	4.36*	1.42, 7.30	4.36*	1.47, 7.25	4.32*	1.42, 7.22
Alcohol intake (g/day)	0.08*	0.00, 0.149	0.07	−0.00, 0.14	0.07	−0.00, 0.14
Calcium intake (10 mg/day)	−0.04*	−0.08, −0.00	−0.04*	0.07, −0.00	−0.04*	−0.07, −0.00
Blood lead (SD)†	−0.13	−1.35, 1.09				
Tibia lead (SD)†			1.37*	0.02, 2.73		
Patella lead (SD)†					0.57	−0.71, 1.84
Model R^2	0.0956		0.1015		0.0950	

* $p < 0.05$

† Parameter estimates are based on 1 standard deviation (SD) in blood lead level (4.03 µg/dl), tibia lead level (13.65 µg/g), and patella lead level (19.55 µg/g).

dependent variable; a linear relationship between the dependent and each independent variable; error terms with constant spread and Normally distributed; and the independent variables not perfectly correlated with each other. How can we check that these assumptions are satisfied?

- *A metric continuous dependent variable.* Refer to Chapter 1 if you are unsure how to identify a metric continuous variable.

- *A linear relationship between the dependent variable and each independent variable.* Easiest to investigate by plotting the dependent variable against each of the independent variables; the scatter should lie approximately around a straight line.[11] The other possibility is to plot the residual values against the *fitted* values of the independent variable (bmi in our example). These are the values the estimated regression equation would give for mean bmi, for every combination of values of HIP and WST. The scatter should be evenly spread around zero, with no discernible pattern, such as in Figure 17.7(a).

- *The residuals have constant spread across the range of values of the independent variable.* Check with a plot of the residual values against the *fitted* values of bmi. The spread of the residuals should be fairly constant around the zero value, across the range of fitted values of the independent variable. Figure 17.7(b) is an example of non-constant variance. The spread appears to increase as the value of the independent variable increases. Figure 17.7(c) is an example of both non-linearity and non-constant variance.

- *The residuals are Normally distributed for each fitted value of the independent variable.* This assumption can be checked with a histogram of the residuals. For our bmi example, the histogram in Figure 17.10 indicates that, apart from a rather worrying outlier, the distribution is Normal. You might want to identify which woman this outlier represents and check her data for anomalies.

- *The independent variables are not perfectly correlated with each other.* Unfortunately, this is not an easy assumption to check. Some degree of correlation is almost certain to exist among some of the independent variables.

Exercise 17.8 (a) Explain briefly each of the basic assumptions of the multiple linear regression model. (b) With the aid of sketches where appropriate, explain how we can test that these assumptions are satisfied.

---

[11]Notice that we only have to establish this property of linearity for the metric independent variables in the model. Any binary variables are linear by default – they only have two points, which can be joined with a straight line. Any ordinal independent variables will have to be expressed as binary dummies – again linear by default for the same reason.

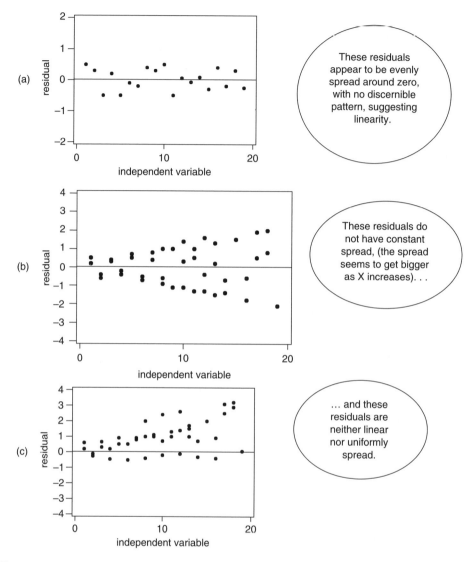

Figure 17.7 Testing the basic assumptions of the linear regression model by plotting the residuals against the fitted values of the regression equation

An example from practice

Let's apply the above ideas to check the basic assumptions of the ordinary least squares method as applied to the multiple linear regression of body mass index (bmi) on hip circumference (HIP) and waist circumference (WST), which we considered earlier. Recall that the model was:

$$bmi = b_0 + b_1 \times HIP + b_2 \times WST$$

and that both HIP and WST were found to be statistically significant explainers of the variation in bmi.

The first assumption is that bmi is a metric continuous dependent variable, which it is. The second assumption is that the relationship between bmi and HIP and bmi and WST should be linear. If we draw a scatterplot of bmi against each of these variables, we get the scatterplots shown in Figure 17.8. These indicate a reasonable degree of linearity in each case. Notice though that the spread in bmi appear to get larger as WST increases.

The third assumption is that the residuals have constant spread over the range of fitted values of the model. Figure 17.9 is a plot of these residuals against the fitted values of bmi. This third assumption appears not to be completely satisfied. The spread of residual values appear to increase as the fitted bmi value increases. This may be an indication that an important independent variable is missing from the model. However, the distribution of points above and below the zero line seems reasonably symmetric, supporting the linearity assumption demonstrated in the scatterplots.

The fourth assumption of the Normality of the residuals is checked with the histogram of the residuals, see Figure 17.10. These do appear to be reasonably Normal, although there is some suggestion of positive skew.

Thus all of the basic assumptions appear to be reasonably well satisfied (apart from the multi-colinearity assumption which we have not tested), and the ordinary least squares regression estimates b_1 and b_2 of the population parameters β_1 and β_2, are the 'best' we can get, i.e. they fit the data at least as well as any other estimates.[12]

Multiple linear regression is popular in clinical research. Much more popular though, for reasons which will become clear in the next chapter, is logistic regression.

Analysis of variance

Analysis of variance (ANOVA) is a procedure that aims to deal with the same problems as linear regression analysis, and many medical statistics books contain at least one chapter describing ANOVA. It has a history in the social sciences, particularly psychology. However, regression and ANOVA are simply two sides of the same coin – the *generalised linear model*. As Andy Field (2000) says:

> Anova is fine for simple designs, but becomes impossibly cumbersome in more complex situations. The regression model extends very logically to these more complex designs, without getting bogged down in mathematics. Finally, the method (Anova) becomes extremely unmanageable in some circumstances, such as unequal sample sizes. The regression method makes these situations considerably more simple.

In view of the fact that anything ANOVA can do, regression can also do, and, for me anyway, do it in a way that's conceptually easier, I am not going to discuss ANOVA in this book. If you are interested in exploring ANOVA in more detail, you could do worse than read Andy Field's book, or that of Altman (1991).

---

[12]There are other methods of estimating the values of the regression parameters, which I don't have the space to consider. However, provided the basic assumptions are satisfied, none will be better than the ordinary least squares estimators.

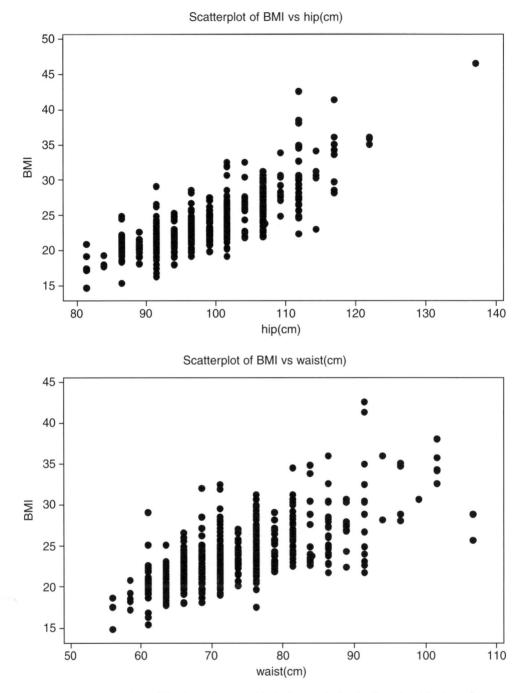

Figure 17.8 Scatterplots of the dependent variable body mass index (bmi) against hip circumference (HIP) – top plot – and waist circumference (WST) – bottom plot. As you can see, both plots indicate a more-or-less linear relationship

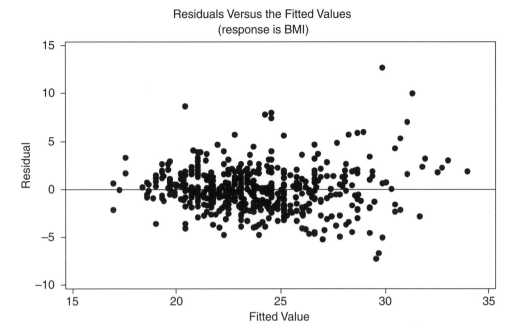

Figure 17.9 A plot of the residuals versus the fitted bmi values, as a check of the basic assumptions of the linear regression model

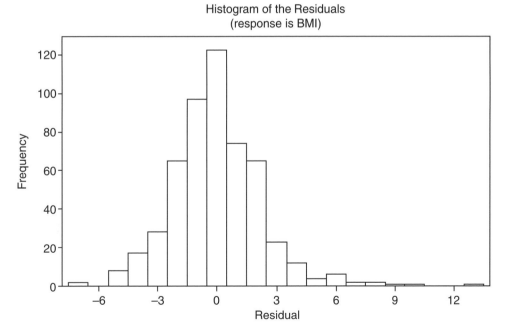

Figure 17.10 A plot of the residuals in the body mass index example, showing reasonable Normality, and thus satisfying the fourth assumption governing the use of the ordinary least squares estimation method

18

Curvy models: logistic regression

Learning objectives

When you have finished this chapter you should be able to:

- Explain why a linear regression model is not appropriate if the dependent variable is binary.

- Explain what the logit transformation is and what it achieves.

- Write down the logic regression equation.

- Explain the concept of linearity and outline how this can be tested for and dealt with.

- Explain how estimates of the odds ratios can be derived directly from the regression parameters.

- Describe how the statistical significance of the population odds ratio is determined.

- Interpret output from SPSS and Minitab logistic regression programs.

A second health warning!

Although the maths underlying the logistic regression model is perhaps more complicated than that in linear regression, once more a brief description of the underlying idea is necessary if you are to gain some understanding of the procedure and be able to interpret logistic computer outputs sensibly.

Binary dependent variables

In linear regression the dependent or outcome variable must be metric continuous. In clinical research, however, the outcome variable in a relationship will very often be dichotomous or *binary*, i.e. will take only *two* different values: alive or dead; malignant or benign; male or female and so on. In addition, variables that are not naturally binary can often be made so. For example, birthweight might be coded 'less than 2500 g', and '2500 g or more', Apgar scores coded 'less than 7', '7 or more', etc. In this chapter I want to show how a binary dependent variable makes the linear regression model inappropriate.

Finding an appropriate model when the outcome variable is binary

If you are trying to find an appropriate model to describe the relationship between two variables Y and X, when Y, the dependent variable, is continuous, you can draw a scatterplot of Y against X (Figure 17.2 is a good example) and if this has a linear shape you can model the relationship with the linear regression model. However, when the outcome variable is binary, this graphical approach is not particularly helpful.

For example, suppose you are interested in using the breast cancer/stress data from the study referred to in Table 1.6, to investigate the relationship between the outcome variable 'diagnosis', and the independent variable 'age'. Diagnosis is, of course, a binary variable with two values: $Y = 1$ (malignant) or $Y = 0$ (benign). If we plot *diagnosis* against *age*, we get the scatterplot shown in Figure 18.1, from which it's pretty well impossible to draw any definite conclusions about the nature of the relationship.

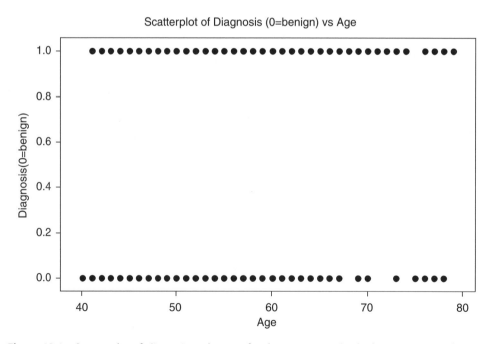

Figure 18.1 Scatter plot of *diagnosis* against *age* for the 332 women in the breast cancer and stress study referred to in Table 1.6

Table 18.1 Proportion of women with malignant lump in each age group

Proportion with malignant lump, i.e. $Y = 1$. Or the probability that $Y=1$, i.e. $P(Y=1)$	Midpoint of age group
0.140	45
0.226	55
0.635	65
0.727	75

The problem is that the large variability in age, in both the malignant and benign groups, obscures the difference in age (if any) *between* them. However, if you *group* the age data: 40-49, 50-59, etc., and then calculate the *proportion* of women with a malignant diagnosis (i.e. with $Y = 1$) in each group, this will reduce the variability, but preserve the underlying relationship between the two variables. The results of doing this are shown in Table 18.1.

Notice that I've labelled the first column as the 'Proportion with $Y = 1$, *or* the Probability that $Y = 1$, written as $P(Y = 1)$'. Here's why. In linear regression, you will recall that the dependent variable is the *mean* of Y for a given X. But what about a binary dependent variable? Can we find something analogous to the mean? As it happens, the mean of a set of binary, zero or one, values is the same as the *proportion* of ones,[1] so an appropriate equivalent version of the binary dependent variable would seem to be 'Proportion of $(Y = 1)$s'.

But proportions can be interpreted as probabilities (see Chapter 8). So the dependent variable becomes the 'Probability that $Y = 1$', or $P(Y = 1)$, for a given value of X. For example the probability of a malignant diagnosis $(Y = 1)$ for all of those women aged 40, which we can write as, $P(Y = 1)$ given $X = 40$.

You can see in Table 18.1, the proportion with malignant breast lumps (the probability that $Y = 1$) increases with age, but does it increase linearly? A scatterplot of the proportion with malignant lumps, $Y = 1$, against group age midpoints is shown in Figure 18.2, which does suggest *some* sort of relationship between the two variables. But it's definitely *not* linear, so a *linear* regression model won't work. In fact, the curve has more of an elongated S shape, so what we need is a mathematical equation that will give such an S-shaped curve.

There are several possibilities, but the *logistic* model is the model of choice. Not only because it produces an S-shaped curve, which we want, but, critically, it has a meaningful clinical interpretation. Moreover, the value of $P(Y = 1)$ is restricted by the maths of the logistic model to lie between zero and one, which is what we want, since it's a probability.

The logistic regression model

The simple[2] *population* logistic regression equation is:

$$P(Y = 1) = (e^{\beta_0 + \beta_1 X})/(1 + e^{\beta_0 + \beta_1 X}) \tag{1}$$

---

[1] For example, the mean of the five values: 0, 1, 1, 0, 0 is 2/5 = 0.4, which is the same as the proportion of 1s, i.e. 2 in 5 or 0.4.
[2] 'Simple' because there is only one independent variable – so far.

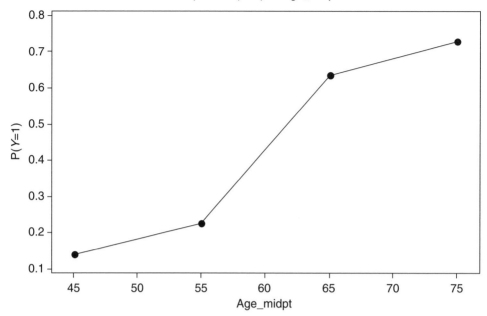

Figure 18.2 Scatterplot of the proportion of women with a malignant diagnosis ($Y = 1$) against midpoints of age group

which we estimate with the *sample* logistic regression equation:

$$P(Y = 1) = (e^{b0+b1X})/(1 + e^{b0+b1X}) \tag{2}$$

by determining the values of the estimators b_0 and b_1. We'll come back to this problem in a moment. Note that e is the exponential operator, equal to 2.7183, and has nothing to do with the residual term in linear regression. As you can see, the logistic regression model is mathematically a bit more complicated than the linear regression model.

The outcome variable, $P(Y = 1)$, is the probability that $Y = 1$ (the lump is malignant), for some given value of the independent variable X. There is no restriction on the type of *independent* variable, which can be nominal, ordinal or metric.

As an example, let's return to our breast cancer study (Figure 1.6). Our outcome variable is *diagnosis*, where $Y = 1$ (malignant) or $Y = 0$ (benign). We'll start with one independent variable – *ever used an oral contraceptive pill* (OCP), Yes $= 1$, or No $= 0$. We are going to treat OCP use as a possible risk factor for receiving a malignant diagnosis. This gives us the sample regression model:

$$P(Y = 1) = (e^{b0+b1 \times OCP})/(1 + e^{b0+b1 \times OCP}) \tag{3}$$

So all we've got to do to determine the probability that a woman picked at random from the sample will get a malignant diagnosis ($Y = 1$), with or without OCP use, is to calculate the values of b_0 and b_1 somehow, and then put them in the logistic regression equation, with OCP $= 0$, or OCP $= 1$.

Estimating the parameter values

Whereas the linear regression models use the method of ordinary least squares to estimate the regression parameters β_0 and β_1, logistic regression models use what is called *maximum likelihood estimation*. Essentially this means choosing the population which is *most likely* to have generated the sample results observed. Figure 18.3 and Figure 18.4, respectively, show the output from SPSS's and Minitab's logistic regression program for the above OCP model.

SPSS's and Minitab's logistic regression program both give $b_0 = -0.2877$ and $b_1 = -0.9507$. If we substitute these values into the logistic regression model of Equation (3), we get:[3]

$$\text{if OCP} = 0 \text{ (has never used OCP), } P(Y = 1) = 0.4286$$

$$\text{if OCP} = 1 \text{ (has used OCP), then } P(Y = 1) = 0.2247$$

So a woman who has never used an oral contraceptive pill has a probability of getting a malignant diagnosis nearly twice that of a woman who *has* used an oral contraceptive. Rather than being a risk factor for a malignant diagnosis, in this sample the use of oral contraceptives seems to confer some protection against a breast lump being malignant.

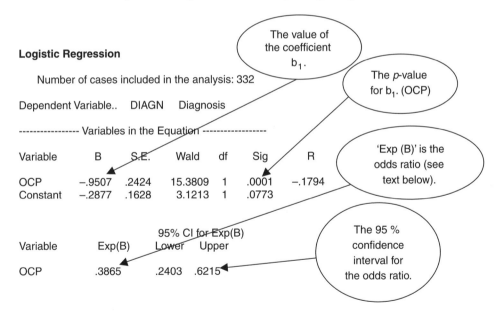

Figure 18.3 Abbreviated output from SPSS for a logistic regression with *diagnosis* as the dependent variable, and *use of oral contraceptive pill* (OCP) as the independent variable or risk factor

---

[3] You'll first need to work out the values of $(b_0 + b_1 \times \text{OCP})$, then $(1 + b_0 + b_1 \times \text{OCP})$, then raise e to each of these powers. Then divide the former by the latter.

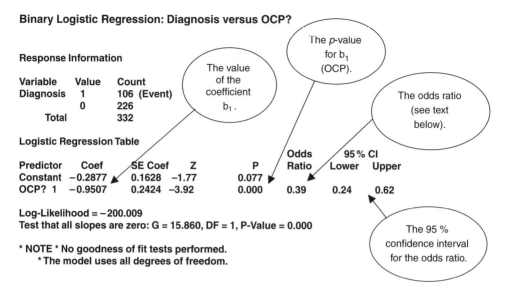

Figure 18.4 Output from Minitab for a logistic regression with *Diagnosis* as the dependent variable and *Use of Oral Contraceptive Pill* (OCP) as the independent variable or risk factor

The odds ratio

The great attraction of the logistic regression model is that it readily produces odds ratios. But how? There's quite a lot of maths involved, but eventually we can get to the following result:

$$\text{Odds ratio} = e^{b0+b1}/e^{b0} = e^{b1}\ ^4$$

It is this ability to produce odds ratios that has made the logistic regression model so popular in clinical studies. Thus to find the odds ratio all you need to do is raise e to the power b_1, easily done on a decent calculator.

For example, in our Diagnosis/OCP model, $b_0 = -0.2877$ and $b_1 = -0.9507$, so the odds ratio for a malignant diagnosis for woman using OCP compared to women not using OCP is:

$$\text{Odds ratio} = e^{-0.9507} = 0.386$$

In other words, a woman who has used OCP has only about a third of the odds of getting a malignant diagnosis as a woman who has not used OCP. This result seems to confirm our earlier result that use of OCP provides some protection against a malignancy. Of course we don't know whether this result is due to chance or whether this represents a real statistically

[4] Making use of the rule: $X^a/X^b = X^{a-b}$.

significant result in the population. To answer this question we will need either a confidence interval for β_1 or a p-value. I'll deal with this question shortly.

Exercise 18.1   Explain why, in terms of the risk of using OCP and the probability of getting a malignant diagnosis, that the values $P(Y = 1) = 0.4286$ when OCP $= 0$, and $P(Y = 1) = 0.2247$, when OCP $= 1$, are compatible with an odds ratio $= 0.386$ for a malignant diagnosis, among women using OCP compared to women not using OCP.

Interpreting the regression coefficient

In linear regression, the coefficient b_1 represents the increase in Y for a unit increase in X. We are not so much interested in the meaning of b_1 in the logistic regression model, except to note that if the independent variable is ordinal or metric, then you might be more interested in the effect on the odds ratio of changes of *greater* than one unit. For example, if the independent variable is age, then the effect on the odds ratio of an increase in age of one year may not be as useful as say a change of 10 years. In these circumstances, if the change in age is c years, then the change in the odds ratio is e^{cb_1}.

Exercise 18.2   (a) In linear regression we can plot Y against X to determine whether the relationship between the two variables is linear. Explain why this approach is not particularly helpful when Y is a binary variable. What approach might be more useful? (b) Is age significant? (c) Figure 18.5 shows the output from Minitab for the regression of *diagnosis* on *age* for the breast cancer example. Use the Minitab values to write down the estimated logistic regression model. (d) Calculate the probability that the diagnosis will be malignant, $P(Y = 1)$, for women aged: (i) 45; (ii) 50. (e) Calculate $[1 - P(Y = 1)]$ in each case, and hence calculate the odds ratio for a malignant diagnosis in women aged 45 compared to women aged 50. Explain your result. (f) Confirm that the antilog$_e$ of the coefficient on *age* is equal to the odds ratio. (g) What effect does an increase in *age* of 10 years have on the odds ratio?

Logistic Regression Table. Dependent variable is Diagnosis.

Predictor	Coef	SE Coef	Z	P	Odds Ratio	95% CI Lower	Upper
Constant	−6.4672	0.7632	−8.47	0.000			
Age	0.10231	0.01326	7.72	0.000	1.11	1.08	1.14

Figure 18.5   Output from Minitab for the logistic regression of *diagnosis* on *age*

Statistical inference in the logistic regression model

As you saw in Chapter 11, if the population odds ratio is equal to 1, then the risk factor in question has no effect on the odds for any particular outcome; that is, the variable concerned is *not* a statistically significant risk (or benefit). We can use either the *p*-value or the confidence interval to decide whether any departures from a value of 1 for the odds ratio is due merely to chance or is an indication of statistical significance.

In fact, in Figure 18.4, the 95 per cent confidence interval for the odds ratio for OCP use is (0.24 to 0.62), and since this does not include 1, the odds ratio is statistically significant in terms of receiving a malignant diagnosis. In addition the *p*-value = 0.000, so a lot less than 0.05. However, we still need to be cautious about this result because it represents only a crude odds ratio, which, in reality, would need to be adjusted for other possible confounding variables, such as age. We can make this adjustment in logistic regression just as easily as in the linear regression model, simply by including the variables we want to adjust for on the right-hand side of the model.

Notice that Minitab, Figure 18.4, uses the z distribution to provide a *p*-value, whereas SPSS, Figure 18.3, uses the *Wald statistic*, which can be shown to have a z distribution in the appropriate circumstances.

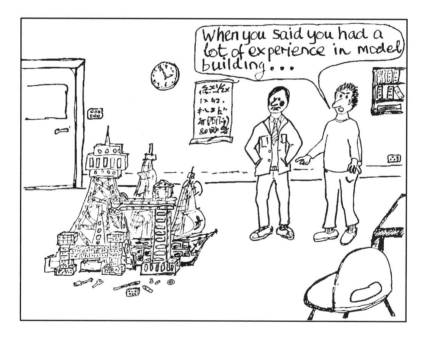

Exercise 18.3   Figure 18.6 shows the output from SPSS for the regression of *diagnosis* on *body mass index* (BMI). Comment on the statistical significance of body mass index as a risk factor for receiving a malignant diagnosis.

		B	Wald	Sig.	Exp(B)	95.0% CI for EXP(B)	
						Lower	Upper
Step 1(a)	BMI	.082	10.943	.001	1.085	1.034	1.139
	Constant	−2.859	19.313	.000	.057		

Figure 18.6 The output from SPSS for the regression of *diagnosis* on *body mass index* (some columns are missing)

The multiple logistic regression model

In my explanation of the odds ratio above I used a simple logistic regression model, i.e. one with a single independent variable (OCP), because this offers the simplest treatment. However, the result we got, that the odds ratio is equal to e^{b_1}, applies to *each* coefficient if there is more than one independent variable, i.e. e^{b_2}, e^{b_3}, etc. The usual situation is to have a risk factor variable plus a number of confounder variables (the usual suspects – age, sex, etc.). Suppose, for example, that you decided to include *age* and *body mass index* (BMI) along with OCP as independent variables. Equation (1) would then become:

$$P(Y = 1) = (e^{\beta 0 + \beta_1 \times \text{OCP} + \beta_2 \times \text{age} + \beta_3 \times \text{BMI}})/(1 + e^{\beta 0 + \beta_1 \times \text{OCP} + \beta_2 \times \text{age} + \beta_3 \times \text{BMI}})$$

$P(Y = 1)$ is still of course the probability that the woman will receive a malignant diagnosis, $Y = 1$. The odds ratio for *age* is e^{b_2}; the odds ratio for BMI is e^{b_3}. Moreover, as with linear regression, each of these odds ratios is *adjusted* for any possible interaction between the independent variables.

As an example, output from Minitab for the above multiple regression model of *diagnosis* against *use of oral contraceptives* (OCP), *age* and *body mass index* (BMI), is shown in Figure 18.7.

> **Exercise 18.4**   Comment on what is revealed in the output in Figure 18.7 about the relationship between diagnosis and the three independent variables shown.

Building the model

The strategy for model building in the logistic regression model is similar to that for linear regression:

- Make a list of candidate independent variables.

- For any nominal or ordinal variables in the list construct a contingency table and perform a chi-squared test.[5] Make a note of the *p*-value.

---

[5] Provided the number of categories isn't too big for the size of your sample – you don't want any empty cells or low expected values (see Chapter 14)

Binary Logistic Regression: Diagnosis versus OCP, Age, BMI

```
Variable              Value  Count
Diagnosis(0=benign)   1        106   (Event)
                      0        224
                      Total    330
```

```
Logistic Regression Table
                                                    Odds      95% CI
Predictor     Coef       SE Coef      z      P      Ratio  Lower  Upper
Constant    -9.24814     1.30391    -7.09  0.000

OCP          0.356767    0.329147    1.08  0.278    1.43   0.75   2.72
Age          0.111670    0.0164348   6.79  0.000    1.12   1.08   1.15
BMI          0.0812739   0.0275908   2.95  0.003    1.08   1.03   1.14
```

```
Goodness-of-Fit Tests

Method            Chi-Square   DF      P
Pearson           329.603      321   0.358
Deviance          328.516      321   0.374
Hosmer-Lemeshow     2.581        8   0.958
```

Figure 18.7 Minitab output for the model *diagnosis* against OCP, *age* and BMI

- For any metric variables, perform either a two-sample t test, or a univariate logistic regression; note the *p*-value in either case.

- Pick out all those variables in the list whose *p*-value is 0.25 or less. Select the variable with the smallest *p*-value (if there is more than one with the smallest *p*-value pick one arbitrarily) to be your first independent variable. This is your starting model.

- Finally, add variables to your model one at a time, each time examining the *p*-values for statistical significance. If a variable, when added to the model, is not statistically significant, drop it, unless there are noticeable changes in coefficient values, which is indicative of confounding.

Goodness-of-fit

In the linear regression model you used R^2 to measure goodness-of-fit. In the logistic regression model measuring goodness-of-fit is much more complicated, and can involve graphical as well as numeric measures. Two numeric measures that can be used are the *deviance coefficient* and the *Hosmer-Lemeshow statistic*. Very briefly, both of these have a chi-squared distribution, and we can use the resulting *p*-value to reject, or not, the null hypothesis that the model *provides a good fit*. The graphical methods are quite complex and you should consult more specialist sources for further information on this and other aspects of this complex procedure. Hosmer and Lemeshow (1989) is an excellent source.

Exercise 18.5   Use the Hosmer-Lemeshow goodness-of-fit statistic in the output of Figure 18.7 to comment on the goodness-of-fit of the model shown.

Linear and logistic regression modelling are two methods from a more general class of methods known collectively as *multivariable* statistics. *Multivariate* statistics on the other hand, is a set of procedures applicable where there is more than one dependent variable, and includes methods such as principal components analysis, multidimensional scaling, cluster and discriminant analysis, and more. Of these, principal components analysis appears most often in the clinical literature, but even so is not very common. Unfortunately, there is no space to discuss any of these methods.

IX

Two More Chapters

19

Measuring survival

Learning objectives

When you have finished this chapter you should be able to:

- Explain what censoring means.

- Calculate Kaplan-Meier survival probabilities.

- Draw a Kaplan-Meier survival curve.

- Use the Kaplan-Meier curve to estimate median survival time (if possible).

- Explain the use of the log-rank test to determine if the survival experience of two or more groups is significantly different.

- Explain the role of the hazard ratio in comparing the relative survival experience of two groups.

- Outline the general idea behind Cox proportional hazards regression and interpret the results from such a regression.

Introduction

Imagine that you have a patient who has overdosed on paracetamol. A spouse asks you what their chances of 'coming through it' are. Or suppose a patient with breast cancer wants to

Medical Statistics from Scratch, Second Edition   David Bowers
© 2008 John Wiley & Sons, Ltd

know which of two possible treatments offers the best chance of survival. You can answer questions like these with the help of a procedure known as *survival analysis*. The basis of this method is the measurement of the time from some *intervention* or *procedure* to some *event of interest*.

For example, if you were studying survival after mastectomy for breast cancer (the procedure), you would want to know how long each woman survived following surgery. Here, the event of interest would be death. For practical reasons you usually have to limit the duration of the study, for example, to one year, or five years, etc. Very often you will want to compare the survival experiences of two groups of patients; for example women having a mastectomy, with women having less radical surgery.

Censored data

One particular problem, which makes this type of analysis tricky, is that you often don't observe the event of interest in *all* of the subjects. For example, after five years, by no means all of the women will have died following the mastectomy. We don't know how long these particular patients will live after the end of the study period, only that they are still alive when the study period ends. In addition, some patients may withdraw from the study during the study period; they may move away, or simply refuse further participation, or die from a cause unrelated to the study. These types of incomplete data are said to be *censored*.

A final problem is that not all patients may enter the study at the same time. Fortunately, methods have been developed to deal with these difficulties. One of which, known as the *Kaplan–Meier method*, gives us a table of survival probabilities which can be charted as the Kaplan-Meier chart. The two questions that are often of the greatest interest are:

- What's the probability of a patient surviving for some given period of time?

- What's the *comparative* survival experience of two groups of patients?

A simple example of survival in a single group

Look at the data in Table 19.1, which shows survival data (in months) for a group of 12 patients diagnosed with a brain tumour, who were followed up for 12 months.

Table 19.1 shows that seven patients died, two left the study prematurely and three survived. This means that you have seven definite and five censored survival times. We can represent the survival times in the last column of Table 19.1 graphically, as in Figure 19.1, where the survival times are arranged in *ascending* order.

Calculating survival probabilities and the proportion surviving: the Kaplan-Meier table

The Kaplan-Meier method requires a Kaplan-Meier table like Table 19.2, with, strictly speaking, rows *only* for time periods when a death occurs (shown in bold in the table). However, I have

Table 19.1 Survival times (months) over a 12-month study period, of 12 patients diagnosed with brain tumour. *Indicates censored data (patient survived, S, or left study prematurely, P). The *actual* survival time for these patients is not known

Patient	Month of entry to study (0 indicates present at beginning of study)	Time after study start date to death or censoring (months)	Outcomes: Died (D), Survived (S) or left study prematurely (P)	Survival times
1	0	12	S*	12
2	0	12	S*	12
3	0	11	D	11
4	0	8	D	8
5	1	6	P*	5
6	2	12	S*	10
7	2	4	D	2
8	2	5	D	3
9	2	9	D	7
10	3	9	P*	6
11	3	8	D	5
12	3	7	D	4

included all 12 rows in the table to help illustrate the method more clearly. The second column tells us how many people were still alive, n, at the beginning of each month, t. This will equal the total initial number of patients in the study, minus both the total number of deaths and the total number of premature withdrawals up to the beginning of the month. Column 4 records the number of deaths d in each month. Column 5 records the total number at risk during the month, r. By dividing column 4 by column 5, we get d/r, the probability that a patient still alive at the beginning of the month will die during it (which is equivalent to the *proportion* of patients dying in that month). The value of d/r is shown in column 6.

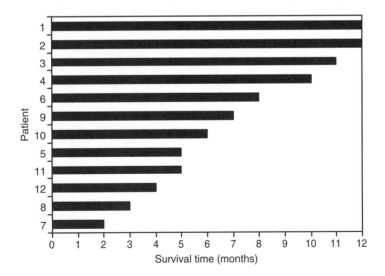

Figure 19.1 Chart of survival times (in ascending order) from Table 19.1

Table 19.2 Calculation of Kaplan-Meier survival probabilities

1 Month	2 Number still in study at start of month t	3 Withdrawn prematurely during month t	4 Deaths in month t	5 Number at risk in month t	6 Probability of death in month t	7 Probability of surviving month t	8 Cumulative probability of surviving to month t
t	n	w	d	r	d/r	$p = 1 - d/r$	S
1	12	0	0	12	0	1	1
2	12	0	0	12	0	1	1
3	12	0	0	12	0	0	1
4	12	0	1	11	$1/11 = 0.091$	0.909	0.909
5	11	0	1	10	$1/10 = 0.100$	0.900	0.818
6	10	1	0	9	0	1	1
7	9	0	1	8	$1/8 = 0.125$	0.875	0.716
8	8	0	2	6	$2/6 = 0.333$	0.667	0.478
9	6	1	1	4	$1/4 = 0.250$	0.750	0.358
10	4	0	0	4	0	1	1
11	4	0	1	3	$1/3 = 0.333$	0.667	0.239
12	3	0	0	3	0	1	1

Since d/r is the probability of dying during a time period, then $(1 - d/r)$ must be the probability of surviving to the end of the time period. This survival probability is shown in column 7. To calculate the probability of surviving *all* of the preceding time periods *and* the current time period, you must successively multiply the probabilities in column 7 together (ignoring any 0's). The resultant cumulative probabilities, labelled S, are shown in column 8. For example, the value for S of 0.818 in row 5 is $1 \times 1 \times 1 \times 0.909 \times 0.900$. These column 8 values are the *Kaplan-Meier survival probabilities*.

Table 19.2 indicates that the probability of a patient surviving to the end of the third month is 1, to the end of the fourth month is 0.909, and so on, and for the full 12 months after the diagnosis is 0.239.

We can also interpret these values as *proportions*. For example, 0.909 of the patients (or 90.9 per cent, will survive to the end of the fourth month. About a quarter (23.9 per cent) will survive the full 12 months. We can generalise these results to the *population* of patients of whom this sample is representative, and who have the same type of brain tumour, at the same stage of development, and receive the same level of care. In addition, we may want to adjust for possible confounding variables such as age, sex, etc. We'll deal with this question later.

The Kaplan-Meier chart

If you plot the cumulative survival probabilities in the last column of Table 19.2 against time, you get the *Kaplan-Meier curve*, shown in Figure 19.2. Notice that the survival 'curve' looks like a staircase, albeit with uneven steps. Every time there is a death, the curve steps down. Since there are seven deaths, there are seven steps down.[1]

---

[1] Notice there is a double step down at period 8 because of the two deaths.

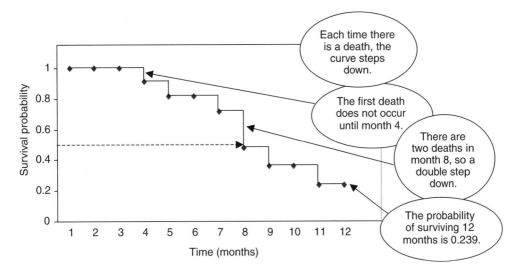

Figure 19.2 The Kaplan-Meier survival curve drawn from the data in Table 19.2 (the dotted line indicates median proportion surviving – see text below)

Exercise 19.1   The data in Table 19.3 shows the survival times (in days) of eight patients with acute myocardial infarction, treated with a new reperfusion drug Explase, as part of a fibrinolytic regimen. Patients were followed up for 14 days. Calculate survival probabilities and plot Kaplan-Meier survival curves. Comment on your results.

Table 19.3   The survival times (in days) of eight patients with acute myocardial infarction. Patients were followed up for 14 days

Patient	Day of entry to study (0 indicates present at beginning of study)	Time after study start date to death or censoring (days)	Outcomes: Died (D), Survived (S) or Left study prematurely (P)
1	0	3	D
2	0	14	S
3	0	8	D
4	0	12	P
5	1	14	S
6	2	13	D
7	2	14	S
8	2	14	S

Determining median survival time

One of the consequences of not knowing the actual survival times of all of those subjects who survive beyond the end of the study period is that we cannot calculate the mean survival time of the whole group. However, if you interpret the probabilities on the vertical axis of a Kaplan-Meier chart as proportions or percentages, you can often easily determine *median* survival times. It is that value which corresponds to a probability of 0.5 (i.e. 50 per cent). In Figure 19.2, the median survival time is 8 months. At this time, half of the patients still survived. Obviously the survival time of any proportion of the sample can be determined in this same way, including the interquartile range values, provided that the Kaplan-Meier curve goes down far enough (unfortunately it often doesn't).

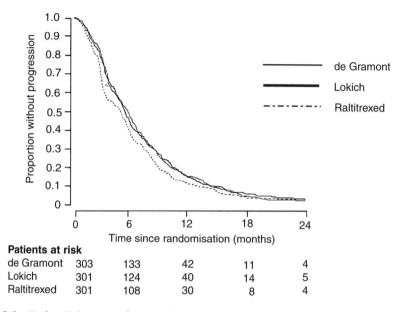

Figure 19.3   Kaplan-Meier curves for overall survival for three groups of patients in a comparison of three chemotherapy regimes in the treatment of colorectal cancer. Reprinted from *The Lancet*, 2002, **359**, 1559 with permission from Elsevier

Exercise 19.2   Figure 19.3 shows Kaplan-Meier curves for progression-free survival, for three groups of patients in a comparison of three chemotherapy regimes used for the treatment of colorectal cancer (Maughan *et al.* 2002). The three regimes were: the de Gramont regimen; the Lokich regimen; and Raltitrexed. What were the approximate median survival times for progression-free survival with each of the three regimes?

Comparing survival with two groups

Although the survival curve for a single group may sometimes be of interest, much more usual is the desire to compare the survival experience of two or more groups. For example, Figure 19.4 is taken from a study of chemotherapy for the treatment of bladder cancer (Medical Research Council Advanced Bladder Working Group 1999). One group of patients ($n = 485$) was randomly assigned to receive conventional radical surgery (cystectomy) or radiotherapy, while a second group ($n = 491$) received the conventional treatment *plus* chemotherapy. The

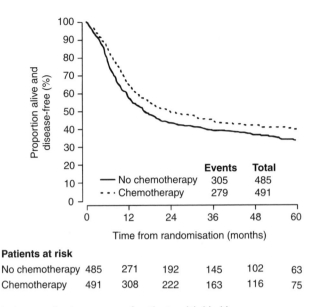

Figure 19.4 Survival curves for two groups of patients with bladder cancer, one group given conventional surgery or radiotherapy, the other group given the conventional treatment *plus* chemotherapy. Reprinted coutresy of Elsevier (*The Lancet*, 1999, Vol No. **354**, p. 533–9)

question asked, 'Was the survival experience of the chemotherapy group any better over the five year follow up?'

The two Kaplan-Meier curves seem to show that the proportions surviving in the chemotherapy group was larger than those in the conventional group throughout the duration of the study, since the survival curve for the former was higher than that of the latter. In fact, the authors of this study report *median* values for disease-free survival of 20 months for the chemotherapy group and 16.5 months for the no-chemotherapy group. The 95 per cent confidence interval for the difference in medians was (0.5 to 7.0) months, so the difference in medians was statistically significant.

Notice that the authors have provided a table showing the numbers at risk at each time interval. This is to remind us that the smaller numbers of survivors towards the end of a trial produce less reliable results. As a direct consequence of this effect, you should not assume that just because the gap between two survival curves gets progressively larger (as it is often seen to do), that this is *necessarily* due to an actual divergence in the survival experiences in the two groups. It might well be caused simply by the low numbers of subjects still at risk. This can make the ends of the curves unreliable.

The log-rank test

If you want to compare the *overall* survival experience of two (or more) groups of patients (rather than say comparing just the median survival times as we did above), then one possible approach is to use the non-parametric *log-rank test*. Essentially, the null hypothesis to be tested is that the two samples (the two groups) are from the same population as far as their survival experience is concerned. In other words there is *no difference* in the survival experiences.

The log-rank test of this hypothesis uses a comparison of observed with expected events (deaths, say), given that the null hypothesis is true.[2] If the *p* value is less than 0.05 you can reject the null hypothesis and conclude that there is a statistically significant difference between the survival experience of the groups. You can then use the Kaplan-Meier curves to decide which group had the significantly better survival. A limitation of the log-rank test is that it cannot be used to explore the influence on survival of more than one variable, i.e. the possibility of confounders – for this you need Cox's proportional regression, which we'll come to shortly.

The authors in the bladder cancer study reported a log-rank test *p* value of 0.019 for the difference in survival times at *three years*, but unfortunately don't give the results of the test over the whole five year duration of the study.

Exercise 19.3 What do you conclude about the statistical significance of the difference in three year survival times of the chemotherapy and non-chemotherapy groups from the results given in the previous paragraph?

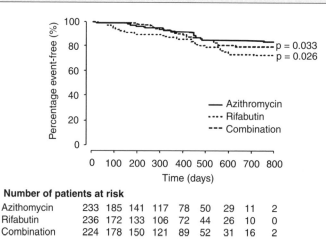

Number of patients at risk

Azithomycin	233	185	141	117	78	50	29	11	2
Rifabutin	236	172	133	106	72	44	26	10	0
Combination	224	178	150	121	89	52	31	16	2

Figure 19.5 Kaplan-Meier curves from a study to assess the clinical efficacy of azithromycin for prophylaxis of *Pneumocystitis* carinii pneumonia in HIV-1 infected patients. Reprinted courtesy of Elsevier (*The Lancet*, 1999, Vol No. **354**, p. 1891–5)

An example of the log-rank test in practice

Figure 19.5 shows the Kaplan-Meier curves from a study to assess the clinical efficacy of azithromycin for prophylaxis of *Pneumocystitis* carinii pneumonia in HIV-1 infected patients (Dunne *et al.* 1999). Patients were randomly assigned to one of three treatment groups: the first group given azithromycin, the second rifabutin and the third a combination of both drugs. The figure shows the event-free (no *Pneumocystitis* carinii pneumonia) survival experiences over an 800 day period for the three treatment groups.

---

[2] You may have spotted the similarity with the chi-squared test considered earlier in the book. In fact the calculations are exactly the same.

The log-rank test was used to test the hypothesis that there is no difference in the percentage event-free between the azithromycin and rifabutin groups (p value $= 0.033$), and between the azithromycin and the combination groups (p-value $= 0.026$). The authors concluded that azithromycin as prophylaxis for *Pneumocystitis* carinii pneumonia, provides additional protection over and above standard *Pneumocystitis* carinii pneumonia prophylaxis. However, these results should be treated with caution because of the very small size of the survivor group towards the end of the study.

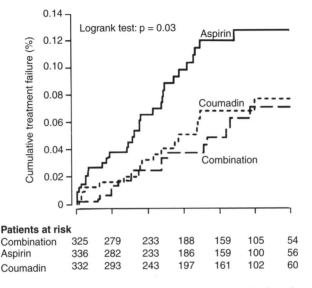

Figure 19.6 Kaplan-Meier curves of percentage number of subsequent ischaemic events from a randomised controlled trial into the relative effectiveness of aspirin and oral anticoagulants (coumadin), used for antiplatelet treatment, following myocardial infarction. Reprinted courtesy of Elsevier (*The Lancet* 2002, **360**, 109–14, Fig. 3, p. 111)

Exercise 19.4   Figure 19.6 shows the Kaplan-Meier curves for the percentage number of ischaemic events from a randomised controlled trial into the relative effectiveness of aspirin and oral anticoagulants (coumadin) for antiplatelet treatment following myocardial infarction (van Es *et al.* 2002). The object was to investigate which of these two drugs is more effective for the long-term reduction of subsequent ischaemic events, and whether the combination of the two drugs offers greater benefit than either drug alone. Is there a statistically significant difference in mortality between the three possible treatments? Which treatment seems to offer the best survival?

The hazard ratio

The log-rank test is limited by the fact that it is just that – a test. It will tell you if there is a significant difference between the survival experience of two (or more) groups, but does not *quantify* that difference. For this we need what is called the *hazard ratio* (based on the ratio of observed and expected events for the two groups), along with which we can calculate a confidence interval. As a matter of interest, the authors of the bladder cancer study reported, for those alive and disease free, a hazard ratio of 0.82, with a 95 per cent confidence interval of (0.70 to 0.97). We can interpret this result to mean that the group who had chemotherapy had a risk of dying in the study period of only 82 per cent compared to the risk for the non-chemotherapy group, and this difference was statistically significant (confidence interval does not include 1).

Exercise 19.5   The survival curves shown in Figure 19.4 from the bladder cancer study are for subjects who are alive *and* disease free. For subjects who were alive but not necessarily disease free, the authors report the following results. What do these results tell you?

Comparison of the survival time in the two groups gave a hazard ratio of 0.85 [95 per cent CI of (0.71 to 1.02)]. The absolute difference in 3-year survival was 5.5 per cent, 50.0 per cent in the chemotherapy group, 55.5 per cent in the non-chemotherapy group [95 per cent CI of (-0.5 to 11.0)]. The median survival time for the chemotherapy group was 44 months and for the no-chemotherapy group was 37.5 months [95 per cent CI of (-0.5 to 15)].

The proportional hazards (or Cox's) regression model

Although researchers can use the log-rank test to distinguish survival between two groups, the test only provides a *p* value; it would be more useful to have an estimate of any difference in survival, along with the corresponding confidence interval. The hazard ratio mentioned above provides this, but neither the log-rank test nor the simple hazard ratio allow for adjustment for possible confounding variables, which may significantly affect survival. For this we can use an approach known as *proportional hazards (or Cox's) regression*. This procedure will provide both estimates and confidence intervals for variables that affect survival, and enable researchers to adjust for confounders. We will discuss briefly the principle underlying the method, and the meaning of some of the terms used.

The focus of *proportional hazards regression* is the *hazard*. The hazard is akin to a failure rate. If the end-point is death, for example, then the hazard is the rate at which individuals die at some point during the course of a study. The hazard can go up or down over time, and the distribution of hazards over the length of a study is known as the *hazard function*. You won't see authors quote the hazard regression function or equation, but for those interested it looks like this:

$$\text{Hazard} = h_0 + e^{(\beta_1 X_1 + \beta_2 X_2 + \ldots)}$$

h_0 is the baseline hazard and is of little importance. The explanatory or independent variables can be any mixture of nominal, ordinal or metric, and nominal variables can be 'dummied', as described in Chapter 17 and Chapter 18. The same variable selection procedures as in linear or logistic regression models can also be used, i.e. either automated or by hand.

The most interesting property of this model is that e^{β_1}, e^{β_2}, etc. give us the *hazard ratios*, or HRs, for the variables X_1, X_2, and so on (notice the obvious similarity with the odds ratios in logistic regression). The hazard ratios are essentially *risk ratios*, but called hazard ratios in the context of survival studies. For example, in a study of the survival of women with breast cancer, the variable X_1 might be 'micrometastases present (Y/N)'. In which case, the hazard ratio HR_1 (the risk of death for a patient when micrometastases are present compared to that for a patient where they are absent, is equal to e^{b_1}. All of this is only true if the relative effect (essentially the *ratio*) of the hazard on the two groups (for example, the relative effect of micrometastases on the survival of each group) remains constant over the whole course of the study.

An application from practice

As an example of proportional hazards regression, Table 19.4 is taken from a study into the relative survival of two groups of patients with non-metastatic colon cancer; one group having open colectomy (OC), the other laparoscopy-assisted colectomy (LAC) (Lacy *et al.* 2002). The figure shows hazard ratios and their confidence intervals: for the probability of being free of recurrence; for overall survival; and for cancer-related survival, after the patients were stratified according to tumour stage.

So, for example, patients with lymph-node metastasis do only about a third as well in terms of being recurrence-free over the course of the study compared to patients without lymph-node metastasis (hazard ratio = 0.31), and this difference is statistically significant since the confidence interval does not include 1 (and the *p* value of 0.0006 is < 0.05). Patients with lymph-node metastasis also compare badly with non-metastasis patients in terms of both

Table 19.4 Results of a Cox proportional hazards regression analysis comparing the survival of patients with laparoscopy-assisted colectomy versus open colectomy, for the treatment of non-metastatic colon cancer. Reproduced courtesy of Elsevier (*The Lancet*, 2002, Vol No. **359**, page 2224–30

	Hazard ratio (95% CI)	p
Probability of being free of recurrence		
Lymph-node metastasis (presence *vs* absence)	0.31 (0.16–0.60)	0.0006
Surgical procedure (OC *vs* LAC)	0.39 (0.19–0.82)	0.012
Preoperative serum CEA concentrations ($\geq$4 ng/mL *vs* <4 ng/mL)	0.43 (0.22–0.87)	0.018
Overall survival		
Surgical procedure (OC *vs* LAC)	0.48 (0.23–1.01)	0.052
Lymph-node metastasis (presence *vs* absence)	0.49 (0.25–0.98)	0.044
Cancer-related survival		
Lymph-node metastasis (presence *vs* absence)	0.29 (0.12–0.67)	0.004
Surgical procedure (OC *vs* LAC)	0.38 (0.16–0.91)	0.029

Type of surgical procedure, laparoscopy-assisted vs open colectomy, is significantly beneficial in terms of recurrence-free and cancer-related survival, but not in terms of overall survival.

OC = open colectomy; LAC = laparoscopy-assisted colectomy; CEA = carcinoembryonic antigen.

overall survival (only about half as well, HR = 0.49), and cancer-related survival (just over a quarter as well, HR = 0.29). Both of these results are statistically significant. Note that type of surgery; laparoscopy-assisted versus open colectomy, is not statistically significant in terms of overall survival as the confidence interval of (0.23 to 1.01) includes 1.

Table 19.5 Hazard ratios due to a number of risk factors in a univariate (unadjusted), and multivariate (adjusted) cohort analysis of the risk to HIV+ women of vulvovaginal and perianal condylomata acuminata and intraepithelial neoplasia. Reproduced courtesy of Elsevier (*The Lancet*, 2002, Vol No. **359**, page 108–14

	Number of women	Univariate analysis[*] Hazard ratio (95% CI)	p	Multivariate analysis[†] Adusted hazard ratio (95% CI)	p
Risk factor					
HIV-1 infection	726	17.0 (4.07–70.9)	0.0007	6.96 (1.51–32.2)	0.01
CD4 T lymphocyte count[‡]	707	3.38 (2.24–5.10)	<0.0001	1.66 (1.03–2.69)	0.04
Human papillomavirus infection	699	4.86 (2.21–10.7)	0.0006	3.76 (1.67–8.43)	0.0013
History of injecting two or more drugs three or more times per week	726	3.09 (1.57–6.07)	0.003	2.32 (1.14–4.71)	0.02
Less than a highschool education	725	2.15 (1.09–4.22)	0.03	1.99 (1.00–3.98)	0.05
Cigarette smoking at enrolment	726	0.84 (0.43–1.64)	0.61	0.71 (0.35–1.44)	0.34
Age <35 years at enrolment	726	1.85 (0.93–3.68)	0.08		
Currently unmarried	726	2.48 (0.96–6.38)	0.06		
Annual income <US$ 10 000	711	1.15 (0.56–2.34)	0.71		
First sex at <16 years of age	723	1.33 (0.69–2.59)	0.40		
>7 lifetime sex partners	722	1.40 (0.71–2.79)	0.33		
History of prostitution	722	1.83 (0.90–3.74)	0.10		
History of ever injecting drugs	726	1.74 (0.90–3.39)	0.10		
History of sexually transmitted disease[§]	654	1.58 (0.72–3.45)	0.25		

[*]In univariate analysis, vulvovaginal lesion was the outcome variable.
[†]355 HIV-1-positive and 325 HIV-1-negative women were included in the multivariate analysis, with vulvovaginal or perianal lesion as the outcome variable and HIV-1 infection, CD4 T lymphocyte count, human papillomavirus infection, less than a highschool education, cigarette smoking, and history of injection of two or more drugs three or more times per week as covariates.
[‡] HIV-1 negative women were presumed to have a CD4 count >500 cell/, μL.
[§] Does not include a history of genital warts.

Exercise 19.6   Table 19.5 shows the hazard ratios (unadjusted and adjusted) due to a number of risk factors in a cohort analysis of the risk to HIV+ women of vulvovaginal and perianal condylomata acuminata and intraepithelial neoplasia (Conley *et al.* 2002). Interpret the multivariate results. How do these differ from the univariate results?

Checking the proportional hazards assumption

The proportional hazards assumption can be checked graphically using what is known as the *log-log* plot. Unfortunately, this procedure is beyond the scope of this book.

20

Systematic review and meta-analysis

Learning objectives

When you have finished this chapter you should be able to:

- Provide a broad outline of the idea of systematic review.

- Outline a typical search procedure.

- Describe what is meant by publication bias and its implications.

- Describe how we can use the funnel plot to examine for the presence of publication bias.

- Explain the importance of heterogeneity across studies and how the L'Abbé plot can be used in this context.

- Explain the meaning of meta-analysis.

- Outline the role of the Mantel-Haenszel procedure in combining studies.

- Describe what a forest plot is and how it is used.

Medical Statistics from Scratch, Second Edition David Bowers
© 2008 John Wiley & Sons, Ltd

Introduction

If you have a patient with a particular condition and you want to know the current consensus on the most effective treatment, then you could perhaps ask the opinions of colleagues (although they may know no more than you) or maybe look through some pharmaceutical publicity material. Or read all the relevant journals lying around your clinic or office. Better still, if you have access to one of the clinical databases, such as Medline, then the job will be that much easier; in fact, anything like an adequate search is almost impossible otherwise. If you want your search to capture everything written on your topic then you will need a systematic approach. This process of searching for all relevant studies (or trials) is known as a *systematic review.*

However you do your systematic review, you are likely to encounter some difficulties:

- Many of the studies you turn up will be based on smallish samples. As you know, small samples may well produce unreliable results.

- Partly as a consequence of the above problem, many of the studies come to different and conflicting conclusions.

- There will be some studies that you simply do not find. Perhaps because they are published in obscure and/or non-English-language journals, or are not published at all (for example, internal pharmaceutical company reports, or research dissertations). This shortfall may lead to what is known as publication bias.

To some extent you can address the first two of these problems by combining all of these individual studies into one large study, as you will see later (a process called *meta-analysis*), and you will also want to deal with the potential for publication bias. But let's start with a brief description of systematic review.

Systematic review

The basis of a systematic review is a comprehensive search that aims to identify all similar and relevant studies that satisfy a pre-defined set of *inclusion and exclusion criteria*. As an example, the following extract from a systematic review and meta-analysis of studies of dietary intervention to lower blood cholesterol, shows the inclusion and exclusion criteria, together with a brief description of the search procedure (Tang *et al.* 1998).

Methods

Identification of trials and extraction of data

We aimed to identify all unconfounded randomised trials of dietary advice to lower cholesterol concentration in free-living subjects published before 1996. Trials were eligible for

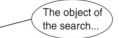
The object of the search...

inclusion if there were at least two groups, of which one could be considered a control group; treatment assignment was by random allocation; the intervention was a global dietary modification (changes to various food components of the diet to achieve the desired targets); and lipid concentration were measured before and after the intervention.

Trials of diets to reduce fat intake in women considered to be at risk of breast cancer were included because the diets were similar to those aimed at lowering cholesterol concentration. We excluded trials of specific supplementation diets (such as those with particular oils or margarine, garlic, plant sterol, or fibre supplements, etc.), multifactorial intervention trials, trials aimed primarily at lowering body weight or blood pressure, and trials whose interventions lasted less than four weeks. Trials based on randomisation of workplace or general practice were also excluded.

To identify these trials we identified four electronic databases (Medline, Human Nutrition, EMBASE, and Allied and Alternative Medicine). These databases included trials published after 1966. We also identified trials by hand searching the American Journal of Human Nutrition by scrutinising the references of review articles and of each relevant randomised trial, and by consulting experts on the subject.

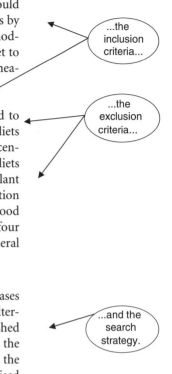

...the inclusion criteria...

...the exclusion criteria...

...and the search strategy.

Reports that appeared only in non-English language journals were examined with the help of translators. Trials were categorised according to their approximate target diet into four groups.

The end result of a systematic review then, is a list of studies, each one of which provides a value for the specified outcome measure. In the above example, this outcome measure was the percentage difference in mean total blood cholesterol between the intervention (dietary advice) group and the control group. Examination of this list of outcome values may provide the required insights into treatment effectiveness.

Exercise 20.1   Briefly outline the systematic review procedure and some of the problems that may arise.

The forest plot

The list of studies produced by the systematic review is often accompanied by what is known as a *forest plot*. This plot has study outcome on the vertical axis, usually arranged by size of study (i.e. by sample size), and the outcome measure on the horizontal axis. The outcome measure might be odds or risk ratios, means or proportions, or their differences, and so on. There are a number of ways of displaying the data. For example, by using a box with a horizontal line through it, whose length represents the width of the 95 per cent confidence interval for whatever outcome measure is being used. Or with a diamond, whose width represents the 95 per cent confidence interval. The area of each box or diamond should be proportional to its sample size. As an example, the forest plot for the cholesterol study referred to above is shown in Figure 20.1.

Here the 22 individual studies, each represented by a black square whose size is proportional to sample size, are divided into four groups according to their approximate target diet (we don't need to go into the details). The aggregated mean percentage reduction in cholesterol (with a 95 per cent confidence interval) for each of these groups is represented by a white square, whose size is proportional to the sample size of the aggregated individual studies. The large white square at the bottom of the plot is the aggregated value for all the studies combined. I'll come back to this shortly.

The horizontal axis represents mean percentage change in blood cholesterol. As you can see, 21 of the 22 studies show a reduction in percentage cholesterol (the study fourth from the top lies exactly on the zero, or no difference, line). However, in seven of the studies the confidence interval crosses the zero line, indicating that the reduction in cholesterol is not statistically significant. The remaining 15 studies show a statistically significant reduction (95 per cent confidence interval does not cross the zero line), as do all four group summary values. Thus there appears to be plenty of evidence that dietary interventions of the type included here do manage to achieve statistically significant reductions in total blood cholesterol.

Exercise 20.2   The results in Table 20.1 show the outcomes (relative risk for proportion of subjects with side effects), from each of six randomised trials comparing antibiotic with placebo for treating acute cough in adults (Fahey *et al.* 1998). Draw a forest plot of this data and comment briefly on what it shows. Note: relative risks greater than 1 favour the placebo (i.e. fewer side effects).

Table 20.1   The outcomes (relative risk for proportion of subjects with side effects), from each of six randomised trials comparing antibiotic with placebo for treating acute cough in adults. Reproduced from *BMJ* 1998, **316**: 906–10. Figure 4, p. 909. Figures 2 and 3, p. 908, courtesy of BMJ Publishing Group

Study	Sample size	Relative risk (95 % CI)
Briskfield *et al.*	50	0.51 (0.20 to 1.32)
Dunlay *et al.*	57	7.59 (0.43 to 134.81)
Franks and Gleiner	54	3.48 (0.39 to 31.38)
King *et al.*	71	2.30 (0.93 to 5.70)
Stott and West	207	1.49 (0.63 to 3.48)
Verheij *et al.*	158	1.71 (0.80 to 3.67)
Total	597	1.51 (0.86 to 2.64)

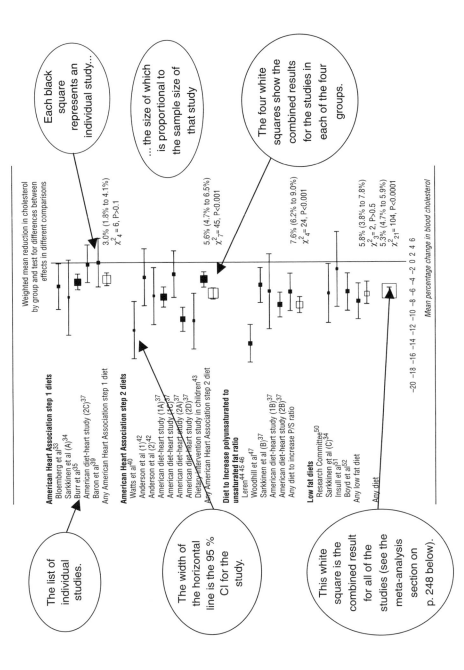

Figure 20.1 Forest plot for the dietary intervention and blood cholesterol study. Mean percentage changes (with 95 per cent confidence intervals) in blood total cholesterol concentration. Reproduced from *BMJ* 1998, **316**: 1213–20, courtesy of BMJ Publishing Group

Publication and other biases

The success of any systematic review depends critically on how thorough and wide-ranging the search for relevant studies is. One frequently quoted difficulty is that of *publication bias*, which can arise from a number of sources:

- The tendency for journals to favour the acceptance of studies showing *positive* outcomes at the expense of those with negative outcomes.

- The tendency for authors to favour the submission to journals of studies showing *positive* outcomes at the expense of those with negative outcomes.

- Studies with positive results are more likely to be published in English language journals giving them a better chance of capture in the search process.

- Studies with positive results are more likely to be cited, giving them a better chance of capture in the search process.

- Studies with positive results are more likely to be published in more than one journal, giving them a better chance of capture in the search process.

- Some studies are never submitted for publication. For example, those that fail to show a positive result, those by pharmaceutical companies (particularly if the results are unfavourable), graduate dissertations and so on.

In the light of all this it is important that possible presence of publication bias should be addressed. One possibility is to use what is known as a *funnel plot*.

The funnel plot

In a funnel plot the *size* of the study is shown on the vertical axis and the size of the treatment's effect (for example, as measured by an odds or risk ratio, or a difference in means, etc.) is shown on the horizontal axis. In the absence of bias the funnel plot should have the shape of a *symmetric* upturned cone or funnel. Larger studies shown at the top of the funnel will be more precise (their results will not be so spread out), smaller studies, shown towards the bottom less precise, and therefore more spread out. These differences produce the funnel shape. However, if the funnel is asymmetrical, for example, if parts of the funnel are missing or poorly represented – and this will usually be near the bottom of the funnel where the smaller studies are located – then this is suggestive of bias of one form or another.[1]

---

[1] There are a number of other possible causes of bias in systematic reviews. Those interested should look, for example, at Egger and Davey Smith (1998), where other possible biases are discussed.

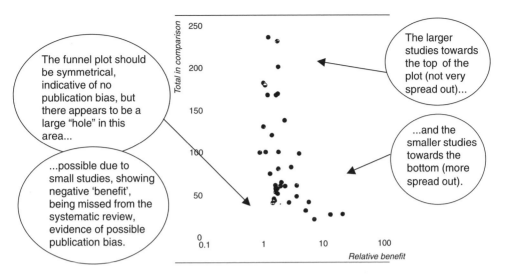

Figure 20.2 Funnel plot used to check for publication bias in a systematic review of the effectiveness of topically applied non-steroidal anti-inflammatory drugs. The asymmetry of the funnel is an indication of publication bias (see text). Reproduced from *BMJ*, Jan 1998; **316**: 333–338, courtesy of BMJ Publishing Group

As an example, Figure 20.2 is a funnel plot from a systematic review of the effectiveness of topically applied non-steroidal anti-inflammatory drugs in acute and chronic pain conditions (Moore *et al.* 1998). Relative benefit (risk ratio) is shown on the horizontal axis. Each point in the figure represents one of the studies. Values to the left of the value of 1 on the horizontal axis show negative 'benefit', values to the right, positive benefit.

The asymmetry in the funnel is quite marked, with a noticeable absence of small studies showing negative 'benefit' (risk ratio less than 1). The authors comment:

> The funnel plot might be interpreted as showing publication bias. The tendency for smaller trials to produce a larger analgesic effect might be construed as supporting the absence of trials showing no difference between topical non-steroidal and placebo. We made strenuous efforts to unearth unpublished data and contacted all pharmaceutical companies in the United Kingdom that we identified as producing non-steroidal products. One company made unpublished data available to us, but the others did not feel able to do so.

Exercise 20.3 a) Outline the major sources of publication bias. (b) Figure 20.3 shows a funnel plot from a systematic review of trials of beta blockers in secondary prevention after myocardial infarction (Egger and Davey Smith 1998). The plot has odds ratio (horizontal axis) against sample size. Comment on the evidence for publication bias.

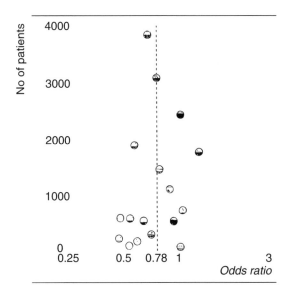

Figure 20.3 Funnel plot from a systematic review of trials of beta blockers in secondary prevention after myocardial infarction. Reproduced from *BMJ* 1998, **316**: 61–6. Figure 2, p. 64, courtesy of BMJ Publishing Group

Combining the studies

Meta-analysis is the process of combining a number of separate studies to produce one 'super-study'. So, for example, we might have three separate studies, with sample sizes of 40, 80 and 150. When combined, we get a super-study with a sample size of 270. The assumption of the meta-analysis is that this super-study will provide a more reliable and precise overall result for the output variable in question, than do any of the smaller individual studies. We can use the *Mantel-Haenszel* procedure to combine the studies.[2] Before studies can be combined, however, they must satisfy the *homogeneity* criterion. A few words about that first, before we look at an example of meta-analysis.

Homogeneity among studies

Even when a set of potentially similar studies has been identified, authors have to make sure they are similar, or *homogeneous*, enough to be combined. For example, they should have similar subjects, have the same type and level of intervention, the same output measure, the same treatment effect and so on. Only if studies are *homogeneous* in this way can they be properly combined. Studies which don't have this quality are said to suffer from *heterogeneity*. The underlying assumption (i.e. the null hypothesis) of meta-analysis is that all of the studies measure the same effect in the same population, and that any differences between them is due to chance alone. When the results are combined the chance element cancels out.

---

[2] Note that this is not to be confused with the Mantel-Haenszel test for heterogeneity.

You might find the comments on heterogeneity by the authors of the diet and cholesterol study quoted earlier illuminating (Tang, *et al.* 1998):

Heterogeneity between study effects

The design and results of these dietary studies differed greatly. They were conducted over 30 years and varied in their aims, in the intensity and type of intervention, and in the different baseline characteristics of the subjects included. Completeness and duration of follow up also differed. Unsurprisingly, the heterogeneity between their effects on blood cholesterol concentration was also significant. Among the longer trials some, but not all, of the heterogeneity between the effects on blood cholesterol concentration seemed to be due to the type of diet recommended. Deciding which trials should be included in which groups is open to different interpretation and, although we tried to be consistent, for some trials the target diets either were not clearly stated or did not fit neatly into recognised categories such as the step 1 and 2 diets. It is important to be cautious in interpreting meta-analysis when there is evidence of significant heterogeneity; although there was no evidence that the overall results were influenced by trials with outlying values.

The homogeneity assumption should be tested. One possibility is for the authors to provide readers with a *L'Abbé plot*. The L'Abbé plot displays *outcomes* from a number of studies, with the percentage of successes (or reduction in risk, etc.) with the treatment group on the vertical axis, and same measure for the control/placebo group on the horizontal axis. The 45° line is thus the boundary between effective and non-effective treatment. Values above the line show beneficial results. If possible, varying sized plotting points proportional to sample size should be shown. The more compact the plot, the more homogeneous the studies.

As an example, Figure 20.4 is a L'Abbé plot showing outcomes from 37 placebo-controlled trials of topical non-steroidal anti-inflammatory drugs in acute (●), and chronic (■), pain

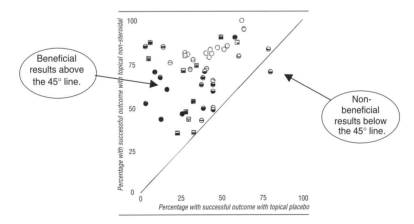

Figure 20.4 L'Abbé plot showing outcomes from 37 placebo-controlled trials of topical non-steroidal anti-inflammatory drugs in acute (●) and chronic (■) pain conditions. The compactness of the plotted points is a measure of homogeneity across the studies. Reproduced from *BMJ*, Jan 1998; **316**: 333–338, courtesy of BMJ Publishing Group

conditions (Moore *et al.* 1998). In this plot, the authors have not plotted the points in proportion to sample size. Whether the degree of spread of the points in Figure 20.4 is indicative of homogeneity among the studies is a matter of judgement, which can only be made by those experienced in the interpretation of these charts. Note that the *overall* meta-analytic result can also be plotted on this same plot (but is not shown in Figure 20.4).

Mantel-Haenszel test for heterogeneity

A more commonly used alternative is the *Mantel-Haenszel test for heterogeneity*, which uses the chi-squared distribution (see Chapter 14). The null hypothesis is that the studies are homogeneous. An example of its use is given in Table 20.2, which is taken from a study that 'aimed to identify and evaluate all published randomised trials of hospital versus general practice care for people with diabetes' (Griffin 1998). The author's Table 2 presents a summary of the weighted (by sample size) mean differences, for a number of different outcomes. The author's Table 3 presents similar information for different outcomes in terms of the odds ratio. The p-values for the Mantel-Haenszel test (using chi-squared) are given in the last column. Only one set of studies (Referral to chiropody, p-value < 0.005) displays evidence of heterogeneity, but since this comprised only two studies, the result is somewhat meaningless.

Meta-analysis and the Mantel-Haenszel procedure

If the studies pass the homogeneity test then we can combine them using the Mantel-Haenszel procedure, to produce the meta-analysis; this will give us an overall value for the outcome in question. The procedure is often accompanied by a forest plot, showing the individual studies, together with the combined result, as in the next example.

This is a report of a meta-analysis of randomised controlled trials to compare antibiotic with placebo, for acute cough in adults, referred to above (Fahey *et al.* 1998). The focus was on placebo-controlled trials, which reported two specific outcomes: the proportion of subjects reporting productive cough; and the proportion of subjects reporting no improvement at follow-up.[3] Figure 20.5 shows the forest plots for these two acute cough outcomes, in terms of the risk ratios (called by the authors 'relative risks') in favour of the specific outcome.

The overall net outcome effect is shown with a diamond shape here (one for each of the two outcomes). The area of the diamond is proportional to the total number of studies represented, and the width the 95 per cent confidence interval. Values to the left of an odds ratio of 1 (bottom axis) show reductions in fatalities among cases, those to the right an increase in fatality (compared to control groups).

The Mantel-Haenszel procedure was used to produce the final result shown at the bottom of the forest plot in Figure 20.5. The aggregate relative risks are 0.85 for productive cough and 0.62 for no improvement at follow-up. These appear to show reductions in the risk for both conditions and favour the antibiotic over the placebo. However, since both have 95 per cent confidence intervals which include 1, neither is in fact significant, confirmed by the fact that

---

[3] There was a third outcome concerned with side-effects which is not considered here. See Exercise 20.2 above.

Table 20.2 The Mantel-Haenszel test for heterogeneity across studies, with a number of different outcomes in the diabetes care study. The null hypothesis is that the studies are homogeneous. Only one outcome (chiropody) has significant heterogeneity. Reproduced from *BMJ* 1998, **317:** 390–6. Table 2, p. 392, courtesy of BMJ Publishing Group

Outcome	Weighted difference in mean values (95% CI)		χ^2 test of between trial heterogeneity	P value
	Favours prompted GP care	Favours hospital care		
Glycated haemoglobin (%) (3 trials, n = 535)	−0.28 (−0.59 to 0.03)		3.90	>0.10
Systolic blood pressure (mm Hg) (2 trials, n = 369)		1.62 (−3.30 to 6.53)	2.56	>0.10
Diastolic blood pressure (mm Hg) (2 trials, n = 369)		0.56 (−1.69 to 2.80)	0.10	>0.75
Frequency of review (per patient per year) (2 trials, n = 402)	0.27 (0.07 to 0.46)		0.59	>0.30
Frequency of glycated haemoglobin test (per patient per year) (2 trials, n = 402)	1.60 (1.45 to 1.75)		0.05	>0.80

Outcome	Odds ratios (95% CI)		χ^2 test of between trial heterogeneity	P value
	Favours prompted GP care	Favours hospital care		
Mortality (2 trials, n = 455)		1.06 (0.53 to 2.11)	0.0	1.0
Losses to follow up (3 trials, n = 589)	0.37 (0.22 to 0.61)		1.63	>0.30
Referral to chiropody (2 trials, n = 399)	2.51 (1.59 to 3.97)		9.77	<0.005
Referral to dietitian (2 trials, n = 399)		0.61 (0.40 to 0.92)	0.56	>0.30

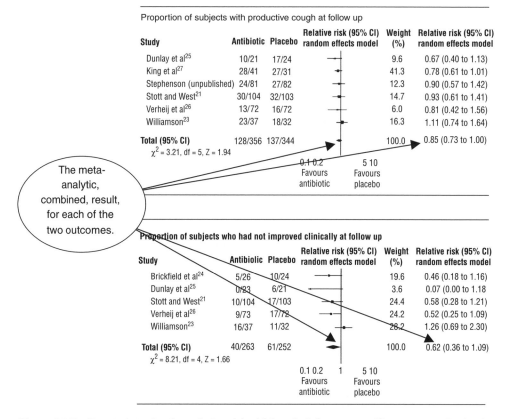

Figure 20.5 Forest plots showing relative risks (risk ratios) for two specific outcomes; *Productive cough*, and *No improvement at follow-up*, in a systematic review of antibiotic versus placebo for acute cough in adults. Reproduced from *BMJ* 1998, **316**: 906–10. Figure 4, p. 909. Figures 2 and 3, p. 908, courtesy of BMJ Publishing Group

both diamonds cross the line where relative risk = 1. In other words, the efficacy of antibiotic over placebo for acute cough in this population is not established by this meta-analysis.

However, look back at Figure 20.1, the forest plot for the dietary intervention and blood cholesterol meta-analysis. Here you will see at the bottom of the figure, the box representing the overall aggregated mean per cent reduction in cholesterol (labelled 'Any diet'), which shows a reduction of 5.3 per cent. This box does not cross the per cent change line, so this is a statistically significant result, confirmed by the 95 per cent confidence interval of (4.7 per cent to 5.9 per cent).

Exercise 20.4 (a) Explain why homogeneity across studies is important before a meta-analysis is performed. (b) What methods are available for the detection of heterogeneity? (c) What advantage over the results of individual studies does a meta-analysis provide?

Appendix
Table of random numbers

23157	54859	01837	25993	76249	70886	95230	36744
05545	55043	10537	43508	90611	83744	10962	21343
14871	60350	32404	36223	50051	00322	11543	80834
38976	74951	94051	75853	78805	90194	32428	71695
97312	61718	99755	30870	94251	25841	54882	10513
11742	69381	44339	30872	32797	33118	22647	06850
43361	28859	11016	45623	93009	00499	43640	74036
93806	20478	38268	04491	55751	18932	58475	52571
49540	13181	08429	84187	69538	29661	77738	09527
36768	72633	37948	21569	41959	68670	45274	83880
07092	52392	24627	12067	06558	45344	67338	45320
43310	01081	44863	80307	52555	16148	89742	94647
61570	06360	06173	63775	63148	95123	35017	46993
31352	83799	10779	18941	31579	76448	62584	86919
57048	86526	27795	93692	90529	56546	35065	32254
09243	44200	68721	07137	30729	75756	09298	27650
97957	35018	40894	88329	52230	82521	22532	61587
93732	59570	43781	98885	56671	66826	95996	44569
72621	11225	00922	68264	35666	59434	71687	58167
61020	74418	45371	20794	95917	37866	99536	19378
97839	85474	33055	91718	45473	54144	22034	23000
89160	97192	22232	90637	35055	45489	88438	16361
25966	88220	62871	79265	02823	52862	84919	54883
81443	31719	05049	54806	74690	07567	65017	16543
11322	54931	42362	34386	08624	97687	46245	23245

Medical Statistics from Scratch, Second Edition   David Bowers
© 2008 John Wiley & Sons, Ltd

Solutions to Exercises

Note: Although I have provided complete solutions to the calculating parts of the exercises, I have offered only brief comments where a commentary is required. This is deliberate, firstly because I don't want to write the book again in terms of the solutions and secondly tutors might want to tease these answers from the students themselves, perhaps as part of a wider discussion.

1.1 Ethnicity, sex, marital status, type of operation, smoking status, etc.

1.2 Apgar scale, Waterlow scale, Edinburgh Post-natal Depressions scale, Beck Depression Inventory, SF36, Apache, etc.

1.3 GCS produces ordinal data, which are not real numbers, so can't be added or divided.

1.4 Height, temp., cholesterol, body mass index, age, time, etc.

1.5 Number of deaths, number of angina attacks, number of operations performed, number of stillbirths, etc.

1.6 A continuous metric variable has an infinite or uncountable number of possible values. A discrete metric variable has a limited, countable number of possible values. (a) 7 (0, 1, 2, . . . , 6). (b) Not possible to do this, since number of possible weights is infinite.

1.7 VAS data is ordinal, because these are subjective judgements, which are not measured but assessed, and will probably vary from patient to patient and moment to moment. So it's not possible to calculate *average* if by this is meant adding up four values and dividing by four, because ordinal data are not real numbers.

1.8 Age, MC. Social class, O. No. of children, MD. Age at 1st child, MC. Age at menarche, MC. Menopausal state, O. Age at menopause, MC. Lifetime use of oral contraceptives, N. No. years taking oral contraceptives, MC. No. months breastfeeding, MC. Lifetime use of hrt, MC. Years of hrt, MC. Family history of ovarian cancer, N. Family history of breast cancer, N. Units of alcohol, MD. No. cigs per day, MD. Body mass index, MC. (key: N = nominal; O = ordinal; MD = metric discrete; MC = metric cont.).

1.9 Maternal age, MC, but given here in ordinal groups. Parity, MD. No. cigs daily, MD. Multiple pregnancy, N. Pre-eclampsia, N. Cesarean, N.

Medical Statistics from Scratch, Second Edition   David Bowers
© 2008 John Wiley & Sons, Ltd

1.10   Age, MC. Sex, N. Number of rooms in home, MD. Length of hair, O. Colour of hair, N. Texture of hair, N. Pruritus, N. Excoriations, N. Live lice, O. Viable nits, O.

2.1

Cause of injury	Frequency (number of patients)	Relative frequency (% of patients)
Falls	46	61.33
Crush	20	26.67
Motor vehicle crash	6	8.00
Other	3	4.00

2.2

Satisfaction with nursing care	Frequency (number of patients)	Relative frequency (% of patients)
Very satisfied	121	25.5
Satisfied	161	33.9
Neutral	90	18.9
Dissatisfied	51	10.7
Very dissatisfied	52	10.9

2.3

% mortality	tally	Frequency
10.0–14.9	HHH ////	9
15.0–19.9	HHH ///	8
20.0–24.9	HHH	5
25.0–29.9	///	3
30.0–34.9	/	1

Observation: Most ICUs have percentage mortality under 20 per cent.

2.4

Parity	Frequency	% frequency
0	5	12.50
1	6	15.00
2	14	35.00
3	10	25.00
4	3	7.5
5	1	2.5
6	0	0
7	0	0
8	1	2.5

Most women have a parity between 1 and 3, with the largest percentage of women (35 per cent) having a parity of 1.

2.5 (a)

GCS score	Frequency (no. of patients)	Cumulative frequency (cumulative no. of patients)	Relative frequency (% of patients)	Cumulative relative frequency. (Cumulative % of patients)
3	10	10	6.49	6.49
4	5	15	3.25	9.74
5	6	21	3.90	13.64
6	2	23	1.30	14.94
7	12	35	7.79	22.73
8	15	50	9.74	32.47
9	18	68	11.69	44.16
10	14	82	9.09	53.25
11	15	97	9.74	62.99
12	21	118	13.64	76.63
13	13	131	8.44	85.07
14	17	148	11.04	96.11
15	6	154	3.90	100.00

(b) 53.25 per cent

2.6

(a) Better to have parity as the columns and diagnosis as the rows.

Diagnosis	Parity (no.)		
	≤ 2	>2	totals
Benign	22	10	32
Malignant	4	4	8
totals	26	14	40

(b)

Diagnosis	Parity (%)	
	≤ 2	>2
Benign	84.6	71.4
Malignant	15.4	28.6
totals	100.0	100.0

(c) Only 15.4 per cent of those with a parity of 2 or less had a malignant diagnosis, compared to nearly twice as many with a parity of 3 or more. Low levels of parity seem to favour a benign diagnosis.

2.7

OCP	Cases (n = 106)	Controls ($n = 226$)
Yes	38	61
No	62	39
totals	100	100

Comment: Only 38 per cent of those receiving a malignant diagnosis (the cases) had at some time used OCP, whereas 61 per cent of the controls (receiving a benign diagnosis), had used OCP. This suggests that a woman who had used OCP is more likely to receive a benign diagnosis. This is not a contingency table. There are two distinct groups of patients, those with a malignant diagnosis and those with a benign diagnosis.

3.1 Most common type of stroke is non-disabling large-artery in both groups. Second most common is disabling large artery in both groups.

3.2

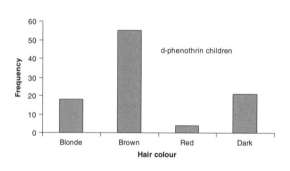

3.3

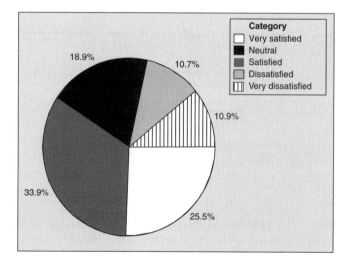

3.4

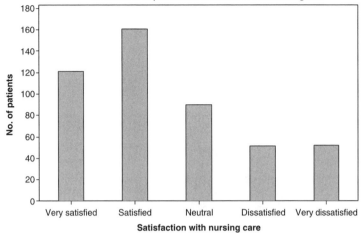

3.5

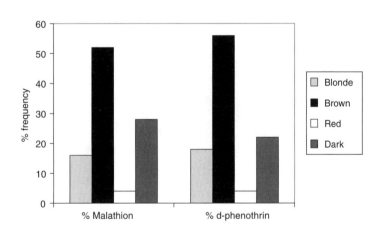

3.6 Stacked bar chart

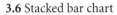

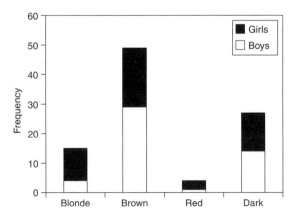

3.7 Schools have very few cases, most only one (20 schools). The majority of the rest have under 10 cases. One school exceptionally has 23 cases.

3.8 Most men have SP levels between four and four and a half, with progressively fewer and fewer men with less and more SP than this. There is a longish tail of higher values (up towards six).

3.9

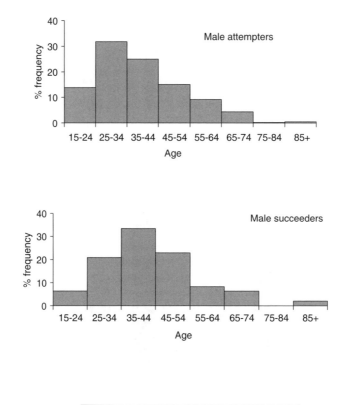

3.10

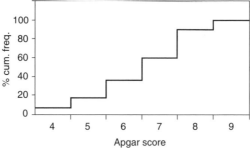

3.11 (a) In both groups minimum cholesterol levels are about 4 mmol/l, maximum levels about 11 mmol/l, but the control group showed slightly higher cholesterol levels throughout. About half the patients had a cholesterol level of 6 mmol/l and half more.

(b)

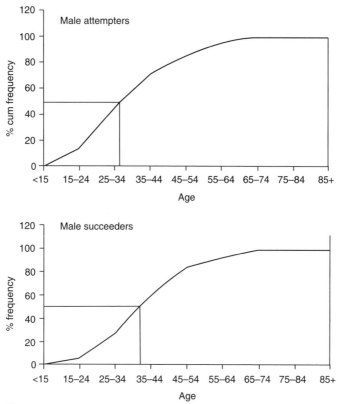

About 26 and 33

Comment: although this data is grouped we can see that half of the male attempters were younger than the youngest half of the male succeeders.

4.1 (a) highest is 70–79, (b) lowest is <15.

4.2 Less skewed.

4.3 (a) Negative. (b) The distribution is positively skewed, but only shows the lowest 95 per cent of values.

4.4 For attempters, the majority of both men and women are aged between 25 and 35. For succeeders, the majority are between 25 and 54. In all cases the distributions are positively skewed.

5.1 (a) Proportion breast fed $= 67/149 = 0.4497$; percentage $= 0.4497 \times 100 = 44.97\,\%$.
(b) Proportion bottle fed $= 93/182 = 0.5110$; percentage $= 0.5110 \times 100 = 51.10\,\%$.

5.2 (a) Prevalence of genital chlamydia $= (23/890) \times 100 = 2.58\,\%$.
(b) Incidence of SIDS per year $= 10/10000$.

Incidence rate *per thousand* live births per year $= 10/10 = 1$ SIDS death per 1000 live births per year.

5.3   (a) Cases and controls, modal class = II. (b) Satisfied. (c) PSF = 0.

5.4   Falls.

5.5   (a) Putting the percentage mortality values in ascending order gives:

11.2	12.8	13.5	13.6	13.7	14.0	14.3	14.7	14.9	15.2	16.1	16.3	17.7
1	2	3	4	5	6	7	8	9	10	11	12	13

18.2	18.9	19.3	19.3	20.2	20.4	21.1	22.4	22.8	26.7	27.2	29.4	31.3
14	15	16	17	18	19	20	21	22	23	24	25	26

Since there is an even number of values, the median percentage mortality is the average of the two 'middle' values, i.e. the average of the 13th (17.7) and 14th (18.2) values, i.e. the 13.5th value. The median is thus = (17.7 + 18.2)/2 = 17.95 %. Or you could have used the formula, median = $\frac{1}{2}$ (n + 1)th value; or $\frac{1}{2}$ (26 + 1) = $\frac{1}{2}$ × 27 = 13.5th value, as before.

(b) Attempters. (i) Men. 412 men. So median will be the average of the 206th and 207th values, which are in the 35–44 age group. (ii) Women. 562 women. So median is the average of the 281th and 282th values, which are in the 35–44 age group.
Succeeders.
(i) *Men.* 48 men, so median will be average of the 24th and 25th values, so the median must be in the 35–44 age group. (ii) *Women.* 55 women, so median is value of the middle, 28th, value, so the median must be in the 35–44 age group. You might want to repeat this exercise using the formula.

5.6   (a) mean > median; because of long tail of values to the right (positive skewness). (b) mean > median; positively skewed.

5.7   Mean percentage mortality = 18.66 %, compared to median of 17.95 %. These values are quite similar which suggests that the distribution might be reasonably symmetric (which you could check with a histogram).

5.8   (a) With outliers, mean = 720.4, median = 500, standard deviation = 622.2. (b) Without outliers, mean = 610.6, median = 500, standard deviation = 319.8.

5.9   Using 25th percentile is 1/4 (n + 1)th value, then the 25th percentile = 14.23 %. Using 75th percentile is $\frac{3}{4}$ (n + 1)th value, then the 75th percentile = 21.43 %. So a quarter of the ICUs have a mortality of less than 14.23 %, and a quarter have a mortality above 21.43 %.

5.10   Breast fed, range = 20 to 28 years; bottle fed, range = 20 to 27 years.

5.11   Interquartile range of percentage mortality = (14.23 to 21.43) %. This means that the range of the middle half (50 per cent) of the ICU % mortality rates is from 14.23 per cent to 21.43 per cent.

5.12   Median (iqr) pain = 51 (23.8 to 87.8). The median pain level is 51 out of a maximum of 100, so 50 per cent of subjects had pain levels below 51 and half above 51. The interquartile range indicates that the middle 50 per cent of pain levels lay between 23.8 and 87.8.

5.13   Q2, the median = 6mmol/l; Q1 = 5.5mmol/l; Q3 = 7.0mmol/l; iqr = (5.5 to 7.0) mmol/l.

5.14

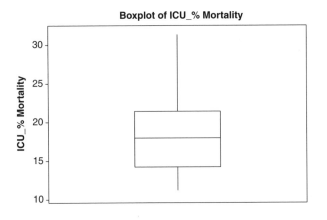

Seems to have a long positive tail and positively skewed (or outliers).

5.15 Median percentage DNA damage higher in the control group - about 12 compared to about eight in survivors. Interquartile range is also slightly larger. Max value much larger in controls (about 25 compared to 15). Minimums similar.

5.16 You can think of this, roughly speaking, as indicating that the average distance of all of these cord platelet count values is 69×10^9/l from the mean value of 306×10^9/l.

5.17 SD = 5.36 %. With a mean of 18.66 per cent (Exercise 5.6), this suggests that the ICU's percentage mortality rates are, on average, 5.36 per cent away from this mean value.

5.18 For data to be Normally distributed, we need to be able to fit in three standard deviations below the mean (and three above it). In all cases it is impossible (by a long way!) to fit three SDs below the mean value without going into negative time. This would suggest that all the distributions are positively skewed.

6.1 The target population is the population at which the research is aimed; this is too large to be studied in any way. The study population is a more attainable but nonetheless still too large to be studied. The sample is a sample, representative of the study population. Consider trying to study the population of people in the UK who are HIV+. This is large population, perhaps many hundreds of thousands. It will be impossible to identify all, or even a reasonable proportion of this population. Many of these people will be transient; many will be undiagnosed. Many will refuse to participate in any research, etc.

6.2 The principal advantage is that a random sample will be representative of the population. The principal drawback is that a sampling frame is needed to take a random sample. Practically, sample frames for any realistic population are virtually impossible to obtain.

6.3 In an observational study, the investigators do not influence in any way the recruitment, treatment or aftercare of subjects, but may simply ask questions, take measurements, observe events and so on. In an experimental study, the investigator takes any active role in some aspect of the study, giving a drug, changing nursing care, etc.

6.4   A sample to determine levels of satisfaction with an endoscopy procedure. A sample to determine the prevalence of pressure sores in elderly patients in hospitals.

6.5   (a) Case-control studies are usually quicker, cheaper and better with rare conditions, than cohort studies. They don't suffer from subject fall-out over time. (b) Selection of suitable controls is often difficult. Problems with reliance on accuracy of patient recall, and medical records. Not good when exposure to risk factor is rare.

6.6   By double-blinding.

6.7   (a) To produce two groups of subjects who are as alike as possible. This will balance all factors, known and unknown, that might differentially affect the response of the two groups to the two treatments or treatment and placebo, and includes controlling for confounders. (b) Any solution to this problem will, of course, depend on the particular set of random numbers used. My random numbers were: 2 3 1 5 (7) 5 4 (8) 5 (9) (0) 1 (8) 3 (7) 2. Since we only have six blocks we can't use the random numbers in parentheses. With blocks of four:

> Block 1, CCTT;   Block 2, CTCT;   Block 3, CTTC;
> Block 4, TCTC;   Block 5, TCCT;   Block 6, TTCC

The first number is 2, so the first four subjects are allocated as block 2: C, T, C and T. The next number is 3, so the next four subjects are allocated: C, T, T and C. Continue this procedure until there are 20 in each group.

6.8   (a) The authors used a cross-section study of schoolchildren who were given a skin-prick test of sensitivity to six common allergens (the outcome variable), to determine atopic status, complimented by a questionnaire completed by parents to elicit pertinent socio-economic factors (including number of siblings). Possible confounders identified by the researchers were family history of atopy, sex, socio-economic status, presence of pets, smoking, and age.

(b) The researchers used a double-blind RCT, with patients (aged 2–15 years) randomised to either CF or PM. To quote, 'A double-dummy techniques was used: patients randomly assigned to CF also received a placebo PM, and patients randomly assigned to PM also received a placebo CF. Drug allocation was determined by a computer-generated list of random numbers.' The clinical outcome variable was the presence or absence of persistent dysentery after three days, and acceptable stool quality[1] and no fever after five days. Confounding is not an issue in RCTs, since the randomisation process is supposed to produce two groups with identical characteristics.

(c) The researchers used a cohort design, following a group of 2185 pregnant women becoming pregnant and having a baby between August 1991 and May 1993. The women were divided into two groups, normotensive and hypertensive. The outcome variable was defined as a birthweight below the 10th decile of expected weight (values from reference tables). Potential confounders were parity, age, socio-economic status, ethnicity, weight and height, smoking status, and use of aspirin.

(d) The researchers used a case-control study, in which cases were women with Down syndrome children, and controls were women selected randomly, having children with no congenital

---

[1] Satisfying a number of criteria.

abnormalities. Controls were matched only on birth year. There were 10 controls for each case! Potential confounding factors were: maternal and paternal ages, marital status (married/unmarried), parity, alcohol consumption (yes/no), prior foetal loss, and race (white/non-white).

(e) The researchers describe their study design as a 'follow-up' study. They selected two groups of patients (and their relatives), one receiving home-based care in one part of a city, the other hospital-based care, in a different part of the city. The relatives were interviewed at 10 days, one month and one year, and given questionnaires to assess the burden they were experiencing, their satisfaction with the service, and the General Health Questionnaire. The patients were assessed after four days, and then weekly and given a number of psychiatric questionnaires (Present State Examination, Morningside Rehabilitation Scale). The results from these various questionnaires constituted the outcome measures.

(f) The researchers used a randomised cross-over design. The subjects were randomised to either the 'regular' treatment arm (two puffs of salbutamol four times daily) or the 'as needed' treatment arm (salbutamol used as needed), each arm lasting two weeks. Patients were asked to record their peak expiratory flow rate (PEFR) morning and evening before inhaler use, the number of asthma episodes, and the number of as-needed salbutamol puffs used for symptom relief.

(g) The researchers summarise their design as follows, 'All new clients referred for counselling by GPs were asked to complete a questionnaire before and after counselling'. This contained: three psychological scales to measure anxiety and depression, self-esteem, and quality of life; and questions on levels of satisfaction with the counselling service. GPs were also asked to complete a questionnaire on their level of satisfaction with the service. The prescribing of anxiolytic/hypnotic and anti-depressant drugs, and the number of referrals to other mental health services in practices with and without counsellors was compared.

7.1 (a) A population parameter is a defining characteristic of a population, for example the mean age of all men dying of lung cancer in England and wales. The population parameter is unknown but can be estimated from a representative sample drawn from this population. (b) A sample will never have exactly the same characteristics as a population because there is always the possibility that those members of a population not included in the sample may in some way be different from those included. (c) Determining the parameters of a target population is the underlying objective, but in practice this may prove to be difficult if not impossible. The study population is the population that, in practice, can be sampled.

7.2   They may be more wealthy or poorer, or older, or ethnically more or less mixed, etc.

8.1   (a) (i) p(benign) $= 226/332 = 0.681$; (ii) p(malignant) $= 106/332 = 0.319$. Notice these two probabilities sum to 1. (b) p(postmenopausal) $= 200/332 = 0.602$; (c) p(>3 children) $= 112/332 = 0.337$.

8.2   (a) p(age <30) $= (0.355 + 0.206 + 0.043) = 0.604$. (b) p(age >29) $= (0.248 + 0.148) = 0.396$.

8.3   (a) 0.99. (b) 0.165

8.4   (a) Men.

Dead	Alcohol consumption (beverages/week)		Totals
	<1	>69	
Yes	195	66	261
No	430	145	575
Totals	625	211	836

(i) Absolute risk of death if consuming <1 beverage per week = 195/625 = 0.312. (ii) Absolute risk of death if consuming >69 beverages per week = 66/211 = 0.313.

(b) Women.

Dead	Alcohol consumption (beverages/week)		Totals
	<1	>69	
Yes	394	1	395
No	2078	19	2097
Totals	2472	20	2492

(i) Absolute risk of death if consuming <1 beverage per week = 394/2472 = 0.159. (ii) Absolute risk of death if consuming >69 beverages per week = 1/20 = 0.050.

Interpretation of results. For men there is approximately the same absolute risk of death among those consuming <1 beverage per week and those consuming >69 beverages per week (0.312 versus 0.313). For women the absolute risk of death if consuming <1 beverage per week is about three times the absolute risk for those consuming >69 beverages per week (0.159 versus 0.050). This perhaps surprising result may be due to the very small numbers consuming >69 beverages per week, which makes the result very unreliable.

8.5   (a) Under 35.

Smoked	Down syndrome baby	
	Yes	No
Yes	112	1411
No	421	5214
Totals	533	6625

(i) The odds that a woman having a Down syndrome baby smoked = 112/421 = 0.2660. (ii) The odds that a woman having a healthy baby smoked = 1411/5214 = 0.2706.

(b) ≥ 35

	Down syndrome baby	
Smoked	Yes	No
Yes	15	108
No	186	611
Totals	201	719

(i) The odds that a woman having a Down syndrome baby, smoked = 15/186 = 0.0806. (ii) The odds that a woman having a healthy baby, smoked = 108/611 = 0.1768.

Interpretation of results. Among the under 35 mothers there is little difference in the odds for Down syndrome between smoking and non-smoking mothers (0.2660 versus 0.2706). Among mothers ≥ 35, the odds for Down syndrome among smoking mothers is about a half the odds for non-smoking mothers (0.0806 versus 0.1768).

8.6 (a) p = 0.0806/(1 + 0.806) = 0.0746; (b) p = 0.1768/(1 + 0.1768) = 0.1502.

8.7 (a) Men: risk ratio of death among those drinking >69 beverages per week compared to those drinking <1 beverage per week = 0.313/0.312 = 1.003. (b) Women: risk ratio = 0.050/ 0.159 = 0.314.

Interpretation of results. For men a risk ratio very close to 1 implies that that there is no increased or decreased risk of death among those drinking <1 compared to those drinking >69 beverages per week. For women, the risk of death among the heavy drinkers appears to be only about a third the risk for light (or none) drinkers. But small numbers in the sample are not reliable.

8.8 (a) Mothers <35. Odds ratio for a woman with a Down syndrome baby having smoked, compared to a woman with a healthy baby = 0.2660/0.2706 = 0.9830. (b) Mothers ≥ 35. Odds ratio = 0.0806/0.1768 = 0.4558.

Interpretation of results. In younger mothers, the odds ratio close to 1 (0.9830) implies that smoking neither increases nor decreases the odds for Down syndrome. In older mothers, the odds ratio of 0.4558, implies that mothers who smoked during pregnancy have under half the odds of having a Down syndrome baby compared to non-smoking mothers.

8.9

	Periodontitis		
Death from CHD	Yes	No	Totals
Yes	151	92	243
No	1635	3450	5085
Totals	1786	3542	5328

Absolute risk of dying from CHD with periodontitis = 151/1786 = 0.084. Absolute risk of dying from CHD with no dental disease = 92/3542 = 0.026. So risk reduction = 0.084 − 0.026 = 0.058. Therefore NNT = 1/0.058 = 17.2, i.e. 18 people.

9.1   The smaller the s.e. of the sample mean, the more precise the estimate of the population mean. In this case the sample mean vitamin E intake of 6.30 mg (non-cases), has a s.e. of 0.05 mg, so we can be 95 per cent confident that the *population* mean vitamin E intake (non-cases) is no further than two s.e.s from this mean, i.e. within ± 0.10 mg. The largest s.e., 5.06 mg, and therefore the least precise estimate of the population mean, is that for vitamin C (cases).

9.2   (a) Cases. Sample mean age = 61.6 y, sample s.d. = 10.9 y, $n = 106$. Thus s.e.$(\bar{x}) =$ $10.9/\sqrt{106} = 1.059$. The 95 per cent confidence interval is therefore: ($61.6 \pm 2 \times 1.059$), or (59.582 to 63.718) years. (b) Controls. Sample mean age = 51.0 y, sample s.d. = 8.5 y, $n = 226$. Thus s.e.$(\bar{x}) = 8.5/\sqrt{226} = 0.565$. The 95 per cent confidence interval is therefore: ($51.0 \pm 2 \times$ 0.565), or (49.870 to 52.13) years. The fact that the two CIs don't overlap means that we can be 95 per cent confident that the two population mean ages are significantly different.

9.3   For the integrated care group, over 12 months the sample mean number of admissions is 0.15. The 95 per cent confidence interval means we can be 95 per cent confident that the interval from 0.11 to 0.19 will contain the population mean number of visits for the population of which this is a representative sample. For the conventional care group the sample mean number of visits is lower, 0.11, and the 95 per cent confidence interval means we can be 95 per cent confident that the interval from 0.08 to 0.15 will contain the population mean number of visits.

9.4 $p = 0.290$, s.e.$(p) = \sqrt{\dfrac{0.29(1 - 0.29)}{226}} = 0.030$. 95 % CI is:

$$(0.290 - 2 \times 0.030 \text{ to } 0.290 + 2 \times 0.030) = (0.230 \text{ to } 0.350)$$

So we can be 95 per cent confident that the interval from 0.230 to 0.350 (or 23.0 to 35.0 per cent), will contain the population proportion of women who are pre-menopausal.

9.5   For all three time periods the median differences in pain levels are reasonably similar (38, 31 and 35), as are the 95 per cent confidence intervals, which all overlap, indicating no statistically significant difference between the two groups at any time period.

10.1   Three of the confidence intervals include zero, so there is no statistically significant difference in population mean infant weights between non-smoking and smoking mothers. The confidence interval for the difference in the mean weight of non-smoking mothers and mothers smoking 1–9 cigarettes per day, (-118 to -10) g, for boys, does *not* include zero, so this difference in population mean weights is statistically significant.

10.2   That for the radius, which has the narrowest confidence interval.

10.3   Because overlapping confidence intervals imply that the difference is not statistically significant.

10.4   The difference in sample median alcohol intakes is 5.4 g. The 95 per cent confidence interval of (1.2 to 9.9) g, does not include zero, so we can be 95 per cent confident that the population difference in median alcohol intake is statistically significant and lies somewhere between 1.2 g and 9.9 g.

11.1   For *gingivitis*, the confidence intervals for both CHD and *mortality* contain 1, so difference in risk compared to no disease is not statistically significant. For *periodontitis* neither confidence interval includes 1, so the difference in risk is statistically significant. For *no teeth*, the confidence interval for CHD includes 1, so not statistically significant, but for *mortality*, the confidence interval does not include 1, so the difference in risk compared to no disease is statistically significant.

11.2 (a) Age and sex are notorious as confounders of many other variables, and adjustment for them is nearly always advisable. (b) With no exercise taken as the referent state, the odds ratio for all three age groups are less than 1, suggesting perhaps that exercise at any age reduces the odds for a stroke. However, only exercise taken between 15 and 40 has a statistically significant effect, since the confidence interval for the 40–55 year-old group, (0.3 to 1.5), includes 1. Note, by the way, that a 25-year-old and a 40-year-old individual could each be allocated to either one of two groups. The groups are not well defined.

11.3 The following risk factors are statistically significant for increasing the risk of thromboembolic events: being aged ≤ 19; having any parity other than 1; smoking ≥ 10 cigarettes per day; having multiple pregnancy; having pre-eclampsia; having a cesarean. The latter two appear to increase the risk the most.

12.1 (a) Is the proportion of women using the clinic same as proportion of men, i.e. 0.5? (b) $H_0: \pi = 0.5$ (π is population proportion of women using clinic). (c) Yes, reject because the p-value is less than 0.05. The proportion of women is *not* 0.5, i.e not the same as men. (d) No, don't reject because the p-value is *not* less than 0.05. The proportion of women using the clinic is the same as men.

12.2 Since both p-values (0.25 and 0.32) exceed 0.05, then there is no statistically significant difference in the two means.

12.3 Mean age, mean age at menopause, and mean body mass index are statistically significant, since their p-values are all less than 0.05. The other four variables show no statistically significant difference since their p-values are all greater than 0.05.

12.4 (a) A false positive is when the null hypothesis is rejected when it shouldn't have been, because it is true, i.e. an effect is detected when there isn't one. (b) A false negative is when the null hypothesis is not rejected when it should have been, because it is false, i.e. a real effect is not detected.

12.5 (a) We want to minimise the probability of a type I error, i.e. a false positive. For example, we might have a test, the results of which, if positive, will lead to an unnecessary intrusive intervention. (b) Because if α is made very small, β would be become unacceptably large because of the trade-off between the two measures.

12.6 (a) (i) $n = (2 \times 12^2/10^2) \times 10.5 = 31$; (ii) $n = (2 \times 12^2/10^2) \times 14.9 = 43$; (iii) $n = (2 \times 12^2/10^2) \times 11.7 = 34$. (b) (i) $n = [(0.4 \times 0.6 + 0.20 \times 0.80)/0.20^2] \times 10.5 = 105$; (ii) $n = [(0.4 \times 0.6 + 0.20 \times 0.80)/0.20^2] \times 14.9 = 149$; (iii) $n = [(0.4 \times 0.6 + 0.20 \times 0.80)/0.20^2] \times 11.7 = 117$.

12.7 $P_a = 0.70$. $P_b = 0.80$, so $(P_b - P_a) = -0.10$. Therefore, (a) $n = [(0.70 \times 0.30 + 0.80 \times 0.20)/ -0.10^2] \times 7.8 = 289$; (b) $n = [(0.70 \times 0.30 + 0.80 \times 0.20)/ -0.10^2] \times 14.9 = 551$.

13.1 There are only two statistically significant risk factors, both of which show higher risks for the alteplase patients (i.e. rr < 1); CAPG, rr $= 0.884$, p-value $= 0.049$, see table footnote for meaning of CAPG; and a Killip classification > 1; rr $= 0.991$, p-value $= 0.026$. Anaphylaxis is a complication which is almost statistically significant (rr $= 0.376$, p-value $= 0.052$, and we might want to consider it so.

13.2 In the model with the seven variables shown, all are statistically significant except passive smoking from husband, and at work. With only the first five variables included, plus passive smoking from husband and/or at work, makes this last variable statistically significant (p-value $= 0.049$).

14.1 Expected values:

		Apgar < 7		
		Yes	No	Totals
	Yes	3.667	6.333	10
Mother smoked	No	7.333	12.667	20
	Totals	11	19	30

14.2 The test statistic $= \{(8 - 3.667)^2/3.667 + (3 - 7.333)^2/7.333 + (2 - 6.333)^2/6.333 + (17 - 12.667)^2/12.667\} = 12.109$. Since we have a 2×2 table, then we are in the first row of Table 14.3, because $(2 - 1) \times (2 - 1) = 1 \times 1 = 1$, and the critical chi-squared value which must be exceeded to reject the null hypothesis is 3.85. The test statistic value of 12.109 exceeds this value, so the evidence is strong enough for us to reject the null hypothesis of equal proportions of smokers in both Agar groups. There does appear to be a relationship between smoking and Apgar scores.

14.3 (i) No trend across categories of social class, p-value $= 0.094$; (ii) statistically significant trend across the two categories (yes/no) of oral contraceptive use, p-value $= 0.000$; (iii) no trend across categories of alcohol consumption, p-value $= 0.927$; (iv) no trend across categories of cigarette consumption, p-value $= 0.383$.

15.1

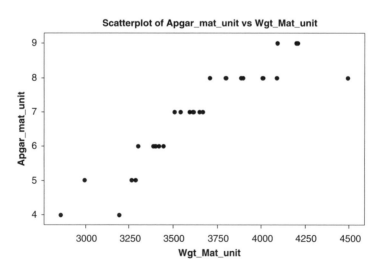

Association seems to be strong and positive.

15.2   The association seems to be strong and positive.

15.3   The association appears to be strong and positive, but does not appear to be linear.

15.4   (a) All are statistically significant. (b) 0.896 for mothers less than two years from birth date. (c) 0.632 for mothers where the baby concerned was $\geq$ 3rd born.

16.1   Yes. No.

16.2   Contingency table:

		Observer 1		
		<16	$\geq$16	Totals
Observer 2	<16	5	2	7
	$\geq$16	0	9	9
Totals		5	11	16

(a) Observed proportional agreement $= (5 + 9)/16 = 0.875$.

(b) Expected values are as follows:

		Observer 1	
		<16	$\geq$16
Observer 2	<16	2.19	4.81
	$\geq$16	2.81	6.19

Expected agreement $= (2.19 + 6.19)/16 = 0.523$. So kappa $= (0.875 - 0.523)/(1 - 0.523) = 0.738$. From Table 16.3, chance adjusted agreement is very good.

17.1   Scatterplot.

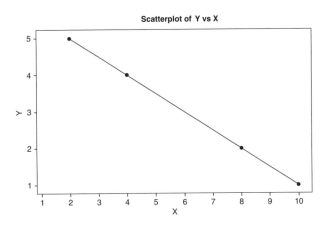

Scatterplot of Y vs X

Equation is: $Y = 6.0 - 0.5X$

17.2 (a) best straight line by eye:

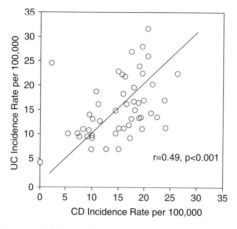

Equation is: $UC = 1 + 0.85 \times CD$. By $+0.85$.

(b) $\%M = 46.886 - 0.620E$. A decrease is % mortality of 0.620 %. (c) % exposed at work $= 12 + 0.92 \times$ % current smokers. 22 %.

17.3 mean BMI $= 41.902$ kg/m^2.

17.4 (a) All p-values < 0.05 so all statistically significant. (b) Will *decrease* bmi by 0.025 for each 1 year increase. (c) Adjusted R^2 was 0.635, now 0.638, so marginal improvement. (i) 18.42; (ii) 10.95.

17.5

Subject	Age	D_1	D_2
1	50	1	0
2	55	0	0
3	35	0	1

17.6 (a) Severity of disability; mental disorders; respiratory system disorders; numbers of residents in private residential homes (all p-values < 0.05). (b) (i) natural log of utilisation time increases by 0.006, or 1.006 minutes (taking antilog). (ii) increase of 0.043 in natural log, or 1.044 minutes. (c) About 11 per cent (see R^2 in table footnote).

17.7 (a) Age; age squared; family history of hypertension; calcium intake. (b) We can be 95 per cent confident that the population regression parameter on *age* is between 0.28 and 0.64. (c) The blood lead model (largest age coefficient value).

17.8 See text.

18.1 Using the formula, odds $=$ probability/(1 $-$ probability) from Chapter 8. When $P(Y = 1) = 0.4286$ when OCP $= 0$, then odds $= 0.7501$. When $P(Y = 1) = 0.2247$, when OCP $= 1$, odds $= 0.2898$. The odds ratio $= 0.2898/0.7501 = 0.386$.

18.2 (a) Because there are only two values for the dependent variable. It would be better to group the variables first and plot proportions in each group. (b) Yes, the confidence interval for odds ratio of (1.08 to 1.14) does not include 1. (c) $P(Y = 1) = e^{(-6.4672 + 0.10231 \times \text{age})}$.

(d)(i) 0.1343. (ii) 0.2707. (e) 0.8657, 0.7299. Odds ratio = 0.4182. A woman aged 45 has only about 41 per cent the odds of a malignant diagnosis as a woman aged 50. (f) The antilog$_e$ of 0.10231 equals 1.108 (rounded to 1.11 by Minitab). (g) 10 × 0.10231 = 1.0231. antilog$_e$ of 1.0231 = 2.78. In other words an increase in age of 10 years increases the odds ratio by 2.78.

18.3 BMI is statistically significant since the p-value is < 0.05 and confidence interval does not include 1.

18.4 OCP is not statistically significant; p-value 0.278 is > 0.05; and confidence interval includes 1. Age and BMI both statistically significant; p-values are < 0.05 and neither confidence interval includes 1.

18.5 The null hypothesis is that the goodness-of-fit is good. The p-value here is 0.958, which is not less than 0.05, so we cannot reject the null hypothesis and conclude that the fit is good.

19.1

1	2	3	4	5	6	7	8
Day	Number still in study at start of day t	Withdrawn prematurely up to day t	Deaths in day t	Number at risk in day t	Probability of death in day t	Probability of surviving day t	Cumulative probability of surviving to day t
t	n	w	d	r	d/r	$p = 1 - d/r$	S
3	8	0	1	8	1/8 = 0.125	0.875	0.875
8	7	0	1	6	1/6 = 0.167	0.833	0.758
13	6	1	1	4	1/4 = 0.25	0.75	0.569

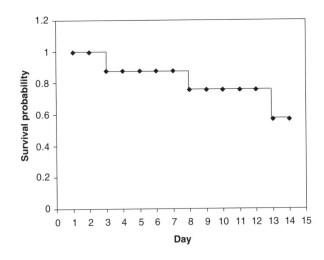

19.2 Raltitrexed; about 5 months. Lokich; about 5$^1\!/_2$ months. de Gramont; about 6 months.

19.3 Since the p-value is < 0.05, then a null hypothesis of no difference in survival times can be rejected.

19.4 The log-rank test *p*-value is 0.03. Since this is < 0.05 we can assume that there is a statistically significant difference between the treatments. The combination seems to work best since it shows the lowest percentage treatment failure.

19.5 All confidence intervals include the value 1 so none are statistically significant.

19.6 In the multivariate (adjusted) results, the first five are all statistically significant since none of the confidence intervals includes 1. This is the same as for the five univariate analyses. The last, cigarette smoking at enrolment, is not statistically significant since this confidence interval does include 1; which is also not statistically significant in the univariate analysis. None of the other variables are statistically significant in the univariate analyses.

20.1 See the text.

20.2 Risk ratio (relative risk) shown by ▲. Size of sample not indicated in this figure.

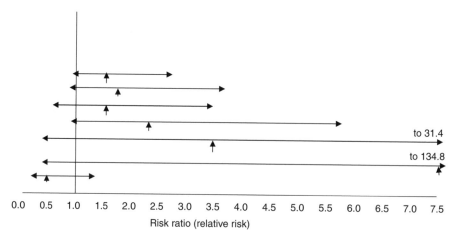

20.3 (a) See the list in the section headed 'Publication and other biases'. (b) On the question of publication bias and this funnel plot the authors comment, 'Visual assessment shows some asymmetry, which indicates that there was selective non-publication of smaller trials with less sizeable benefits. However, in formal statistical analysis the degree of asymmetry is found to be small and non-significant. Bias does not therefore seem to have distorted the findings from this meta-analysis.'

20.4 (a) If studies are not similar in objective, in outcome measure, in design, have similar subjects and so on then it is not sensible to combine them. (b) L'Abbé plots; Mantel-Haenszel test; chi-squared test. (c) A larger combined sample is likely to be more reliable (precise) than a number of smaller samples.

References

Altman, D.G. (1991) *Practical Statistics for Medical Research*. London: Chapman & Hall.

ASSENT-2 (Assessment of the Safety and Efficacy of a New Thrombolytic) Investigators. (1999) *Lancet*, **354**, 716–21.

Blanchard, J.F., Bernstein, C.N., Wajda, A. and Rawsthorne, P. (2001) Small-area variations and sociodemographic correlates for the incidence of Crohn's disease and ulcerative colitis. *Amer. J. Epid.*, **154**, 328–33.

Bland, J.M. and Altman, D.G. Statistical methods for assessing agreement between two clinical measurements. *Lancet*, **I**, 307–10.

Bland, M. (1995) *An Introduction to Medical Statistics*. Oxford: Oxford University Press.

Brueren, M.M., Schouten, H.J.A., de Leeuw, P.W., van Montfrans, G.A. and van Ree JW. (1998) A series of self-measurements by the patient is a reliable alternative to ambulatory blood pressure measurement. *Brit. J. General Practice*, **48**, 1585–9.

Chapman, K.R., Kesten, S. and Szalai, J.P. (1994) Regular vs as-needed inhaled salbutamol in asthma control. *Lancet*, **343**, 1379–83.

Cheng, Y., Schartz, J., Sparrow, D. *et al.* (2001) Bone lead and blood lead levels in relation to baseline blood pressure and the prospective development of hypertension. *Amer. J. Epid.*, **153**, 164–71.

Chi-Ling, C., Gilbert, T.J. and Daling, J.R. (1999) Maternal smoking and Down syndrome: thecon-founding effect of maternal age. *Amer. J. Epid.*, **149**, 442–6.

Chosidow, O., Chastang, C., Brue, C. *et al.* (1994) Controlled study of Malathion and *d*-phenothrin lotions for *Pediculus humanus* var *capitas*-infested schoolchildren. *Lancet*, **344**, 1724–6.

Conley, L.J., Ellerbrock, T.V., Bush, T.J. *et al.* (2002) HIV-1 infection and risk of vulvovaginal and perianal condylomata acuminate and intraepithelial neoplasia: a prospective cohort study. *Lancet*, **359**, 108–14.

Conter, V., Cortinovis, I., Rogari, P. and Riva, L. (1995) Weight growth in infants born to mothers who smoked during pregnancy. *BMJ*, **310**, 768–71.

DeStafano, F., Anda, R.F., Kahn, H.S., Williamson, D.F. and Russell, C.M. (1993) Dental disease and risk of coronary heart disease and mortality. *BMJ*, **306**, 688–91.

Dunne, M.W., Bozzette, S., McCutchan, J.A. *et al.* (1999) Kemper Class activity, Havlir D, for the California Collaborative Treatment Group. Efficacy of Azithromycin in prevention of Pneumocystis carinii pneumonia: a randomised trial. *Lancet*, **354**, 891–5

Egger, M. and Davey Smith, G. (1998) Bias in location and selection of studies. *BMJ*, **316**, 61–6.

Fahey, T., Stocks, N. and Thomas, T. (1998) Quantitative systematic review of randomised controlled trials comparing antibiotic with placebo for acute cough in adults. *BMJ*, **316**, 906–10.

Fall, C.H.D., Vijayakumar, M., Barker, D.J.P., Osmond, C. and Duggleby, S. (1995) Weight in infancy and prevalence of coronary heart disease in adult life. *BMJ*, **310**, 17–9.

Field, A. (2000) *Discovering Statistics Using SPSS for Windows*. London: Sage.

FRISC II (FRagmin and Fast Revascularisation during InStability in Coronary artery disease) Investigators. (1999) Long-term low-molecular-mass heparin in unstable coronary-artery disease: FRISC II prospective randomised multicentre study. *Lancet*, **354**, 701–7.

Goel, V., Iron, K. amd Williams, J.I. (1997) Enthusiasm or uncertainty: small area variations in the use of the mammography services in Ontario, Canada. *J. Epid. Comm. Health*, **51**, 378–82.

Goldhaber, S.Z., Visani, L. and De Rosa, M. (1999) Acute pulmonary embolism: clinical outcomes in the International Cooperative Pulmonary Embolism Registry (ICOPER). *Lancet*, 353, 1386–9.

Grampian Asthma Study of Integrated Care. (1994) Integrated care for asthma: a clinical, social, and economic evaluation. *BMJ*, **308**, 559–64.

Grandjean, P., Bjerve, K.S., Weihe, P. and Steuerwald, U. (2000) Birthweight in a fishing community: significance of essential fatty acids and marine food contaminants. *Int. J. Epid.*, **30**, 1272–7.

Griffin, S. (1998) Diabetes care in general practice: a meta-analysis of randomised control trials. *BMJ*, **317**, 390–6.

Gronbaek, M., Deis, A., Sorensen, T.I.A. *et al.* (1994) Influence of sex, age, body mass index, and smoking on alcohol intake and mortality. *BMJ*, **308**, 302–6.

Grun, L., Tassano-Smith, J., Carder, C. *et al.* (1997) Comparison of two methods of screening for genital chlamydia infection in women attending in general practice: cross sectional survey. BMJ, **315**, 226–30.

He, Y., Lam, T.H., Li, L.S. *et al.* (1994) Passive smoking at work as a risk factor for coronary heart disease in Chinese women who have never smoked. *BMJ*, **308**, 380–4.

Hearn, J. and Higinson, I.J., on behalf of the Palliative Care Core Audit Project Advisory Group. (1998) Development and validation of a core outcome measure for palliative care: the palliative care outcome scale. *Quality in Health Care*, **8**, 219–27.

Hosmer, D.W. and Lemeshow, S. (1989) *Applied Logistic Regression Analysis*. Chichester: John Wiley & Sons, Ltd.

Hu, F.B., Wand, B., Chen, C., Jin, Y., Yang, J., Stampfer, M.J. and Xu X. (2000) Body mass index and cardiovascular risk factors in a rural Chinese population. *Amer. J. Epid.*, **151**, 88–97.

Imperial Cancer Fund OXCHECK Study Group. (1995) Effectiveness of health checks conducted by nurses in primary care: final results of the OXCHECK study. *BMJ*, **310**, 1099–104.

Inzitari, D., Eliasziw, M., Gates, P. *et al.* (2000) The causes and risk of stroke in patients with asymptotic internal-carotid-artery stenosis. *NEJM*, **342**, 1693–9.

Janson, C., Chinn, S., Jarvis, D *et al.*, for the European Community Respiratory Health Survey. (2001) Effect of passive smoking on respiratory symptoms, bronchial responsiveness, lung function, and total serum IgE in the European Community Respiratory Health Survey: a cross-sectional study. *Lancet*, **358**, 2103–9.

Kavanagh, S. and Knapp, M. (1998) The impact on general practitioners of the changing balance of care for elderly people living in an institution. *BMJ*, **317**, 322–7.

Knaus, W.A., Draper, E.A., Wagner, D.P. and Zimmerman, J.E. (1985) APACHE II: A severity of disease classification system. *Critical Care Medicine*, **13**, 818–29.

Lacy, A.M., Garcia-Valdecasas, J.C., Delgado, S. *et al.* (2002) Laparoscipy-assited colectomy versus open colectomy for treatment of non-metastatic colon cancer: a randomised trial. *Lancet*, **359**, 2224–30.

Ladwig, K.H., Roll, G., Breithardt, G., Budde, T., Borggrefe, M. (1994) Post-infarction depression and incomplete recovery 6 months after acute myocardial infarction. *Lancet*, **343**, 20–3.

Leeson, C.P.M., Kattenhorn. J.E. and Lucas, A. (2001) Duration of breast feeding and arterial disability in early adult life: a population based study. *BMJ*, **322**, 643–7.

Lindberg, G., Bingefors, K., Ranstam,J. and Rastam, A.M. (1998) Use of calcium channel blockers and risk of suicide: ecological findings confirmed in population based cohort study. *BMJ*, **316**, 741–5.

Lindelow, M., Hardy, R. and Rodgers, B. (1997) Development of a scale to measure symptoms of anxiety and depression in the general UK population: the psychiatric symptom frequency scale. *J. Epid. Comm. Health*, **51**, 549–57.

Lindqvist, P., Dahlback, M.D. and Marsal, K. (1999) Thrombotic risk during pregnancy: a population study. *Obstetrics and Gynecology*, **94**, 595–9.

Luke, A., Durazo-Arvizu, R., Rotimi, C. *et al.* (1997) Relations between body mass index and body fat in black population samples from Nigeria, Jamaica, and the United States. *Amer. J. Epid.*, **145**, 620–8.

Machin, D., Campbell, M.J., Fayers, P.M. and Pinol, A.P.Y. (1987) *Sample Size Tables for Clinical Studies*. Oxford: Blackwell Scientific.

Maughan, T.S., James, R.D., Kerr, D.J. *et al.*, for the British MRC Colorectal Cancer Working Party. (2002) *Lancet*, **359**, 1555–63.

McCreadie, R., Macdonald, E., Blacklock, C. *et al.* (1998) Dietary intake of schizophrenic patients in Nithsdale, Scotland: case-control study. *BMJ*, **317**, 784–5.

McKee, M. and Hunter, D. (1995) Mortality league tables: do they inform or mislead? *Quality in Health Care*, **4**, 5–12.

Medical Research Council Advanced Bladder Working Party. (1999) Neoadjuvant cisplatin, methotrexate, and vinblastine chemotherapy formuscle-invasive bladder cancer: a randomised controlled trial. *Lancet*, **354**, 533–9.

Michelson, D., Stratakis, C., Hill, L. *et al.* (1995) Bone mineral density in women with depression. *NEJM*, **335**, 1176–81.

Moore, R.A., Tramer, M.R., Carroll, D., Wiffen, P.J. and McQuay, H.J. (1998) Quantitative systematic review of topically applied non-steroidal anti-inflamatory drugs. *BMJ*, **316**, 333–8.

Morris, C.R., Kato, G.J., Poljakovic, M. *et al.* (2005) Dysregulated arginine metabolism, hemolysis-associated pulmonary hypertension, and mortality in sickle cell disease. *JAMA*, **294**, 81–91.

Nikolajsen, L., Ilkjaer, S., Christensen, J.H., Kroner, K. and Jensen, T.S. (1997) Randomised trial of epidural bupivacaine and morphine in prevention of stump and phantom pain in lower-limb amputation. *Lancet*, **350**, 1353–7.

Nordentoft, M., Breum, L., Munck, L.K., Nordestgaard, A.H. and Bjaeldager, P.A.L. (1993) High mortality by natural and unnatural causes: a 10 year follow up study of patients admitted to a poisoning treatment centre after suicide attempts. *BMJ*, **306**, 1637–41.

Olson, J.E., Shu, X.O., Ross, J.A., Pendergrass, T. and Robison, L.L. (1997) Medical record validation of maternity reported birth characteristics and pregnancy-related events: A report from the Children's Cancer Group. *Amer. J. Epid.*, **145**, 58–67.

Prevots, D.R., Watson, J.C., Redd, S.C. and Atkinson, W.A. (1997) Outbreak in highly vaccinated populations: implications for studies of vaccine performance. *Amer. J. Epid.*, **146**, 881–2.

Protheroe, D., Turvey, K., Horgan, K. *et al.* (1999) Stressful life events and difficulties and onset of breast cancer: case-control study. *BMJ*, **319**, 1027–30.

Rainer, T.H., Jacobs, P., Ng, Y.C. *et al.* (2000) Cost effectiveness analysis of intravenous ketorolac and morphine for treating pain after limb injury: double blind randomised controlled trail. *BMJ*, **321**, 1247–51.

Relling, M.V., Rubnitz, J.E., Rivera, G.K. *et al.* (1999) High incidence of secondary brain tumours after radiotherapy and antimetabolites. *Lancet*, **354**, 34–9.

Rodgers, M. and Miller, J.E. (1997) Adequacy of hormone replacement therapy for osteoporosis prevention assessed by serum oestradiol measurement, and the degree of association with menopausal symptoms. *Brit. J. General Practice*, **47**, 161–5.

Rogers, A. and Pilgrim, D. (1991) Service users views of psychiatric nurses. *Brit J Nursing*, **3**, 16–7.

Rowan, K.M., Kerr, J.H., Major, E. *et al.* (1993) Intensive Care Society's APACHE II study in Britain and Ireland – I: Variations in case mix of adult admissions to general intensive care units and impact on outcome. *BMJ*, **307**, 972–81.

Sainio, S., Jarvenpaa, A.-L. and Kekomaki, R. (2000) Thrombocytopenia in termi nfants: a population-based study. *Obstetrics and Gynecology*, **95**, 441–4.

Schrader, H., Stovner, L.J., Helde, G., Sand, T. and Bovin, G. (2001) Prophylactic treatment of migraine with angiotensin converting enzyme inhibitor (lisinopril): randomised, placebo-controlled, cross-over study. *BMJ*, **322**, 19–22.

Shinton, R. and Sagar, G. Lifelong exercise and stroke. *BMJ*, **307**, 231–4.

Staessen, J.A., Byttebier, G., Buntinx, F. *et al.* (1997) Antihypertensive treatment based on conventional or ambulatory blood pressure measurement. *JAMA*, **278**, 1065–72.

Tang, J.L., Armitage, J.M., Lancaster, T. *et al.* (1998) Systematic review of dietary intervention trials to lower blood total cholesterol in free-living subjects. *BMJ*, **316**, 1213–20.

Thomson, A.B., Campbell, A.J., Irvine, D.S. *et al.* (2002) Semen quality and spermatozoal DNA integrity in survivors of childhood cancer: a case-control study. *Lancet*, **360**, 361–6.

Turnbull, D., Holmes, A., Shields, N., *et al.* (1996) Randomised, controlled trial of efficacy of midwife-managed care. *Lancet*, **348**, 213–219.

van Es, R., Jonker, J.J., Verheught, F.W.A., Deckers, J.W. and Grobbee, D.E., for the Antithrombotics in the Secondary Prevention of Events in Coronary Thrombosis-2 (ASPECT-2) Research Group. (2002) Aspirin and coumadin after acute coronary syndromes (the ASPECT-2 study): a randomised controlled trial. *Lancet*, **360**, 109–14.

Wannamethee, S.G., Lever, A.F., Shaper, A.G. and Whincup, P.H. (1997) Serum potassium, cigarette smoking, and mortality in middle-aged men. *Amer. J. Epid.*, **145**, 598–607.

Yong, L.-C., Brown, C.C., Schatzkin, A. *et al.* (1997) Intake of vitamins E, C, and A and risk of lung cancer. *Amer. J. Epid.*, **146**, 231–43.

Zoltie, N. and de Dombal, F.T., on behalf of the Yorkshire Trauma Audit Group. (1993) The hit and miss of ISS and TRISS. *BMJ*, **307**, 906–9.

Index

Medical Statistics from Scratch Second Edition   David Bowers
© 2008 John Wiley & Sons, Ltd

WORKING THE CROWD
Social Media Marketing for Business

Eileen remains on the cutting edge of social media strategy that when implemented returns a measurable return on interest. I would highly recommend her book to any business who wants to deepen their customer interactions through powerful word of mouth marketing strategies.

Kim Matlock
Senior Director, Digital & Consumer Related Marketing, Hard Rock International

Brown's varied experience and analysis of the needs of both small and large businesses for social media makes her advice stand out from the crowded field – and told in the lively voice those hearing her via social media channels have come to know and love.

Betsy Aoki
Senior Program Manager, Social Media, Microsoft

Eileen Brown blends extensive real world business experience with in-depth social media knowledge to create a unique and valuable guide.

Professor Sue Thomas
Institute of Creative Technologies, De Montfort University

It's a good book. If you don't have a social media strategy yet, then reading this one will take you a long way forward. I recommend it to any business wondering about 'the twitter'.

Kate Gregory's Blog

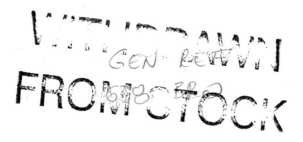

BCS, The Chartered Institute for IT

Our mission as BCS, The Chartered Institute for IT, is to enable the information society. We promote wider social and economic progress through the advancement of information technology science and practice. We bring together industry, academics, practitioners and government to share knowledge, promote new thinking, inform the design of new curricula, shape public policy and inform the public.

Our vision is to be a world-class organisation for IT. Our 70,000 strong membership includes practitioners, businesses, academics and students in the UK and internationally. We deliver a range of professional development tools for practitioners and employees. A leading IT qualification body, we offer a range of widely recognised qualifications.

Further Information

BCS The Chartered Institute for IT, First Floor, Block D, North Star House, North Star Avenue, Swindon, SN2 1FA, United Kingdom.
T +44 (0) 1793 417 424
F +44 (0) 1793 417 444
www.bcs.org/contactus

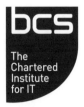

WORKING THE CROWD
Social Media Marketing for Business

Eileen Brown

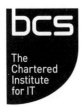

Published by British Informatics Society Limited (BISL), a wholly owned subsidiary of BCS, The Chartered Institute for IT, First Floor, Block D, North Star House, North Star Avenue, Swindon, SN2 1FA, United Kingdom.
www.bcs.org

ISBN 978-906124-71-7

British Cataloguing in Publication Data.
A CIP catalogue record for this book is available at the British Library.

Disclaimer:
The views expressed in this book are of the author(s) and do not necessarily reflect the views of BISL or BCS except where explicitly stated as such. Although every care has been taken by the authors and BISL in the preparation of the publication, no warranty is given by the authors or BISL as publisher as to the accuracy or completeness of the information contained within it and neither the authors nor BISL shall be responsible or liable for any loss or damage whatsoever arising by virtue of such information or any instructions or advice contained within this publication or by any of the aforementioned.

Typeset by Lapiz Digital Services, Chennai, India.
Printed at CPI Antony Rowe, Chippenham, UK.

This book is for my husband Steve, who keeps hold of the loop of my yo-yo string

CONTENTS

LIST OF FIGURES

AUTHOR

Eileen Brown is CEO of Amastra: a company which helps you achieve your aspirations using offline and online social methods. She has been in a variety of roles in the IT industry since 1993. After spending 10 years in the Merchant Navy as Shell Tankers' first female Deck Officer, Eileen managed a fleet of ships in a container shipping company, before moving to IT support, then training and management at a training provider in London, technical consultancy at HP and Manager of the IT Pro Evangelist team at Microsoft.

Eileen helps you achieve your goals using social media and Web 2.0 to find and engage with customers, identify your influencers and gain advocates for your brand. She works with you to improve perception about your brand and create a vibrant community, using Social Media to amplify your message and improve the quality of your connection to your customers to increase satisfaction.

She is an accomplished and well-known international speaker and expert on Social Media, Online Branding, Web 2.0 and Unified Communications and is a key advocate for the advancement of Women in Technology. She explores the art of the possible, looking at how technology is changing the world we live in, simplifying work and making staff more productive.

Eileen is a member of the IoD, the BCS, and a fellow of the RSA. She is part of the BCS Strategic panel for Women in IT, sits on the BCS Committee for the Essex region and is the Chair of the Intellect Women in Technology Committee. However, her life isn't spent entirely at her laptop. Away from work, she makes jam and chutney in awesome quantities, tends her flock of chickens, grows organic vegetables and fruit and races around the countryside in her home-built 6.6 litre cobra replica car. Whenever she encounters warmer waters, she scuba dives as much as possible to get away from the phone...

ACKNOWLEDGEMENTS

I'd like to thank all of the people who gave me feedback during the writing of the book and kept me on track as I started to wander. Kay Ewbank read through the chapters and told me how much I preferred commas to full stops in my sentences. Shorter sentences. Shorter sentences. Kate Burton talked to me about book structure and flow, and Mary Branscombe talked to me about vision. Matthew Flynn was very encouraging and patient throughout the process, answering my daft questions and explaining how the publishing process actually works. He also caught my fondness for the grocer's apostrophe at an early stage. Ian Murphy spent ages explaining how books are published and how to get over writer's block when it hits really hard. Betsy Aoki gave me some great tips about making the book more human so that it didn't read entirely like a textbook. Thanks, Betsy, for believing in me.

And Steve supplied me with food, wine and words of encouragement when I started to flag, and managed the running of my home life whilst I researched and wrote. Thank you all.

GLOSSARY

If you've never heard of social media, social networking or social marketing, here are a few of the main terms and phrases that I use throughout the book. I'll explain more of the terms as we move through the chapters, so this isn't an exhaustive list at all.

Aggregation   Software or a website that collects information from several sources for use in one place.

Application programming interface   Enables a software application to interact with other software programs.

Blog   An online chronological diary of entries written by a user or group of users and searchable online.

Folksonomy   The users of a site classify web page information in ways that are useful to them and do not necessarily use the formal taxonomy assigned by the web page designer.

Generation Y   People born between 1980 and 2000.

Hub   The centre of activity of a social group. This can be applied to personal relationships, or to a computer network device which connects multiple devices together to act as a single segment of the network.

Influencer   Anyone who has the ability to change people's perception about a concept, idea or product leading to a change in online behaviour and buying decisions.

Location aware applications   Applications on a mobile device that use the coordinates provided by the mobile network to locate the position of the device.

Mashup   An application on the web containing data from one or more sources which creates a new web service.

Microblogging   Creating a shortened form of a blog entry.

Online brand Your online presence and information on the web.

Social distance A person who is connected to you not directly, but indirectly through another person, has a greater social distance from you than someone who is directly connected to you.

Social engagement Effectively connecting with people in an online two-way dialogue.

Social graph A way of creating a map or a graph showing all of your online connections, their relationship to you and to each other. This will show people who are loosely connected to you via another person and thus have a greater social distance from you.

Social media A collection of web pages and applications that are designed to allow users to interact with their friends.

Social networking Interacting with your friends and your friends of friends online.

Social tools Any website that allows interaction and conversation between its users. Another name for social media.

Strong tie A close interpersonal relationship with an online connection.

Syndication Website material that is made available to multiple other sites.

Viral effect Spreading a marketing message across multiple types media using the network of friends and friends of friends.

Virtual worlds A computer based simulation of a world or environment where users can interact with each other online to play games and inhabit the environment.

Walled garden A site which is for its members alone and that doesn't permit interactivity with users from another site.

Weak tie An occasional connection to someone with whom you wouldn't claim to have more than a casual relationship.

Web 2.0 Web applications and websites that are built to allow interaction, information sharing and uploading of user generated content.

Wiki An editable web page that can have multiple authors.

1 WHY DO WE WANT A SOCIAL MEDIA STRATEGY?

Implementing a social media strategy in your organisation will dramatically change the way you do business.

If you want to connect with your customers and discover what they think about your brand, social media will help. If you want to change perceptions about your company, or improve your customer service, social media will help. If you want to find out who the influencers and advocates are and get them to broadcast your message on your behalf, then social media will identify the key people in your network whom you should engage with. For you as an individual, if you want to be strategic in your networking goals and you intend to extend your connections by meeting more people, social media will help you reach more people than you ever thought was possible.

With social media in your business, you have a great opportunity to learn more from those around you and discover new information from your extended network. In the right social networks you could discover what you're missing out on in your career, and could create an opening to broaden your perspectives and job prospects. This massive extended virtual network gives you the chance to progress in your professional life using a wider set of connections. You can find a business mentor, advertise your presence or build the relationship to close that deal.

Using social software inside an organisation will also help you achieve an increase in productivity and a reduction in your long term costs.

Companies have spent large sums of money on collaboration software, and yet they don't utilise their investment effectively. There are still multiple islands of data stored in huge storage area networks, which are effectively dead data. Without an effective search mechanism inside a company, without updates, audit notifications and user interaction, this data ages, becomes obsolete and dies. With software providing effective collaboration and interaction securely inside companies, this data has the potential to remain dynamic, engaging and an asset to the company. This social computing environment can then benefit teams, organisations and positively impact the company's customers.

So what does the phenomenal growth in social media interaction mean for your business? With iPod application downloads hitting an astonishing 1 billion in 9 months, what does that mean for Apple's business? What could this mean for your future revenue stream? What potential can you tap into by using this new way of communicating to your advantage?

There have been many articles and discussions about social media and social networking and the potential opportunities they can bring to companies. There are myriad benefits for corporations that choose to leverage this form of communication and use the **conversation** as a digital marketing tool to help them with community engagement or to present the opportunity to increase revenue and market share.

> One of the cardinal rules of social networking is that it's all about giving rather than receiving.

You contribute to the greater sum of knowledge by adding your perspective, know-how, advice, anecdotal stories or links to other sources of knowledge. And there are myriad ways that you can share this information. There are so many tools with odd names that define the term 'social media'. Among them are blogs, moblogging, wikis, tagging, bookmarking, massively multiplayer online role-playing games (MMORPGs), tweets, podcasts, screencasting, vlogs, video, videoblogging, phlogs, video uploads, video sharing, status updates and virtual worlds (I'll explain all of these terms later). Where on earth do you start? Which mechanism is right for your corporate social strategy and which do you need to avoid? What is the process to use for a successful strategy? Where is your plan?

There are several steps to think of in order to achieve success with social networking both inside and outside the organisation.

> These steps are not meant to be used in isolation if a successful strategy is to be followed.

Digital engagement allows us to solve a specific business problem, to connect more effectively with our customers, to listen to their challenges, to help them and to gain advocates who are brand evangelists. Knowing what challenges you want to overcome helps you to set the first part of your strategy in motion, and having a clear plan in place for your business helps you on the first few steps on your journey.

SOCIALLY CONNECTED

I discovered IT quite late in life compared to most of my peers. I'd never considered computing as a career when I was at school, I had gained limited experience with very basic computer programming on a computer science O-level class. I learned binary and I tried to get my head around very basic computing concepts.

I remember the delight I felt on writing my first FOR NEXT loop that actually worked when the program was initiated. I was obviously more of a technician than a scholar. I didn't want to learn about Babbage's engine, I was much keener to learn how the mechanical parts of the computer read the punch tape and converted the tape into characters. I also had other plans for my career. I left school after taking my O levels as I had decided to pursue something completely different and was determined to follow my goal.

I joined the Merchant Navy as a deck cadet on a four-year apprenticeship with Shell Tankers and completely forgot all about computers. Instead I immersed myself in learning how to navigate an oil tanker, load and discharge cargo and maintain the ship's physical condition with gallons of gloss paint and a chipping hammer. In the late 1970s satellite navigation systems were rare, and even if they were installed on board, they were only accurate to about 1 mile. Instead we relied on using logarithmic tables, sextants and the haversine formula to complete our navigation calculations and mark the ship's position by the stars and the sun. I passed my exams, becoming the first female deck officer to sail with Shell Tankers, and I had fulfilled my childhood dream.

I left the sea and joined a container shipping company, working in their office as a containership planner. If the vessel was late in port, due to bad weather or cargo loading delays, then it naturally followed that she would arrive later in every other port on her journey. Cargo space on the vessel was sold by the shipping agents up to 3 months in advance; containers were loaded and delivered to a specific schedule to meet the vessel. It was vital that the shipping agents were well aware of any delays to the vessel's arrival time.

There was a personal computer (PC) on every floor of the shipping company, running Windows 3.11, WordStar and Lotus 123 version 2. It tended to be used to print memos created in the DOS version of WordStar which were occasionally faxed to the ship captains. One day I had an epiphany. I worked out that I could transfer my paper based ships schedule to the spreadsheet in Lotus 123, I could update an entry in one cell of the spreadsheet. Each port in the route could be updated with the new date of either arrival or departure. The spreadsheet would automatically adjust the rest of the schedule for the next 3 months whilst still maintaining the actual historical record of arrival and departure dates. It seems so obvious now, but back then, amongst the team of container planners who had been working using manual methods for years, it was a total revelation.

> This simple spreadsheet simplified working across the whole team and made us much more productive.

My love affair with technology and social collaboration began. I realised that I was really good at teaching users about technical – and not so technical – concepts. I loved finding out and explaining how things worked.

I accepted a job as a technical trainer at a Microsoft training provider in London and I suddenly realised that I'd found my niche in technology. I became

a Microsoft Certified Professional (MCP) on NT 3.51. I became a Microsoft Certified Trainer (MCT). I then became a Microsoft Certified Systems Engineer (MCSE) with the Internet certification to the acronym (MCSE+I) shortly afterwards.

I then decided to move on to another challenge. I joined Hewlett-Packard as a presales consultant before joining Microsoft as a technical specialist in the Enterprise team.

My skills gained with AS400 systems in the shipping company proved valuable to the presales specialist team. I spent a couple of years talking to enterprise customers about Windows Server before moving to the Evangelism team to talk about technology to the IT Pro audience. The IT Pro team consisted of four evangelists, an architect and a manager – a very small team who had to reach an audience of around 1 million IT professionals in the UK. Our main metrics were to improve audience satisfaction and reach. But apart from the *TechNet* newsletter and the Microsoft website, how would we connect with people we didn't already know?

We started to use social media, specifically blogging, to reach out and talk about what was happening with technology. Back in 2004, YouTube hadn't yet been purchased by Google so we hosted our own 'blogcasts' – short how-to videos and demos of technology with our voiceover, hosted on a server and linked to from our blogs. We used the technical community to record other blogcasts for us and propagate information on their community sites.

> This free sharing of information was mutually beneficial to both the team and the technical community. The resulting videos also benefited users who wanted to learn more about technology.

The community could raise their online profile and demonstrate their technical know-how to their followers, and the team weren't so stretched in resources to produce these videos. I'd discovered the value of using the extended network to benefit both parties.

I became manager of the team in 2005, working on new ways to connect with different audiences in a global market using different types of social media mechanisms and tools. I stayed at Microsoft until 2009 when I left to start out on my own. I could then really focus on the things that connect people.

ONLINE AND FACE TO FACE NETWORKING

I'd been fascinated with social media for a while, but when someone asked me whether social networking was any different from networking physically with people, I realised that there are a lot of similarities in the way I behave online and offline. A lot of the face to face meetings I've had are with people I originally started to connect with online. I've met my virtual connections at a 'tweetup'

(a Twitter meetup) or at an online business networking event, and sometimes I've moved forward to meet them in person. Some of these connections will turn into valuable business relationships, others will be tenuous connections or ties to other people. These casual connections communicate infrequently with me online. When I'm at a face to face networking or business event, I collect business cards, some from people who turn out to be valuable connections and some from people I will never hear from again. However, I've been amazed by some fantastic and inspirational people at physical events, and with a little effort to make contact and really connect this has turned up some valuable business and personal contacts for me both online and offline. I've made some great online connections after physical networking events and I stay in touch with these people much more often than I would have done after a traditional business card exchange.

Face to face networking, according to the Harvard Business school, 'is about building a portfolio of relationships that will help you to continue to develop your career'. These relationships will thrive if you know what is going on around you. The same applies to online networking too.

> If you want to progress in business, don't wait to be discovered. Make sure you have a great online profile and a positive brand.

Keeping close tabs on what is going on, being an active contributor, with valid opinions, information and advice, will raise your profile and help you progress in your career.

I network in lots of different ways – face to face, on the phone, via email, text, online and by using social media. This form of online networking keeps me in touch with so many more people than just email or phone does. I get a huge buzz from connecting people who can help each other out. It gives me a great satisfaction to actually make that connection. So it's not all about my work.

Your world of friends and family, colleagues and business connections is defined by the people you are connected to. Some of your friends know each other; some of your friends are isolated in your social circle. Some of your connections will be farther out in distance from your close family. Some will be people in your address book whom you hardly ever see, others will be connected to you in some way on a daily basis. You can map your connections in the form of a graph. This is your 'social graph', with your more distant connections mapping to the outskirts of the graph. This 'social distance' defines the limits of your graph. But it can provide the gateway to join you to other graphs.

There are tools that leverage the connections in your own social graph and online sites that make it really easy to connect with your friends and the friends of your friends. These online tools make it simple to meet and connect with people in similar situations who can then make more people aware of you and your capabilities. You can make connections across the board with senior colleagues, competitors, and local business people – even with politicians perhaps? It is possible. You want

to meet people who can help you – but where can you find them? There are online connections with your colleagues and IT peers, your friends and family and your friends' friends. There are professional associations and networks, vendors and consultants who could be connected to you. It really does seem like social networking has become an amazing business enabler.

I've been immersed in collaborative technology for over 15 years and it has changed my perspective about the world around me. I've used social networking tools from time to time since I started in IT, and it was only when I started thinking about which social media mechanisms I use inside and outside my workplace, especially when I travel, that I realised just how much it was a key part of my life.

I've been a lurker, a listener, a broadcaster, a conversationalist and an influencer. I've asked for help in forums, talked to strangers using chat software and created videos to help people out. I've shared interesting and not so interesting facts, initially by email to my friends, latterly through my blog, and now on Twitter, Facebook, LinkedIn, YouTube and SlideShare. I've used several different types of tools to syndicate my news and information across other sites so that contacts in different realms can keep in touch. I have a fairly consistent online brand, and searches for eileenb, my online brand profile name, get the searcher to all of the sites I intend it to. But it's my own social behaviour that makes me curious.

Why do I continue this level of interaction with my virtual friends and connections, lots of whom I've never met? What drives this altruistic behaviour, this desire of mine to help others? Is this a desire to connect or communicate, inform or engage? Do I want to convert others to my way of thinking by regularly interacting with my circle of friends, colleagues and connections? Or do I want to try and persuade my friends in my immediate network to tell their friends who are outside my directly connected network about the latest and greatest in technology? What drives my behaviour?

To find out why I do this, I began to take a closer look at the mechanisms behind it. I wanted to find out why it has become such a key part of the digital marketing, community and advertising strategy. I wanted to understand why this mechanism effectively connects you with your customers, amplifies your message and engages your audience. I wanted to know how this network – the 'word of mouth network', or the '**world** of mouth network' – has become such a powerful tool to use in business in the 21st century.

2 THE NEW WAY OF COMMUNICATING

Social media is not something that will burst like the South Sea bubble or the dotcom bubble. This is not something that will pass you or your company by. Social computing has far reaching effects that will permeate every business, reaching all job roles. It is worldwide and pervasive. So what are you doing about it?

Everyone seems to be talking about push–pull marketing, with tools and sites offering get-rich-quick schemes and easy ways to increase your followers. Why has there been so much exposure for this new way of communication? To consider this, we need to look at the key drivers for us to connect with others online.

We need to connect – with another entity across the town, the country, the world. Our need to interact virtually with each other has driven a massive explosion of Web 2.0 applications, designed to help you connect, communicate, snoop and stalk. But it is becoming harder to function effectively in today's technology-obsessed world without effort or seeming to become an Internet geek. The Web 2.0 world can be looked at from many different angles. You can watch the effect that Web 2.0 has had on ordinary consumers and the way they now interact with the web.

Watching how social networks grow across different environments has resulted in a fundamental change in society, technology and business practices.

We begin by looking at how people interact in social groups, both face to face and online, looking at how Generation Y behave on social networking sites and how their behaviour differs from that of the baby boomers. We look at how the conversation between consumers and companies has changed over time into a two-way dialogue and how some companies have benefited from this effect. We then look back to when online social conversation began and how the early bulletin boards, chat rooms and multi-user dungeons have evolved into forums, instant messaging and MMORPGs. We also look at the evolution of the Internet for consumers, the rise of Internet service providers and proprietary forum software such as CompuServe and AOL. We see how walled gardens prevented cross-network interaction and how browsers worked to get around this issue. We then look at how the concept of Web 2.0 changed the way that users interacted with websites and companies, and how social networks grew to take advantage of

this interaction. Finally, we discuss the influencers inside the organisation and explain how these influencers connect, network and propagate information across business groups. We see how adding extra information to the conversation encourages dialogue to flow more readily and effectively builds your network.

IS THIS THE NEW FAD FOR THE 21ST CENTURY?

People like to live in groups – family groups, work groups, hobby groups, sport groups. Since the dawn of time we have connected with each other to grow food, eat, form families, procreate, declare our religious allegiance and fight wars. So, with the advent of PCs and the Internet, what has changed? Nothing, as it turns out. We connect to others to form groups. But nowadays there are digital groups as well as groups for our usual day to day human to human interaction.

> People on the Internet tend to interact with each other in social, trusting and communal ways, and this is what makes the explosion of digital interactivity and interconnectedness so powerful.

From the early days of online activity, before CompuServe, people have interacted with each other electronically. I remember how CompuServe issued a series of numbers to represent user names, and I struggled to connect my 300 baud modem to the Internet by dialling the CompuServe access number on my phone and placing the handset into the soft rubber cradle on the modem hardware device. In the early 1990s, the advent of forums, newsgroups and Internet Relay Chat led to an explosion in interaction with the Web. With Web 2.0 we have been trying to connect digitally in much the same way. There are gardening forums, recipes, dating sites, pornography, religious sites and virtual gaming worlds. We are striving to connect in the same social groups and achieve the same personal goals – but now we want to do it online.

Social networking, and thereby social media, lies at the heart of these connections – and by creating, maintaining and cultivating valuable interactions with the connections in your local and remote hubs, your networks can grow and thrive.

> Companies that have an effective social engagement strategy in place, with a manageable timescale and structured implementation plan, can find their customers, identify who the movers and shakers are, and connect effectively with them.

They can watch who is active in the markets they want to go into, check the sentiments of their audiences' messages and listen for their challenges. Relationships can be built carefully on a one to one basis. Detractors can be turned into advocates, who can be encouraged with an appropriate programme to become key enthusiasts broadcasting and amplifying your message on your behalf.

So is the great conversation just the new buzzword of the new millennium? Or is it actually the biggest shift in human behaviour since the industrial revolution? For this we need to look at the new 'generations'. Baby boomers include people who were born after the Second World War between 1945 and about 1962. Generation X includes people who were born from 1963 to approximately 1979. Generation Y, or the Millennial Generation, includes those born from 1980 to 2000. Generation Z are those who have been born in the 21st century. The Generation Y population now, in 2010, outnumbers the baby boomer population, and 96% of the Generation Y crowd have joined some sort of social network for interaction. These social networks are changing the way we communicate in a fundamental way. We no longer search for news – the news now finds us. Soon we will no longer search for products or services – these products and services will find us via social media.

They key thing here is not that we communicate digitally, rather the particular ways we do so.

> You can't pick the 'winning' medium and ignore what your friends and colleagues are using.

Different mechanisms of communicating using conversational tools may bubble up to the top in popularity for a time, but the fundamental concepts behind how we use these products to communicate are the same throughout each network. These engagement applications are here to stay. Of course, the actual applications themselves will morph into something else, applications for mobile phones will come to prominence, and new technologies that use social media to connect will appear. Old and poorly designed applications will fade into obscurity. We're living in the age of the perpetual beta, and we need to learn to evolve with these technologies and adapt to take advantage of this new way of working. Our challenge is to learn how to adapt to the new way of working in a dynamic and rapidly changing world and work out how social media actually works for us as an individual, colleague, parent and friend.

This fundamental shift in the way we communicate has the ability to transcend boundaries. Barack Obama conducted his presidential election campaign on Twitter and YouTube. He successfully encouraged a significant number of Americans to vote for him, who would not normally have bothered to follow the campaign or vote. He continued this effective online presence with a conference in March 2009 answering questions using a voting style popular on the information channel Digg. He even appears to have a LinkedIn profile. On a more personal level, the video of Susan Boyle, an ordinary contestant on a UK talent show with an extraordinary voice, has been viewed over 120 million times on YouTube, catapulting her into the limelight and millionaire status within 6 months of her first appearance.

For corporate users, embracing this change can be beneficial in more ways than one. A common criticism from consumers is that companies don't listen to them, don't care about the people who buy their goods. Customers feel that once the

goods or services have been purchased, the customer care programmes are poor or non-existent. Companies are often vilified for bringing out 'new and improved' products after poor market research and with little consideration for the customer. They are accused of launching new products that are not ready for the market, that don't fit customer requirements, or fail customers' expectations. On the other hand, there are some companies whose fan base is the envy of the market. Think of the passion that Apple invokes across the technology sector, with new products announced to a joyful fan base and queues of potential purchasers camped out outside the Apple store, desperate to be one of the first to own one of the shiny new gadgets. Think of the hoards of Harley-Davidson aficionados, some of whom are happy to have the brand as a tattoo on their bodies – a permanent reminder of their loyalty. Think of the consumers who will only drink Starbucks coffee and eschew all other brands. Think of the image of Rolls Royce, of Perrier, of Gucci and Coca-Cola.

But what if your company doesn't have this level of loyalty, dedication and support from your customers? Ideally you want to grow your market share, win customers' loyalty perhaps from a competitor and improve perception of your company in the marketplace.

> Consider incorporating push–pull conversations into your traditional strategy as a new mechanism for reaching your audience.

You may have considered extending your traditional marketing approach and current online marketing strategy and you may have plans to embrace the world of Web 2.0. The prospect of interacting with your customers, the people who actually buy your products and services, can give you the opportunity to extend your reach into new, global markets, and connect more closely with your online audience.

WHY DO YOU NEED SOCIAL CONNECTIONS?

In his book, *The Tipping Point*,[1] Malcolm Gladwell describes three types of people – connectors, mavens and salesmen:

> Connectors are the people who 'link us up with the world, people with a special gift for bringing the world together. They are "a handful" of people with an extraordinary knack for making friends and acquaintances'. These individuals typically have social networks of over one hundred people. Connectors gain success in 'their ability to span many different worlds as a function of something intrinsic to their personality, some combination of curiosity, self-confidence, sociability, and energy.'
>
> Mavens are 'information specialists', or 'people we rely upon to connect us with new information.' They accumulate knowledge, especially about the marketplace,

and know how to share it with others. 'A Maven is someone who wants to solve other people's problems, generally by solving his own. Mavens start "word-of-mouth epidemics" due to their knowledge, social skills, and ability to communicate, they are information brokers, sharing and trading what they know'.

Salesmen are 'persuaders', charismatic people with powerful negotiation skills. They tend to have an indefinable trait that goes beyond what they say, which makes others want to agree with them.

Each of these categories of people can potentially become your 'first tier' influencers. These are the people that are **directly** connected to you in some way. They follow news about your brand. They discuss your brand with their connections. They want to have a closer dialogue with you. They are all influencers in their own right and, with their own specific skills, can reach out beyond your immediate network to influence others. Your tier 1 influencers can connect to your tier 2 influencers, who can also help to spread the word about your brand.

If you can find people in your immediate network who have these qualities you can start to engage in dialogue with them, cultivate them and give them information.

If you can find some information that is not generally available externally it will be very well received. Mavens will relish these bits of 'special' information – they will broker the information to the connectors and salesmen in their networks, and the message gets out. Each type of information gatherer will connect in some way to the next tier of influencers which may be further away from you in social distance, but closer to others in their own networks.

TIER 1 INFLUENCERS

- Tier 1 influencers typically hang out on user forums, they help out in community sites and they often have the answers the community needs.

- They respond to questions posed on the forum, or, if they are connector types, they will know someone in their network who does have the answer if they don't actually know it themselves.

- They may run user groups or attend them.

- They are forum moderators.

- They run user Q&A portals and participate in chat rooms.

- They are often quick to respond to a question posted on Twitter or Facebook.

- They are significant in your 'fan-out' evangelism efforts.

Fan-out messaging works like this. I tell two people, who each tell two people, who each tell two people, who each tell two people. My original message has fanned out and has reached 30 new potential customers – or, more importantly, potential influencers for my brand. These influencers and their connections are vital in getting your message out on your behalf. They retweet your interesting news on Twitter, they link to your blog from their own blog and they share useful links on Facebook. This network rebroadcasts and amplifies your message for you.

Tier 1 influencers are often early adopters. They buy the latest gadget, phone and eBook reader. They beta-test new releases of software and often have the latest and greatest laptop. They demonstrate their new hardware to anyone who will watch. They download the latest Twitter client and tweet endlessly about it. I remember the hype about the first iPhone. When it was released in the US in June 2007, hundreds of keen consumers queued for up to 12 hours outside the Apple store to be among the first to own it. They broadcast this to their friends through blogs, Facebook and Twitter. These influencers created a buzz about the device which ensured that a huge amount of people got to hear about it through the reports in the newswires. Now, the iPhone is the most popular mobile device in the US.[2] Apple has the ability to cause ripples around the online world with its new products, as the rumours about the alleged theft of their prototype 4G iPhone showed in April 2010.

Large companies have structured rewards and incentives programmes for influencers who are not usually motivated by financial incentives, but who thrive on knowledge gathering, community and recognition. IBM maintains an Influencer programme for its consultants and integrators, and another for its Partner Resellers. Microsoft has its Most Valuable Professionals programme and Intel has an innovative Intel Insiders programme. This new programme gained an award for innovation in new media in its second year of operation from the Society for New Communications Research in December 2009. Ferrari has a well established community of fans, most of whom have never owned a Ferrari but who continue to give the brand prominence throughout the world. For other examples of brand loyalists, enthusiasts and advocates, you only need to think of Nike, Burberry, Harley-Davidson, Marmite and Calvin Klein.

If you get your key influencers right then your tier 1 and your tier 2 influencers will do the job of getting your message out for you.

If you maintain a close relationship with your tier 1 influencers they will reward you by broadcasting your message for you. Software beta testers willingly try out incomplete software products for the chance to further their knowledge and appear more technically advanced than their peers. Airlines get loyalty from their travellers with Air Miles programmes and frequent flyer clubs, and supermarkets offer incentives through their loyalty and rewards cards. Coffee shops have simple loyalty cards offering free cake or coffee after a certain number of purchases. Even my local car wash at the back of the DIY store offers to give me my seventh car wash free. Of course I take full advantage of this!

If you invest time in maintaining the relationship with your tier 1 influencers, you will find you have a great circle of loyal advocates to spread the word about your brand. These influencers will greatly increase the amount of coverage when they talk about your product or gizmo, so it's worthwhile talking about it. If you don't think you have the time to invest in talking about your product across your channels, then spending 30 minutes a day promoting your message can still be of benefit if it is done outside your immediate circle of connections.

THE NEW WAY OF MARKETING TO YOUR CUSTOMERS

As social media becomes more prevalent in every part of our lives then so do questions about future trends in technology. What will be the next big thing to catch our attention? Where is social media going and how will it evolve? How will our behaviour change to adapt to this new way of communicating? How will our working patterns change? Will we have to do more with less, or will we become completely overwhelmed with the additional tasks we will have to perform in this Web 2.0 world?

We're experiencing a huge shift in our marketing too. The new way of working involves interaction and conversation, engagement and advocacy. Our approach has got to change to incorporate this. Traditional marketing methods now have to include a digital marketing component as part of the overall strategy. Now the old, push ways of marketing have to evolve and incorporate two-way dialogue which encourages conversation with the new thought leaders. And who are these new thought leaders? Well, they are everyone with access to the Internet and a set of friends, followers and connections.

Our customers, our consumers have become the new marketers who drive the conversation about our brands.

They are the new thought leaders and they will shape the way that the company operates. Ensuring longevity of followers in a marketing campaign will also become a priority. During a campaign there will be much activity and therefore awareness, but as activity decreases after the campaign so awareness declines and follower churn sets in.

The need to continue the conversation is becoming more and more relevant.

Regular engagement and interaction add significant value to the conversation and awareness of the brand. Campaigns should be created with repeat engagement in mind to encourage regular interaction and repeat visits.

Marketing departments will have to switch from their current outbound marketing campaigns and listen to the inbound voices. Traditional advertising behaviours will change from broadcasting **at** the consumer to listening **to** them.

The voice of the consumer will become the only voice to listen to, and companies will need to take advantage of their new listening skills. Subject matter experts will have a much louder influence over companies, as their messages will be amplified by the community. They will become the new influencers, advocates, critics and detractors. Companies will **have** to listen to this new voice.

Intelligent companies will be aware of the groundswell of conversation. They will work with their customers and advocates.

> Intelligent companies will cultivate strong positive relationships by creating and maintaining their influencer connections, and they will reward their customers.

They will do this through a series of rewards programmes and they will showcase these advocates as an extension of the company itself.

Marketers will adopt the new mechanism of communications, and more and more marketing efforts will focus on a dialogue with customers instead of a one-way outbound broadcast in a marketing campaign.

> This will result in consumer brand value and perception changes as the two-way dialogue becomes a structured conversation.

Marketing success will no longer be measured in terms of numbers reached, as sentiment and the **two-way conversation** will be considered important.

Social media sites already offer great opportunities to engage with and influence customers in ways that are different from traditional marketing approaches.

> This engagement with sentiment that can be captured almost in real time can offer a baseline for customer perception and identify key influencers.

Many social campaigns, however, currently have mixed results due to the lack of time investment and social presence.

The needs of different audiences should be also taken into account when planning campaigns. Groups of consumers, prosumers (professionals who use technology to do their job), technologists, influencers and hobbyists all have different requirements from a campaign and these behaviours should be taken into account when targets are set.

SUMMARY

- Social media is the new way of communicating online. It will not go away, so you need to adapt your working practices to take advantage of the new conversation.
- Having an effective social media plan in place helps you to effectively connect with your customers.
- Consider implementing push–pull conversations into your strategy.
- There are three types of communicators: connectors, mavens and salesmen. These are your influencers.
- Consider creating an incentives plan for your influencers.
- Intelligent companies will cultivate strong relationships with their influencers and enjoy a shift in perceptions of the company.
- Companies need to invest time and effort in their social media planning.

3   YOUR SOCIAL MEDIA SUCCESS PLAN

There are fundamental tenets to the way to behave in the new world of conversation, and having a good implementation plan in place is essential. There are things you can put in place so you can be successful in social media, and there are behaviours you can adopt so that people will communicate with you.

HOW TO BE SUCCESSFUL WITH SOCIAL MEDIA

- Know where your audience is.
- Don't fish in stagnant water – go where the fresh water flows. Choose dynamic sites with plenty of interaction.
- Give more than you receive. Contribute and interact to engage in dialogue.
- Become valuable to your readers.
- Be sociable.
- Discover who your online advocates are.
- Build a relationship with your influencers inside organisations.
- Understand your social graph, your key connectors and their social distance from other key connectors.
- Define metrics for success. Don't evaluate the return on your investment by using traditional numerical metrics, but by softer metrics such as comments, sentiment and trends.

Most sales and marketing organisations want some form of return from their actions. They want to be able to see a measurable result. They pay for advertising and want an increase in sales. They hold sales activities and want to have sales. They change their website, run a campaign and want a measurable increase in visitors to the site. Unfortunately social media doesn't work on such a transactional basis. It is fluid and dynamic, it is people-centric and disorganised. The social media revolution is powered by people and that's why it can never be transactional.

Many have jumped onto the social networking scene and not been successful. They have registered with every social media site that they have come across and they have found themselves overwhelmed. They wonder how they are going to manage to keep up with all of the information flowing at them and do their job too. Without a good plan in place it is really difficult to carry out their activities in a consistent way to connect with their audience. There are only so many hours in a day for you to keep up with this onslaught of information and stay sane, so here are some recommendations to help you be productive – not destructive.

KEEPING IT UNDER CONTROL

- Be consistent. Try to maintain a regular pattern in your communications on the web. Burst blogging (or tweeting) techniques are annoying to your audience and add extra load to your day. If you have a relatively easy day, then post-date some of your blog posts so that your readers get a regular update. Aim to tweet regularly too and maintain the connection with your audience.

- Don't get overwhelmed. There are so many different social networking sites out there that it's so easy to become flooded with information. If you spend all day on Twitter, or try to keep up with all of the status updates and changes on Facebook, you won't have any time at all for the rest of the things you need to do. You need to learn to cut out all the unnecessary messages. There are some users who seem to have no life beyond their online presence, and other users who smack of desperation. Try to maintain a happy balance, filter out those messages you don't want to see, and be ruthless with the unfollow button. Do you really need all those friends? Are they valuable connections for your business or automated bots looking for keywords or followers?

- Syndication – is it really necessary? You may have accounts on multiple networking sites and update each of them regularly with the same information. However, there are issues with this approach. If you maintain multiple personas on different sites, and share different kinds of information with different social groups, they may not appreciate business related updates on their personal network with you. Additionally, there might be some friends who follow you on many of your social networking sites and who may not appreciate the same information on each of their sites.

- Don't dismiss forums. People come to forums for advice. Often they are unaware that there are other resources available. If you contribute to forums, make sure you cross-reference your information to your blog. It drives traffic to your blog, and connects up the different resources. You can also point people who ask questions on forums to other social networking sites to help them.

- Be generous. If you have knowledge – share it! There are many, many people out there who are thirsty for knowledge. Share it appropriately. Be professional and courteous. Remember that not everyone has the same level of knowledge as you have, so don't flame them unnecessarily.

- Don't expect instant results. Your followers will visit your blog or follow you on Twitter, Facebook or LinkedIn and come back if they like your content. Don't expect to get thousands and thousands of readers in a day. Expect to build up gradually. Ignore all of those Twitter followers that promise a thousand followers a day. They are automated bots of little value to you. You want to have connections to real human beings.

- Deal appropriately with undesirables. If someone wants to connect with you and you don't want them to, don't feel guilty about denying the connection or blocking the follow on Twitter. Generally the person is not notified that you have rejected the connection, and if you have blocked them, they will not be able to contact you further. Don't encourage abuse by accepting connections you do not want. It's time wasting and demoralising.

- Get connected. Like syndication, your blog has your personality stamped onto it. So advertise it. People **want** to connect with you. Place a link to your blog on every online profile you have. You will drive traffic to your blog. If you have a Twitter account, refer to your Twitter handle wherever possible on online sites.

- Sell if you can, but don't sell directly. If you are selling something, don't be afraid to talk about it, evangelise it, discuss it – but don't allow your desire to sell overwhelm your voice. The constant sell will soon become wearing to your readers who will dismiss you as spam.

- Interact. Social Networking is **not** one-way communication. It's the interactions between the participants that make social networking – social. Take advantage of the connections you make to forge new customer relationships and enlarge your virtual network. People with a common interest will follow you, so will really appreciate the personal connection from you.

Many companies don't ask themselves why they are going to implement a social media plan. Often they feel that they need to introduce some sort of activity and use social media as a broadcast channel only. Having an effective conversational plan in place will make you more successful than having a one-way broadcast mechanism. Incorporating metrics will help you with your conversations with key stakeholders. Here are some things to think about and questions to ask.

THINGS TO CONSIDER IN YOUR SOCIAL MEDIA STRATEGY

- Why do you want to incorporate social media into your business? Who do you want to connect with? What results do you want to achieve? How will you measure success?

- Do you want to use specific individuals in your organisation for outbound communication with your external community, or do you intend to include everyone within the company to help you deliver your message?

- Do you know what platform you intend to use to broadcast your efforts? Do you want to focus your efforts on free networking services such as Twitter, Blogger, Facebook, Wordpress and YouTube?

- Do you want to expose your existing collaboration platform like Lotus Notes or Microsoft SharePoint through the firewall for better customisation of the interface and control?

- Do you want to tie your new online conversational strategy back to your company initiatives? There is significant business value to be gained by engaging with your audience using social media, but you need to make sure you focus on your objectives.

- Have you defined your desired results and timescale to achieve your goals? Have you detailed which metrics you want to achieve, and the tools you need to use to measure your success? These tools are important when you tie your achievements back to your strategy.

- Do you have the key points of your strategy in a crystal clear format which can be explained simply to the decision makers at board level?

- Before you launch your plan, have you listened to the conversation before starting to speak yourself? Your audience may not want to hear what you're telling them. By listening, responding and then joining into the conversation, you'll be well on the way to measurable success.

MEASUREMENTS AND METRICS

When you've decided on the tools you're going to use, make sure that you execute your strategy with a defined goal and a defined timescale, say 6 months or a year. Make this implementation plan realistic and start to introduce each tool gradually. As an example, you could devise a plan that executes for a year and consists of the following steps:

SOCIAL MEDIA ONE-YEAR PLAN

- Engage with multiple blogs, forums and wikis covering issues relating to your product or brand. Comment regularly. Start to create a dialogue.

- Create a blog. Try to blog regularly about interesting and useful topics that your readers would be interested in. Include your blog URL on your email auto-signature and on your website. Aim for 100 blog posts per year with an average of 300–400 views per post. Measure comments on your blog, and aim to comment on other blogs at least once per day. This leads viewers of other blogs back to your blog.

- Create a Technorati account and aim to increase your Technorati influence by tagging your posts so that they are easily discovered.

- Create a Twitter account. Include your blog URL on your Twitter profile; include your website URL on your blog. Talk about your Twitter stream on your blog; perhaps embed tweets from Twitter on your blog. Plan to tweet about twice a day and respond to other Twitter comments. Aim to increase your following

with valuable users who are real people whom you can engage with and not automated bots.

- Create a Facebook page that refers to your blog and your Twitter stream URLs. Start conversations and encourage customers to interact and give feedback to your Facebook page from both Twitter and your blog.

- Start a YouTube channel which points to your blog and Twitter. Upload videos regularly. Encourage dialogue and comments. Answer comments. Refer to your YouTube channel from Facebook, Twitter and your blog.

- Start a channel on UStream (or a similar video streaming service) with embedded Twitter stream for live interaction from your customers. Advertise it on each of your other social media channels and advertise all of your other communications channels on UStream.

- Develop a series of webcasts to help customers with any areas they're struggling with on your product or brand. Publish them on channels such as YouTube, Vimeo, MSN Video and Videojug.

Whatever mechanism you use to measure success, you need to have a set of measures and metrics before you start to execute your strategy. Start with a realistic baseline of your online presence and conversations about you. Set a reasonable timescale for metric measurements to be taken. Create your digital and social media policy, making sure it concurs with employee policy. Train your staff in the use of the tools you intend to use, make sure that they are fully aware of your social media corporate guidelines and policy and ask them to use your chosen channels to communicate. After a reasonable period of time measure your success, tracking any feedback and progress you've made through each of these channels. If you haven't defined your baseline metrics, then you will find it very difficult to measure your return on investment (ROI) and your success with your efforts. Your measures of success could be related to the increase in the number of people who are engaging with you and your brand. You could also benefit from an improvement in your conversations with your customers and advocates due to your closer connection to your customers.

It's a great idea to have a social media corporate policy and a strategy about the types of tools you will use to reach your customers. It's also commendable if your work environment and corporate values encourage your teams to use social software to reach your customers. However, if you have no definable way of measuring the impact that your outreach efforts actually have on your intended audience, your implementation plan will be hard to justify to the budget owners in the company.

As with all of your other business objectives, you need to have a way of effectively gathering data from your customers and measuring your key performance indicators. Unfortunately, as there are many tools used to broadcast your message across all of the social channels, then there isn't one particular metrics tool you can use to track your success. But what sorts of metrics do you want for the result you need to achieve? Do your metrics depend on the number of connections you have on Facebook or LinkedIn? Do you want to track the number of fans on your

Facebook group page or the number of members in your LinkedIn Group? Do you want to measure the number of followers you have on Twitter? Do you count numbers? Or do you want to measure interaction, influence, sentiment, mood or revenue? Whatever your goal happens to be, you need to be able to measure these metrics in a structured way.

Defining your targets

There are many tools, both free and commercial, that you can use to track trends and metrics for your campaign. Facebook's Friend Wheel application measures who is in your social graph and how well connected your tier 1 connections are in Facebook. There are other social graph applications and there are lots of Twitter tools like Twitter Grader and TweetStats that show how highly valued your profile is or whether your topic is trending right now on Twitter. Tracking your chosen metrics means that you will need to watch your online channels regularly. Over time you can get a month on month increase in readers, engagement or links clicked and record any comments that have been written. You can then compare the reach you achieve on these channels with the reach you achieve on your paid media channels which will give you an idea of their ongoing value to you.

NUMBERS OR INTERACTION?

- Do you want to track the increase in the number of people reading your company blog?
- Do you want your blog readers to increase their interaction with you by commenting on your blog?
- Do you want your users to fill in a satisfaction survey twice a year so you can see how your customers perceive your company or your brand?
- Do you want to measure change in perception of your company?
- Do you want increase awareness of your brand or sub-brand?
- Do you want to measure increased interaction of users who visit your website, either by measuring their comments on articles you write, page visits, unique users, or responses to online campaigns?

These metrics, such as page views per visitor, unique visitors and time spent on each page, can easily be analysed by an analytics tool such as StatCounter or Google Analytics. But in order to effectively measure interaction and response to your social media efforts you need to think about using some of the metrics to create your baseline.

SOCIAL MEDIA METRICS

Blogging

Number of subscribers (using Feedburner or similar)
Number of web views

Numbers of RSS hits
Number of comments
Number of trackbacks
Number of reposts
Technorati authority
Volume of conversation

User Forums:

Number of new subscribers
Number of new members
Number of new threads
Number of regular posters per month
Number of posts per day
Number of page views
Number of returning unique users
Number of registered users
Response rate
Top 10 ranked questions
Top 10 thread respondents

Twitter:

Number of followers
Number of conversations to @
Number of retweets
Number of URL click-throughs (using a metrics tracker such as bit.ly)
Range of Influence – your people who follow your followers (you can use a software script to automate the process)

Virtual World

Number of visitors
Number of incoming links to a website
Average time on site

Facebook

Number of page fans (people who like the page)
Number of topic discussions
Number of comments / likes

YouTube

Number of views
Number of channel subscribers
Number of comments
Volume of conversation

Photo sharing sites

Number of comments
Number of views
Ranking

Measuring any one of these metrics can be done within your overall strategy and they can help you to measure your ROI. Metrics can also gauge whether you're being successful in your efforts to execute or whether you're failing. This will give you simple figures to show to the board. Your choice of tools depends very much on your marketing strategy and desired outcomes. Here are some of the popular tools used for analysis and metrics:

- BlogPulse
- Brandwatch
- How Sociable
- Google Insights
- GoogleNews
- Market Sentinel
- Nielsen Buzzmetrics
- Omniture
- Onalytica
- Radian6
- Technorati
- Techrigy
- Trendistic
- Twitcalc
- Twitter Trends
- Visible technologies

This all seems like a really simple way to capture your success with social media, but I must sound a note of warning. Beware of depending on one particular product alone for your metrics, and bear in mind that the social media landscape changes frequently. If you're building an application that can be used on networking sites, be wary of nailing your colours to the mast of another social media tool. The site you built your application for might switch allegiance and start to compete with you for business or mindshare.

The music recommendation service iLike, which provides a music application for Facebook, is heavily dependent on its provider.[3] About 80% of iLike's revenue comes from Facebook. iLike has built its entire business on Facebook, and the company was valued at $20 million when MySpace made an offer to buy it. iLike is very dependent on advertising for business and as it has gathered 50 million registered users from Facebook. The issue here is if you have an application that is heavily dependent on a social site's application programming interface, then you are entirely at the mercy of the social site, which may change its terms of use with little or no notice. If iLike were purchased by MySpace, the rival to Facebook, then it could be very difficult for iLike if Facebook decided to withdraw

support for the service, and this is also true for several other applications that are heavily dependent on their hosting sites. Changing the terms or the technology could paralyse the relationship.

So don't bank on using one developer platform exclusively for your business opportunity. If the site decides to pull the plug on you, where else could you go?

WHAT IS RIGHT FOR YOUR ORGANISATION?

There are so many different options and channels you can consider implementing, that it can be difficult to make a choice. I've created a simple flow chart (Figure 3.1) to show you your options when you're deciding which channels you could use for your business. Primarily, you need to decide what you want to achieve by using social media tools. Do you want to use the channel for the community or do you want to demonstrate your credibility in the industry? For simplicity, the chart only shows Facebook, Twitter, blogging, LinkedIn and YouTube.

Figure 3.1 Social media tools flowchart

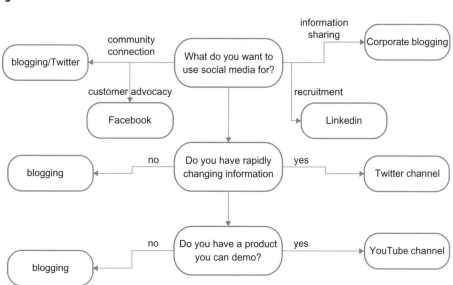

Every company has different outreach requirements and you will use the tools in a different way to achieve a different set of results. All tools can be used for all types of connections to your audience; it's how you use the tools that will make the difference to the way that your customers and partners respond.

Careful consideration of your strategy will also make a big difference to your approach and will help you implement an effective plan. This plan will be closely tied to your corporate objectives with measurable goals and the correct level of investment for the project. Then you will be able to measure your success.

The tools that you use to engage with your customers will be different depending whether your focus is business to business (B2B) or business to consumer (B2C) or you run different campaigns. In Figure 3.2 I've grouped the more popular tools based on their value to the customer in B2B and B2C settings and the impact on your customers if you use them.

Figure 3.2 Tools, their value and impact to the customer

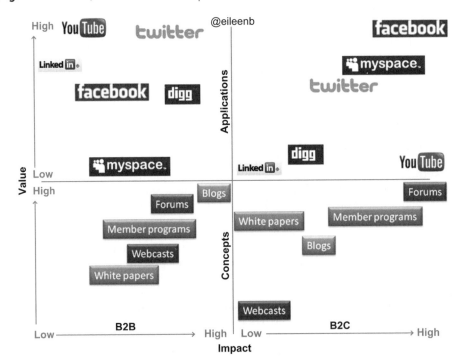

SOCIAL MEDIA IS NOT THE NEW WAY OF COMMUNICATING

Social media is here, and it's here to stay. Our challenge is to take advantage of this and grow both in our home and work lives.

Communicating using these types of tools is not a new concept. It is, however, the buzzword of the moment. There's a plethora of pretty-looking, interactive, engaging applications and hundreds of rival social interaction sites that you can

use to communicate and share information with your network of friends and acquaintances.

> We are, and have always been, social animals who live and work together in groups, and it follows that media has been used for social reasons ever since we lived in caves.

What else are cave paintings for if not to show your fellow cave dwellers just how to handle a buffalo? With the advent of digital communications, it was inevitable that we would find ways to connect with each other online.

From the early days of email, people have been forwarding messages to each other, but the bulletin board changed the way that people interacted. Some of the first applications were built to accommodate communication and sharing. For several decades we have been party to one of the biggest cultural shifts since the industrial revolution and have watched the development of a whole host of types of digital interaction. The range extends beyond Facebook and Twitter to more esoteric offerings such as multi-user dungeons from where World of Warcraft and Second Life can trace their origins. Multi-object-oriented applications are used for text based adventure games and education facilities while instant messaging, chat rooms and bulletin boards are more familiar in the mainstream.

The birth of the bulletin board
One of the earliest bulletin boards was Arpanet, where the first terminals were linked together in California in November 1969. People liked the idea of communicating with each other online. One popular bulletin board in California was the WELL.[4] This was launched in 1985 as the Whole Earth 'Lectronic Link and is still running today.

The US was well ahead of the rest of the world when it came to word of mouth networking, bulletin board and forum software. The early pornographic site, Rusty-N-Edie, had some 124 computers and nearly 6,000 subscribers by 1993. Any subscriber living outside the US had to dial in to the US numbers, paying for an international telephone call (Figure 3.3). The site contained 105,000–110,000 files available for downloading, nearly half of which were graphic image files (GIFs). GIFs from Rusty-N-Edie's bulletin board could be downloaded by the customer to his or her home computer, and could be viewed only with specialised software. Some of these 'adult' photos were the subject of a court case between Rusty-N-Edie and Playboy magazine.[5]

Bulletin boards still exist today. A quick search on the web brought me to Monochrome, and there are several websites devoted to bulletin board archives. These simple interactive 'green screen' technologies allowing real-time interaction between users and message passing are considered to be the foundation upon which social media evolved.

Building walled gardens
Unsurprisingly users wanted to have a new and more engaging way of interacting. CompuServe and AOL provided walled gardens for users.

Figure 3.3 Rusty-N-Edie's bulletin board

```
Éïïï ïïï ïïï ïïï ïïï ïïï ïïï ïïï ïïï ïïï ïïï ïïï ïïï ïïï ïïï ïïï ïïï ïïï ïïï ïïï ïïï ïïï ïïï ïïï ïïï»
 º          This program is brought to you with the blessings        º
 º                  of Rusty n Edie's BBS and its Users.             º
 º                                                                    º
 º      We have the largest collection of Public Domain Software      º
 º        and the largest collection of Adult GIFS & Programs         º
 º                                                                    º
 º          OVER 12 GIGS!!!                       112 LINES!!!        º
 º                                                                    º
 º                       Call 1 216-726-2620                         º
 º                        300 / 1200 / 2400                          º
 º                              or                                    º
 º                       Call 1 216-726-3589                         º
 º        U.S. Robotics Dual Standard 14.4kV32 Compatible            º
 º                              or                                    º
 º                       Call 1 216-726-3619                         º
 º              Hayes V-Series V42 9600 / 19200                      º
 º                              or                                    º
 º                       Call 1 216-726-3620                         º
 º              CompuCom SpeedModem 9600 / 19200                     º
 º                                                                    º
 º          Accessible Via Connect-USA Node RNEBBS                   º
 º              Accessible Via Starlink Node: 4909                   º
 º                                                                    º
 º          WE ARE THE FRIENDLIEST BBS IN THE WORLD!                 º
Èïïï ïïï ïïï ïïï ïïï ïïï ïïï ïïï ïïï ïïï ïïï ïïï ïïï ïïï ïïï ïïï ïïï ïïï ïïï ïïï ïïï ïïï ïïï ïïï¼
```

> Walled gardens are sites where members of that site can chat to other members of that site.

Walled gardens, however, prevent you from communicating with non-members. Users could contribute to bulletin boards within AOL's subscription services which extended its reach outside the United States. AOL first launched in Japan in 1986 and by the early 1990s had thousands of users across the world socially interacting with each other. CompuServe was a very popular service, topping more than 3 million users by 1995, whilst AOL provided online games for the Commodore from 1985 and a graphical chat environment from 1986.

Talking in real time
When you 'talk' to someone on a bulletin board, it's a bit like chatting using mobile phone text messages, and online users wanted something more like a conversation. This need was filled when Internet Relay Chat, was developed.

One of the first examples of news broadcasting using Internet Relay Chat was when it was used to report on the 1991 Soviet *coup d'état* attempt even though there was a media blackout in force at that time.[6] It was used in a similar fashion during the Gulf War, the 1992 US presidential election, and the Oklahoma City bombing in 1995. There are also some examples of weddings being conducted online there! I do wonder whether the happy couples are still married to each other or whether they have announced their separation in a similar community spirited fashion. The idea of Twitter broadcasting news events is certainly not a new concept at all.

As these different streams of communications evolved over time, it became apparent that there were disparate islands of information surrounded by a sea of data. These pieces of information weren't connected to each other at all. CompuServe and AOL forged ahead with their own communities, significantly growing users at a tremendous rate but creating an issue. The main problem with walled gardens is that if you want to interact with your friends who have accounts in other networks, you have to join the other network.

> Walled gardens require all of your contacts to use the same network in order to get value from the connection.

This closed type of interaction only brings benefits to the company that built the network software. Soon browsers such as Netscape circumvented the walled garden approach by providing the mechanism to visit websites around the world. Netscape used graphical user interfaces to present easy to navigate pages with images and files to download. Communication using Network News Transfer Protocol (NNTP) allowed forum software and newsreader software to proliferate, encouraging interaction between disparate members of the new Internet community. NNTP and newsreader software are still used by forum moderators, technical experts and regular contributors to this day. Their main benefit is that they allow offline responses to posted questions on myriad forums covering any topic you'd care to ask about.

Social and non-social software

Fifteen years ago, where did you go to get information about someone to get your work done? You probably tried the library, visited the bookstore, or looked in an encyclopaedia. The information you needed would be stored there and the data was as fresh as the day the book was sent to print. Now let's move forward to today. Where would you go to get that information? You'd go onto the web. Specifically, you'd use a search engine to find the information you need. Some of the data you'll find will be static, and some of the information will be dynamic, up to date and engaging. The web has changed into Web 2.0, it's changed the way you find the things you want and it's become much more interactive and social.

> The way that social media has been adopted is different from the way that other types of 'non-social' software have been used.

If you're working at your PC on desktop applications like Adobe Illustrator, Excel or Word, you do not require validation from your peers in your network or recommendations for you to use the software or find it valuable. You may have heard about the software from someone and decided to try it yourself. Non-social software started to change with the introduction of collaborative applications. Tools like SharePoint, Lotus Notes, Outlook and Instant Messenger introduce the concept of 'others' in your network. You can interact and collaborate with these 'others' in different ways. You can send an email which is instantly delivered or you can update a document on the network which can alert others in your workgroup that the document has changed. You can send an instant message to people across the company and communicate online with your team mates. Collaboration software enables you to interact with 'the others' to efficiently get your work done.

THE GROWTH OF THE WEB 2.0 WORLD

Web 2.0 and social networks exist and thrive because users communicate with each other. They engage in conversations with each other, commenting and responding to information on the web. The conversation started with email, bulletin boards, forums and newsgroups. Now you will probably update your Twitter status and you will talk about what you are doing on Facebook. You can comment on blogs, take a quick online survey or respond to a poll on a website. You can take notes during a webcast and store them online. All of this and more is possible with Web 2.0.

Web 2.0 is a term associated with web applications that allow user interaction.

These applications facilitate interaction, information sharing and collaboration amongst web based communities and social networking sites. For technology influencers, Web 2.0 is about the perpetual beta which is the shift in the way that web applications were developed and deployment. Interaction and feedback between the users and the software designers means that products can continually be updated as the product evolves. The traditional software design life cycle focuses on producing a software product, evaluating and testing it. The product is then launched and used by consumers who often have had no impact on any product design decisions. Web 2.0 allows feedback, interaction and change. Web 2.0 is about constantly changing the technology as people can give feedback on the process by interacting with the software designers and changing the development life cycle.

Consequently Web 2.0 changed the genre of applications. Now there are web applications focused on user centred design, there are sites designed for sharing and there are application mashups. A mashup is a web page or application that combines different sources of data in the form of a service. For example, real-time traffic data in one application can be merged with a mapping application and the merged application used to benefit travellers.

Letting the folks work for you

Web 2.0, with its interaction and dialogue, has brought interoperability and collaboration to the World Wide Web.

The term Web 2.0 is associated with Tim O'Reilly, who ran the O'Reilly Media Web 2.0 conference in 2004. This conference is credited with starting the discussion about the term Web 2.0 in the public forum and brought the idea of the collaborative web alive. Now new genres of services and applications have sprung up: video sharing sites, wikis, blogs, podcasts and forums. Formerly, in what is called the age of Web 1.0, we used static websites and were limited to clicking links to view other static websites. Now Web 2.0 allows users to interact with each other, rate content, edit web pages and modify the style of the page.

Web 2.0, which seemed to rise out of the ashes of the dotcom bubble, brought start-up websites with discussions and interaction between companies and their customers.

This type of interaction is completely different from the way we previously interacted with our friends. I used to use traditional ways of communicating like email and instant messaging to chat to my friends and colleagues. Whenever I found out something new or interesting, I'd send out the link or more probably an attachment to the email and send it to my group of friends. I used forum software to ask technical questions and discuss topics with the online community. Now, I share the link on Twitter or Facebook and I ask my extended network of friends if they have the answer to my questions. I use email distribution lists or forum software as a last resort. How times have changed – and social networking sites have enabled that change for me.

Documents can now be found when you search for terms that are relevant to **you**.

Users now decide how documents are classified or tagged on the web.

These tags, keywords relating to the document or web page, can be grouped together in a 'tag cloud'. A tag cloud is a collection of keywords on a web page indicating which keywords have been marked by more people as relevant descriptions of the document. These tag categories, where the same term was used by several people, started to rise in prominence in the form of tag clouds, where more popular tags appear in larger font sizes. Other users can then see which tag name has been classified by the largest number of community members and can use the new tag name. This collaboration encourages new forms of page grouping as the new type of user generated taxonomy emerges.

Figure 3.4 Tag cloud from my blog, http://eileenbrown.wordpress.com

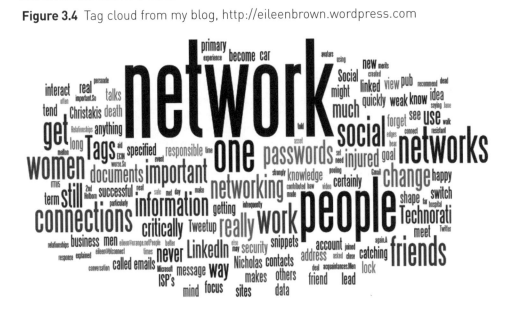

The tag cloud in Figure 3.4 was taken from my blog at http://eileenbrown. wordpress.com. It's easy to see the sort of words I use more often than others in my recent blog entries.

There has been an increase in collaborative technologies that support real-time interactions and user-generated content. Instead of the traditional taxonomy we now have the concept of the folksonomy.

> A folksonomy is something that is classified by 'the folks' instead of an unnamed project team who follow a formal structure for classifying documents.

Folksonomies started to appear as users' tagged content on web pages and assigned categories that were relevant to them. I might classify a topic on the web by a completely different term than you. For example, you might have tagged the story about the Icelandic volcano eruption as 'air travel disruption', whereas I might tag the same eruption as a 'pyroclastic flow'. Others may tag the same eruption with different terms.

This collaborative approach means that anyone can release a partially finished application onto the web, and due to the efforts and feedback of the many, the application can evolve with active participants throughout the development process. This is a fundamental shift in the way that large companies produce software. Their software development cycles were just not agile enough to cope with this level of interaction.

In the world of Web 2.0, applications are developed with massive amounts of input and collaboration from the online community.

With the potential for a whole world of beta testers collaborating with the application developer, the potential in the industry for disruption is huge. The development teams are now participants in an ongoing cyclical process in which the beta testers use the software and offer feedback. Now with careful co-ordination the developers can listen to feedback from their end users, ordinary folks like you and me. They can redesign and develop that software, improve it with iterations of the code, asking for feedback from people like us and bringing the software closer to the needs and requirements of the users.

SOCIALISING AND INTERACTING

For me, Web 2.0 has made socialising with my friends and business colleagues in my existing social networks much easier.

Web 2.0 interaction lets me connect to people outside my immediate network, to bring them closer to me in my social graph.

It also allows me to see what is going on in my second degree network, my friends of friends network. I can stay in touch with colleagues and partners with whom I only tend to work for a few weeks per year. I can find out what my business connections are working on at the moment, which gives me an opportunity to reconnect with them and remind them of my consultancy skills. Social tools such as Facebook, LinkedIn and Twitter allow me to see what the friends of my friends are saying. This makes me want to interact with these connections more frequently, enables me to extend my network and connect to networks outside my social graph.

Web 2.0 provides huge diversity in the way that products are showcased. The ability for organisations to disseminate information via text, video, slides and audio enhances learning in so many ways.

Companies in service industries can use the interaction for better customer dialogue.

Businesses can take advantage of this by providing educational blogs about products and services. The can record 'how to' videos to upload onto YouTube and they can publish audio podcasts for background details and education. Imagine what a revolution this could be for schools and colleges. Teachers could take advantage of the favoured method of learning and teach children using this new media. Pupils could become much more engaged and learning could be enhanced.

Some companies have externally facing wikis for customer comments and feedback on documents; others have forums for help and advice for customers. There are many sites dedicated to helping to educate visitors about medical issues and questions about their wellbeing. There are forums, Q&A documents, and there is even a YouTube channel called FlowTheBook, which is specifically designed for parents to help educate their daughters about menstruation. All of these sites are searchable; they are discoverable and they all give users the ability to interact with the site itself. These sites are much more useful than the medical dictionary sitting on your bookshelf gathering dust.

Creating your organisation's social graph

Some key decision makers and influencers in a network don't play an active part in online activities, but have huge impact throughout their networks.

> These influential decision makers are deep within an organisation and are the 'go to' people when there are problems.

They may be the ideas people when you need to brainstorm, and the people that you can rely on to complete complex tasks. They are valued contacts, trusted advisers, have the ear of the senior executives and are often the hubs of joined networks inside organisations and key to the social graph. These interpersonal ties carry information between people, they can be strong or weak, but they transmit across their networks. Unfortunately, companies don't often know who these valuable people are and waste time repeating work that might not be needed.

A social graph of your organisation, created either manually or using social graphing and mapping tools, can map the number of ties each individual has, whether weak or strong, and indicate which people within your organisation are central to its connectedness. Three or four questions could be asked and the answers mapped out graphically. If you have well connected people, the graph could look very much like a hub and spoke network diagram, or perhaps even a fully meshed network topology. For example, some of the questions that you could ask are:

Your organisational social graph

- Who do you go to within your company for reliable and accurate information?
- Who would you trust to get a complex project completed?
- Who helps you connect to the resource you need?

These graphs, once created, can potentially show a network hidden within your organisation which is totally different than the type of network that may be mapped out by the organisational structure. These charts don't map to hierarchy – far from it. Often middle managers and individual contributors who need to

communicate and connect with multiple groups across an organisation, share information and disseminate information through their many communicated ties.

> Their relative importance to an organisation depends on the number of strong and weak ties they have.

Strong ties are people in your network with whom you have a good relationship. Weak ties are your casual acquaintances, people you know vaguely, but don't have a regular connection to.

Some people seem to know hundreds of people, albeit casually, whereas others have deeper relationships with fewer people. How do people manage these relationships? A recent posting on Facebook said: 'The human mind can only deal with about 200 close relationships. If you have more than 200 friends on Facebook it doesn't mean you are popular, it means your quality control is bad, or your ego is too big.'

There does appear to be a limit to the number of friends you can have. A British anthropologist, Robin Dunbar, hypothesised that there is a theoretical limit to the number of people with whom we can maintain stable social relationships. This number is set at 150. Tools such as Facebook allow you to greatly extend this number using weak ties.

YOUR STRONG AND WEAK TIES

Strong ties can guide you towards other strong networking hubs, and they tend to indicate powerful networks, with very well connected individuals at the hub.

> Unusual information tends to flow better between the weaker ties in your network.

Your strong ties probably have access to the same information that you have. These ties are in the same network as you are and they are less likely pass information around. This same information, however, may be news to the weaker ties in your organisation.

> People connected to you by weaker ties are more likely to propagate the information to people outside your network.

Some individuals are very well connected to other people who work in tightly connected groups like a network hub. These hubs have both strong and weak ties connecting them to other parts of the network. These routing hubs maintain relationships with key central characters and they keep the flow of information inside an organisation moving efficiently.

Mapping your organisation out in this way can identify potential communication issues within your organisation.

The mapping can often highlight positive connections and it can strengthen communications flow. Breaking down the disparate islands of information within an organisation by using either human connections or collaboration software such as email, a document management system or a wiki can improve the information flow within a company and streamline processes.

People hubs, routers and endpoints

To understand how social media can be of benefit inside the organisation, we need to look at how real networking works and why it is useful for some people and not others. To think about the human network, I'd like you to think about hardware hubs and routers. If you think about your circle of friends you'll notice that some people have a tendency to be natural hubs. These people have a collection of friends that feed them information and ask their advice. Other friends seem to behave as routers. These people don't often have the information you need when you ask them a question but they usually know someone who does. Others in your circle of friends are endpoints. They usually ask all the questions. So let's consider endpoints.

Endpoints (or nodes, if we're staying with the technology analogy) need information.

They often don't have connections to enough people in the workplace to be able to network efficiently and get the information they need. This is especially true in larger organisations. Endpoints tend to ask questions of hubs so that they can get the information they need. Sometimes they may need to be connected to others in the organisation that may be able to help.

Hubs tend to have lots and lots of connections in the organisation.

These connections might be strong ties or weak ties. There may be connections to several people throughout the network who can provide the answer to anyone who comes for information. If a hub doesn't have the answer directly, they will often know someone who does have the answer. This third party may be someone with whom the hub has an infrequent or casual relationship – a weak tie. Perhaps this connection may be someone whom the hub has only met once but recognises the potential value of the relationship and connects whenever they need to.

When a hub doesn't have the answer to the question, but knows someone else will be able help then the hub turns into a router.

Routers pass information onto other hubs to find the answer that they need.

An endpoint will sometimes find they connect to a hub, are passed through another hub (who may or may not have the answer) and on until the correct person
is found. Hubs and routers are the best connected people inside an organisation,
and endpoints might try to find out who their primary hubs are. Having a good
strong connection with the hubs in your organisation is a great way to encourage
effective knowledge flow. The best and strongest connections are between hubs
and routers themselves. If we're still staying with the hardware and networking
topology analogy, you might be thinking about a fully meshed diagram by now.
These are the most valuable connections you can make. Are you a hub yourself?
Are you a routing hub? I class myself as a routing hub. I have lots of connections
that I maintain a relationship with and I often pass people onwards if I don't
have the answer myself.

The only problem with this model is that endpoints often feel that they have
nothing of value to offer a hub. Endpoints only seem to want information and
they don't tend to contribute information to the network. Hubs and routers thrive
on two-way information flow and will be reluctant to maintain two-way connections where they don't benefit from the relationship. Hubs and routers get the
most value from other hubs and routers.

If you think you're an endpoint and want to grow your connections, how can you
become a hub? I use the 'extra fact' to give out a hook.

When you start to connect with someone, try to give a little bit more information
than you receive.

In an opening conversation when someone asks how you are – don't just say
'I'm fine, thank you'. Try to give a little bit of extra information to open up the
conversation which will encourage dialogue with the other person. Perhaps you
could say 'I'm fine, thank you, although I'm totally delighted to have completed
the public folder phase and I'm now onto phase 2 of my Exchange migration project' (or something similar). This could potentially open up a dialogue about you as
a person and your current project. Perhaps you might find another Exchange
specialist in a pinstripe suit. The topic isn't all that important; engaging someone
in conversation is.

Sharing a little personal information often opens up the dialogue and encourages
the other person to interact with you. This starts your two-way conversation and
starts to strengthen the tie. With your collections of new ties, strong and weak,
you'll start to be a little hub – and your personal network inside the business will
start to grow.

So what kind of tools should you use to communicate in the new world of engagement? Do you start with a blog, or do you start your own video channel? It seems

overwhelming and it seems very transient. Should you bother at all and wait for this craze to go away?

SUMMARY

- Create an effective and comprehensive social media plan.
- Metrics really matter. Create a baseline and record metrics and measurements.
- Walled gardens need to connect to the outside world for the benefit of their users.
- Use folksonomies for a better understanding of how your customers classify things.
- Use social media interaction for better customer service opportunities.
- Create your organisation's social graph to find out who your internal influencers are.
- Work out who your hubs, routers and endpoints are.
- Use the 'extra fact' to get your hook.
- Cultivate your strong and your weak ties. Both are valuable.

4 THE TOOLS OF THE NEW WEB

Where do you start to get your message out in the new Web 2.0 world? Which applications, amongst the hundreds available, could you consider? In this chapter, we will start by looking at blogging and how a blog can help to start the conversation between you and your audience. We'll then look at how to consume information on a blog and the various tools you can use to read posts, both online and offline. We'll talk about editing your own web pages, and how wikis can be used as powerful tools both inside and outside the firewall. We'll move onto video and web conferencing software and how virtual meetings can be conducted across the web using low cost or free software. We'll talk about mobile blogging and microblogging, discuss the rise of Twitter and include some techniques to enhance your communication over 140 characters. Finally, we'll look at the other worlds – the virtual worlds that exist and the world of the online gamer – and explore how businesses can take advantage.

THE TOOLS OF WEB 2.0

Social computing tools are feature rich and powerful. They are diverse and help to solve a series of communications problems. They provide information to help connect people. Sites such as Ning and MySpace segregate communities into specialist areas, and blogs, wikis, forums and instant messaging applications enhance the interaction on the sites themselves. They propagate information by word of mouth networking and connections. They earn their revenue through paid-for advertising and sponsorship. They can be used to collate targeted groups. These sites can operate for professional purposes or purely for hobbyists. LinkedIn, which positions itself as a business networking site, is also a great source of job listings and a quick way of looking at candidates' curricula vitae and career histories. Other examples of such sites are Facebook, Bebo, Orkut, KickApps and Friendster.

Planning to incorporate these sites into your plan requires some discipline to manage the updates from each site effectively. Some networking sites have their own alerts built into the software which enable you to receive emails when certain actions are triggered. Part of your implementation plan might include allowing for appropriate timely action whenever an alert is generated.

Corporate blogging

One way that companies can start to communicate with their customers outside their formal public relations (PR) and communications mechanisms is by allowing their employees to broadcast their message to their customers through blogging.

Forward-thinking companies with fresh innovative ideas and good blogging policies in place experience a perception shift amongst their customers. Over time, after interaction with bloggers, customers discover that the company is staffed with real people with families, homes, a sense of humour and not mechanoids without a soul.

Blogging, the publishing of information to a web log, allows information and links to be published onto the web in a dynamic way. Your customers will read what you publish on your blog to get information and advice from you. Posts are published in reverse chronological order so that the latest post is shown at the top of the page. Your readers can add their comments to your blog entries, and other bloggers can link to your blog entry from their own blog.

The mechanism of cross-linking to a blog post on another blog is called a trackback or a pingback and it is a useful way for you to track who reads your content.

Subscribing to blogs

Your readers can subscribe to your blog using RSS. RSS stands for Really Simple Syndication – or Rich Site Summary, according to some site definitions – and is an essential tool for websites that have rapidly changing content. In order to take advantage of the RSS feature on a website, you need a feed reader, or aggregator. Subscribers of your blog consume RSS feeds through a feed aggregator. Offline readers such as Sharpreader and Newsgator allow you to read content when you are not connected to the Internet, or you can use a tool such as Google Reader to read aggregated content when you are online. There are also versions of RSS readers specifically designed for mobile devices. When you subscribe to an RSS feed on a web page, your feed reader periodically scans each URL that you have subscribed to, checks for updated content on the page and, if there is new content, downloads a copy for you to read later. The information also includes extra information in meta-tags, such as the date of publication and the owner of the post and a link back to the original post in case you want to add a comment to the post. The content is actually pulled from the URL by the reader itself although it appears to have been pushed to out to subscribers each time a new post is published or created by the author.

Due to the technical limitations of RSS, it isn't possible to obtain statistics on who is subscribing to your RSS feed, which may be an issue for you if your customer engagement strategy includes measuring specific metrics around subscriber types.

Blog syndication

Feed syndicator tools like Feedburner can keep track of your subscribers.

A feed syndicator allows material to be made available to many other websites and for you to measure each click. They can tell you how many unique new subscribers are reading your posts, which can be a useful mechanism if you need to track audience engagement.

Websites that have content that is updated from time to time should consider placing an RSS Feed button on their web page for users to subscribe to and receive push notifications. Hosted blog sites such as Blogger, Wordpress, TypePad, Joomla and Windows Live Spaces all have these feed notification buttons incorporated.

Business to business blogging

There are personal blogs, there are product blogs. There are corporate blogs, and there are blogs written by cats and dogs. Which one is the right approach? Microsoft has many different bloggers who talk about technology innovation, research, opinion and upcoming product releases. There are thousands of bloggers who blog as individuals, there are product team blogs, and support team blogs. There are blogs written on the main Microsoft sites of http://blogs.msdn.com and http://blogs.technet.com. There are blogs written using Live Spaces, Wordpress, LiveJournal and many more. There's a huge amount of information coming from inside the company, designed to educate, inform and announce news to Microsoft's partners and customers. Microsoft is a good example of B2B blogging. Credibility, authority and authenticity all help the customer or partner make an informed decision about Microsoft's large product set. With the huge amount of information flowing from Microsoft every day, it would not be feasible to aggregate all this information into one main channel. It may be possible for a small company to have one 'voice' when engaging with customers or partners, but for large companies this could not work. Would it even be possible for one blog account to aggregate all of the work people are doing in one company without the blog sounding like a PR message? Any major corporate announcement is generally tied to PR initiatives at a corporate level where perhaps there isn't a place on the website for comments from the readers of that message. With a carefully executed PR strategy around these announcements, and a good corporate policy in place, the voice of the blogger (and the microblogger) can be heard, and it can be a very powerful voice indeed when it is closely aligned with corporate strategy and an effective plan in place.

THE POWER OF COLLECTIVE HUMAN KNOWLEDGE

If the PR announcement generates excitement and buzz, and people want to find out more information about your product, new technique or news disclosure, they will go to your site for information. If the only place to go for information is the

official press site, people may get frustrated at the lack of news other than the official PR release. Having an information channel such as a blog, populated by key people who have information and opinions, gives a human perspective to the PR announcement and encourages dialogue with the company. This leads to a perspective of greater transparency and honesty.

Companies that permit their staff to have a public voice and permit them to broadcast to the outside world through their blogs, often gain benefits from using similar forms of collaboration inside the company. There is a wealth of collaboration tools available for use inside the company network. There are applications with embedded presence for instant updates, alerts for document changes and broadcasts, and collaborative applications such as internal wikis. Collaboration tools like these can ensure that companies can effectively share their intellectual property (IP) safely inside their network boundary and behind their security firewall. Staff realise that often some of the simplest ways for teams to collaborate is through the use of team wikis.

Wikis are a great way to get interaction from customers and partners. Wikipedia, a website which contains over 15 million articles, is a wiki. It can be edited and added to by anyone who wishes to modify details on a page. It is imperative that corporate entities have a presence on Wikipedia giving information about the company. If your company is global, then there is a further opportunity for you to reach customers across the non-English-speaking world by localising versions of the corporate page. Almost 80% of articles in Wikipedia are written in languages other than English. For example, the BCS (search for "British Computer Society" in Wikipedia) has its own page. The page includes history, membership details, and certification and there are links to regional BCS branches throughout the UK.

Wikis, by their design, are made to be edited. Unfortunately, some careless editing of a page may do considerable damage to the body of work already created. This damage, whether intentional or otherwise, means that there needs to be some kind of alert mechanism in place to prevent destruction of work already completed. Wikipedia does have a huge problem with wiki editing, both from reporting of inaccurate information, and people deliberately or otherwise falsifying Wikipedia entries. This malicious editing is termed wiki vandalism. Wikipedia defines vandalism as:

> Removing all or significant parts of a page's content without any reason, or replacing entire pages with nonsense. Sometimes referenced information or important verifiable references are deleted with no valid reason(s) given in the summary. ... An example of blanking edits that could be legitimate would be edits that blank all or part of a biography of a living person.[7]

Some wiki vandalism is difficult to discover, however. False or misleading information in a regular technical document on your intranet may escape detection. This information will probably be plausible. It may appear to be true but is

deliberately designed to obfuscate the true meaning. Misinformation like this could lead to significant issues with knowledge transfers within the company, especially if the mistake has been made deliberately. There must be an effective way to track who is using the wiki, what changes are being made, and by whom. An audit trail is an effective way of recovering your data, especially if an effective alerting system is used. This becomes even more critical when that wiki information is on a site posted on your externally facing website and could be compromised by anyone. In this case, an effective alerts strategy, coupled with proactive monitoring of the site and an effective rollback policy for wiki pages, will alleviate any concerns about unscrupulous vandalism.

To make effective connections with your audience it is important to monitor your feeds and respond to your customers' concerns and comments. Setting alerts on blogs, so that you receive an email every time anyone posts a comment on an entry, will enable you to be responsive. This is good PR for the person who posted the original comment, but it also helps to stop your site being spammed by any bots that are using your blog to draw attention to their own blog. These automated blogs typically exist to drive traffic to their own site, and associated advertisements, and they place a link on your blog in the form of a trackback or link in a comment. These links are used by Google as a measure of how popular these external sites are, and are used to increase the page rank of that site. Again, having an effective alert process in place will enable you to remove the links to these sites before the web crawlers have indexed the site and artificially inflated their site popularity rankings.

TOOLS, TOOLS, TOOLS

Terms and concepts
Outside the firewall, blogs and wikis are just one part of the digital engagement toolset. There are many other tools:

TOOLS AND TERMS

- **Podcast** A digital media file, typically audio, made available for download from a website in a consistent format.

- **Vlogging** Short for 'video blogging', which delivers video or Internet television from blogs and from video sharing sites such as YouTube.

- **Moblogging** A mechanism allowing blog posts to be published from a mobile phone.

- **Phlogging** Short for 'photo blogging', where photos are uploaded from a mobile phone directly to the web for sharing.

- **Screencast** A recording of a computer screen, perhaps showing a demonstration of a feature which is captured in video format using a capture tool and uploaded to the web.

These tools, and many more like them, add to the wealth of news distribution mechanisms which encourage user generated content to be added to the web. With an effective plan for finding your customers, engaging with them and getting them to become advocates for your brand, you can leverage these Web 2.0 tools to your advantage and enhance your business.

There are so many tools to update your networking sites that it could take an age to go through them all to update them. Fortunately, there are information aggregators that allow you to pool relevant information. Some tools, Huddle for example, work well for online collaborative ventures or create online workspaces for virtual team work. Other tools, such as Digg, Reddit and Stumbleupon, relay content, news and information, keeping followers up to date. Some tools like Hunch and Yelp in the US are rating services for people to give feedback on a product or a service, and others like Google Reader are online personal aggregators of news. All of these sites are designed to make things easier to find on the social web, linking videos, blogs and other websites together in one useful place, ready to be tagged, marked as a favourite and commented upon by community.

Video

The value of meeting someone face to face cannot be underestimated if you want to be successful in business. However, there are alternatives such as talking to customers on the telephone or seeing them online. There are many applications available on the web that do this – both for consumers and corporates – and they help people communicate wherever they are. Voice over Internet protocol (VoIP) and a headset together enable seamless audio and video communication from computer to computer. All you need is a computer with audio and a webcam. Popular applications include Adobe Acrobat Connect, GoogleTalk, iChat, Intercall, Meetcam, Microsoft Live Meeting, Radvision, Stickam, Skype, Telepresence, WebEx and Yahoo! Messenger.

Blogs

Blogs are personal, compelling and can be hugely successful in a very short space of time. You can find blogs on almost any topic you care to name.

For example, Judith O'Reilly writes the Wife in the North blog.[8] Judith only started to blog when her husband, who wanted to bring up her children in a country setting away from London, moved the family to Northumberland, 30 minutes from the nearest town. Her husband was kept in London for weeks at a time with his work, so Judith started to blog in 2006 as a way of chronicling how different and challenging her new life was.

Her blog is notable for how quickly she managed to turn her blog into a book deal. Her blog was linked to by Tom Watson MP, an influential parliamentary blogger. Tom's blog was linked to by Iain Dale, another influential blogger. Iain's blog was commented upon by Andrew Sullivan, a writer and columnist. The comment came to the attention of Patrick Walsh, a literary agent based in the UK, who contacted Judith about a book deal. This is a classic example of how effective the word of mouth network can be in getting your message out. Judith was amazed by the attention. She wrote:[9]

Blogging is a strange and wonderful thing. I reached out into cyberspace because I needed to – not in any expectation of a book deal. Better than a book deal, any book deal, have been the kindly comments, e-mails and messages from strangers who aren't strangers any more who said: 'I read you and you made me laugh' and 'I read you and you made me cry'. My book deal isn't so much about money; it is more to do with the fact that blogging is a force to be reckoned with. Ultimately blogging is people willing to commit time, effort and emotion.

Mobile blogging

Moblogging, which is the ability to blog, upload videos or pictures from your mobile phone, has grown significantly over the past few years.

The ability to microblog, or use short status updates, post photos or videos, makes the moblogging concept compelling to the consumer and gives companies a great marketing opportunity to connect at the actual event.

Mobile blogging is popular with tourists, people on the move or people who want to post blog entries as they are happening. The ability to communicate with others at events, posting images of new announcements or items, shows readers what you are seeing at the time you are seeing it. You can post updates to your blog, upload photos, sound bites or video clips whilst you are actually at the event watching the news unfold. You are effectively blogging 'live'.

With the advent of applications for mobile phones such as Twitter and Facebook and location aware applications, you can automatically update your location from your device. This term has evolved to include any status update, image or video update from a mobile device or smart phone.

Microblogging: the shorter blog

Microblogging is defined as a shortened version of blogging, uploading an image or posting a video to a website. The most notable microblogging sites are Tumblr, Plurk, Yammer and Twitter, which has exploded in popularity since its launch in April 2006. More and more business is being conducted online, so the value of Twitter cannot be underestimated. With around 50 million status messages or tweets per day according to the Twitter blog, someone, somewhere, is listening to what you have to say. It's a hugely powerful way of promoting your business, connecting with your customers and creating buzz about your brand. With Twitter, you have up to 140 characters to create and post your message, which is then broadcast to the world. Anyone can follow you without your consent. Everything you tweet appears on your feed stream and anyone can click on the link to follow your status updates. If you want to build privacy into your status updates you can. You can decide to protect your updates so that they can't be seen by everyone. Then, when someone wants to follow you on Twitter, you can decide to permit them to follow you. Therefore only people you have individually authorised can see your Twitter stream.

It's very easy to get started on Twitter. All you need to do is to set up a profile and a unique user name on the site. The user name is used in the URL and takes the form of http://twitter.com/username. No spaces or characters other than underscores are permitted in the name. Users communicate with you directly by including your Twitter username, preceded by the '@' sign in their message, which is called a tweet. This message can be seen by anyone who follows the sender of the original message, so whole conversations can be followed. To privately send a tweet which can be seen by the recipient only you need to precede the tweet by the letter D. This is known as a direct message or DM.

You can customise your profile with extra information about yourself within the 160 character limit which is more than the 140 characters permitted by each Twitter status update. You can upload a photo and include a link to your website or blog. You build lists to group people into categories which can be seen by any-one who sees your profile. You can 'favourite' a particular tweet for your reference. This status message which can also be seen by others if they click on your favourites button on your page. You can tag topics by using a hashtag. A hashtag is a word preceded by the character # which can be searched for. If many people use the same hashtag, it can become a trend for others to use. The search func-tion in Twitter lets you search for phrases, words, hashtags or people.

The retweet
The most powerful mechanism is the art of the retweet. A retweet is when some-one rebroadcasts your original status update to their own followers, amplifying your message. There are three main things you need to think about when you planning a message and want it to be retweeted:

User names:
My own Twitter user name, @eileenb, is eight characters in length out of the available maximum of 140 characters. If I want to create something compelling in my status update to engage the audience and encourage a series of retweets then I need to consider this:

HOW TO GET YOUR STATUS RETWEETED

- I want to make sure that, when my message is rebroadcast, the context of the original message isn't lost. Therefore I need to make sure that my original message is short enough to be rebroadcast.

- The first few characters of my message when it is retweeted by another person looks like this: RT @eileenb. This phrase is 12 characters in length. I've counted one trailing space after the character 'b' for spacing purposes. This gives me 128 remaining characters to create my original message.

- Most third party Twitter clients use the form 'RT' at the start of the message, but that's not the only option available. Some seasoned Twitter users use the term 'via'. However, 'via' uses another character from my allocation and would leave only 127 characters for the message.

This is something to keep in mind when you're planning the update that you want to have retweeted. But what if you intend your message to be broadcast over and over again?

Multiple retweets:
Suppose your carefully crafted message, consisting of a maximum of 124 characters, gets retweeted and the news is so interesting that it gets retweeted again. A retweet appends a further name to the tweet which now looks like this: RT@eileenb @quiggles. This new format uses 22 characters from your original allocation of 140, including the trailing space. The more retweets you get, the more user names are appended to the message, leaving fewer characters for the actual message.

URL shorteners:
Try not to put a shortened URL at the end of your tweet. You may be well within your 140-character limit with the original tweet but after it's been retweeted twice without care, the last few characters may have disappeared from the URL, which could leave you with a URL that looks like

http://tinyurl.com/ydr

instead of the five or six characters you actually need to visit the destination page.

Getting your message rebroadcast
People buy from people and relationships do matter, even if they are relationships that started in 140-character form. Getting people to talk about you is important – as are referrals and retweets. Retweets are a great way of getting the message across and amplifying it throughout the Twitter audience. You'll never get poor content rebroadcast, so it's important to consider the impact of your message and its newsworthiness. Make sure you retweet other interesting pieces of information that you find to propagate to your own followers.

There is an awful lot of 'noise' on Twitter, and it is estimated that out of over 10 million users, only 5% of these accounts are actively posting updates. The average tweet per user is 1, which indicates a large number of unused accounts. Statistics currently show that over 50% of accounts are completely inactive. Your challenge is how to channel the relationship that you have created with your Twitter followers into something worthwhile for your business. It is important to remember that Twitter is like any other communications channel. Make your users feel valuable by responding to them, rebroadcasting their messages and giving them more visibility which will encourage positive responses from them. Asking for help often brings new and valuable connections you hadn't considered before. I have discovered new friends on Twitter. I have been at events and total strangers have introduced themselves to me. They have followed me on Twitter and, due to my friendly style of interaction, they feel they know me personally. When I announce that I'll be at an event and will be at a certain place at a specified time, my virtual friends come and say hello. This turns my existing virtual relationship into a face to face relationship and strengthens bonds. I was at a

trade show a couple of years ago and a man walked up to me extending his hand. 'Hi, I'm Gary', he said. I looked puzzled. 'Quiggles!' he announced. It was really great for me to meet someone with whom I'd been having a conversation for months but had never met.

Of course, with the huge amount of information flowing from Twitter, you need a client application to manage the people you follow and the messages they send. The most popular client application at the moment is Tweetdeck, although other applications like Twhirl and Hootsuite are popular. Applications for mobile devices like Twitterific, Twitterfon and Dabr help you tweet on the move. New applications appear and disappear regularly, so it's always a good idea to see what's hot or not at the moment.

VIRTUAL WORLDS AND GAMING

Large corporations such as Disney, Dell and Coca-Cola have a significant presence within virtual worlds because where users congregate there is an opportunity to do business. There are many forms of virtual worlds. There are worlds where you adopt an online identity and communicate with other users in an online environment whom you may or may not know. There are virtual online worlds like Second Life and World of Warcraft. Second Life enables its users to create a virtual identity and interact with other virtual identities with avatars in an online world.

Businesses have taken the example of user participation in these virtual worlds and have created online environments to engage users further. In Second Life, Apple has created an online store, while Microsoft has created virtual properties and theatres hosting online events. Sun has created a virtual campus for training its staff, and the BBC has hosted virtual music festivals.

Gaming and social interaction sites have a naturally symbiotic relationship that companies can leverage to engage their audience. Similar to virtual worlds, gaming environments feature altruistic games. In Facebook the Farmville MMORPG encourages players to give gifts to their farming neighbours and help out on their neighbours' farms. Co-operating in this way gives the player more experience points and helps them advance through the game. There are competitive MMORPG games such as Halo3, EverQuest and the World of Warcraft. In EverQuest, players participate in specific roles and collaborate with each other to win challenges. Pizza Hut has a business presence in the EverQuest game. All players need to do is type the command "/pizza" whilst they are playing EverQuest II. From within the game, the Pizza Hut website appears so that players can place an order for pizza whilst still playing the game. Companies that provide in-game adverts are not new in these types of online games, but this is the first example of being able to order a real pizza from a virtual world. Gamers don't mind these adverts either. Over 90% of gamers believe that real adverts add realism to the online game. The challenge for the advertiser, though, is that the players, on seeing the same adverts over and over again, soon begin to ignore them. New mechanisms that rotate adverts based on time of day are now being developed.

Even Twitter applications have appeared on the gaming scene. MMORPGs are hugely popular, as the millions of people who play Farmville, Mafia Wars and FishVille would testify. There is an in-game Twitter client for the World of Warcraft game called TweetCraft. World of Warcraft is the fastest selling PC game of all time, with millions of subscribers paying a monthly subscription of around $20. TweetCraft sends and receives messages from Twitter and Twitpic, and the Warcraft add-on receives messages from Twitter.

This collaboration between separate games enhances both of the applications. The ability to send and receive tweets whilst playing a game of World of Warcraft, upload screenshots of your game using TwitPic (a photo sharing site) and auto-matically post tweets about your achievements enhances the game and brings the community on board. You can also use a service such as Steam to digitally down-load games from the Internet, play and collaborate in an online community and engage with each other player socially. This many to many communications mech-anism is similar to that which allows Facebook to encourage gamers to see their friends recent gaming activity. Players can view their friends' groups, achieve-ments and games purchased. This friend network encourages gamers to try new games purchased by their online buddies, adding to Steam's revenue stream.

With the massive and varied choice of applications around, which one should you choose for your business? Should you create your own network for your hobby or join an established group? How many social media sites are there to engage in? What are they used for? Which site is suitable for you in your work, your home life or useful in your thirst for knowledge? Is there really a social networking site for everything imaginable?

SUMMARY

- There are many social media tools. Take time to choose the right ones for your business.
- Business to business blogging is vital to show your credibility, capability and authenticity.
- Use syndication to reduce your workload.
- Consider an external wiki to get input from the community.
- Use video sharing sites for 'how to' videos.
- Use microblogging for short impactful status messages.
- Try to create compelling content that gets retweeted.
- Consider the use of virtual worlds – wherever users congregate online there is an opportunity to do business.

5   NETWORKS

In this chapter we'll talk about some of the other main online interaction sites used for business, community, friends and family. We'll look at hobby sites, location sites and music streaming sites. We'll talk about online classified ad sites which enable you to find almost anything online, we'll talk about how you can buy and sell items. Twitter, the current darling of the digital conversation, has become the news hub of the moment, and we'll try to understand why this is. Finally, we'll look at how Generation Y is changing the way we work and how the way we interact is changing the way companies work. We'll start to look brand strategy and where you can start the conversation and collaboration with your customers.

A SITE FOR EVERY PURPOSE

Wherever you look there appear to be sites for connecting and engaging, yet I've only mentioned a few so far. Instead of researching an exhaustive list containing every different online interaction site I can find, I'll talk about a few. I've grouped some of the more popular online interaction sites below into the types of activities that they tend to be used for. This list isn't exhaustive, however; there are thousands of social networking sites, and the list is changing all the time. Wikipedia has a more comprehensive list and the main countries where these sites are popular, but it too is out of date. Here are the main popular sites at the moment.

Business networks

LinkedIn, with over 55 million registered users throughout the world, is considered the premier business networking site. There are opportunities to get introduced to new connections through your existing network, look for a job, or ask questions from industry experts. These connections can consist of your direct connections, their connections (your second degree connections) and their connections (your third degree connections). LinkedIn is mainly used to find jobs, to recommend others in your network and receive recommendations for your work. Recommendations on your profile are useful if you're looking for a new Recruiters and potential employers use these recommendations to determine how many people have recommended you, and they use the details on your profile to gauge your suitability for a role.

Ecademy is a business community founded in 1998 and claims to have 'millions of users'. It enables business people to connect through online networking. It uses connections from its membership to invite its members to business networking

events and offers one to one meetings between its users. It offers a community that connects, refers and helps one another.

Xing is a business network with over 8 million members. Users connect using the six degrees of separation theory and have the ability to view upcoming events and search for other members. Like other networks, Xing allows them to advertise their skills and request connections across the site.

Ryze has over 500,000 members in specialist groups. It advertises the fact that members can 'rise up' through quality business networking. The site offers interaction, the chance to make connections and grow your networks. It offers networks on topics as diverse as 'A joke a day', 'Women in Networking' and 'MLM (Multi Level Marketing) for serious Network Marketers'.

Community
Ning is a site dedicated to building your own online community site where your users can congregate. These customised sites can be used for social clubs, committees, leisure activities and hobbyist sites. There are options to customise your site and to make it individual and eye-catching for your visitors.

Mumsnet is a site designed for parents. Anyone with children can register on the site and discuss parenting, childcare, contraception and issues of the day. In the run up to the 2010 general election in the UK, each political party was invited to answer questions on the site. Topics ranged from what each party's manifesto for mothers would be to what specific benefits for childcare they could expect to see with the new government.

Friends and family
Facebook, with over 600 million users, is a huge social site for personal and business use. It was initially used as a closed network within a walled garden for students at US universities, but the site was subsequently opened to all in 2005. It categorises users into different networks which can be towns, workplaces, companies or schools. Facebook has a huge number of applications written by developers to enhance the social nature of the site, using games quizzes and other methods to engage. Many companies use Facebook pages for business.

Bebo ('blog early blog often') is a social networking site which has been adopted by younger teens and children to socialise with their friends. They can customise their profiles with modules, quizzes and groups, with the opportunity to include a lifestream platform and timeline. A lifestream is a collection of items uploaded to the site and displayed in chronological order. Items can include video, photos, blog entries, notes and links. Bebo takes the privacy of its users very seriously and subscribes to Internet safety initiatives for children.

Friendster was created in 2002 and was an early attempt to connect friends and family together. It enabled you to meet new people by connecting to the friends of your friends, thereby taking advantage of the second degree network to extend your own circle of friends. It was initially designed to be an online dating site, but there was a rise in people who created fake identities on the site. This increase in

'fakesters' destroyed the ability to effectively connect real people using their social graph. Its popularity has waned in the US, but the site is still growing in Asia and has almost 120 million users.

Hi5 is a popular site for people to connect mainly in Latin America. It allows users to create an online profile, share photos and set up music streams on their profile.

Orkut, which is owned by Google, is very popular in Latin America and especially in Brazil. It is also very popular in India, but less so around the rest of the world. The site can be customised with themes to reflect particular tastes, you can add videos to your profile and employ a ranking scheme to grade your friends on a popularity scale. Orkut has had issues with spam applications in the past, and has been banned in some countries due to the lack of privacy controls, particularly over photos of women and concerns over ethical issues.

Hobby

Shelfari is a site dedicated to book lovers. It is owned by Amazon and allows users to build virtual bookshelves of the books they love. Shelfari allows bibliophiles to engage in discussions with other users and make recommendations on books to read.

Knowledge

Wikipedia is the epitome of social media concepts where the collective knowledge of the community is freely given to benefit all. Wikipedia started in 2001, and thousands of contributors have created a changing encyclopaedia. This dynamic online book is used by over 340 million people per month and is the fifth most read website in the world. There are over 13 million articles, 78% of which are written in languages other than English. The non-profit organisation is supported entirely by donations from its users who, in 2009, gave over $7.5 million to keep the infrastructure running and to try and maintain free access 'to the sum of all human knowledge'.[10]

Location

Foursquare is the current mobile device darling for announcing where you are. It operates in a similar way to Brightkite and Gowalla, which are also location announcing applications designed for mobile devices. It offers location based status updates for you to record the places you have visited. It also offers the opportunity to upload photos from that location and comment on the site. Friends can then receive alerts about your location. Identi.ca also allows you to upload microblog status updates from wherever you are.

Music

MySpace is a very popular site frequented by Generation Y and Z, and with musicians. Musicians have the ability to upload their entire catalogue of songs for download as MP3 files and to create playlists of their songs. Artists like Lilly Allen and Sean Kingston were initially discovered on MySpace, and many more have come to prominence from this site. The site appeals to teens and young adults due to the ability to heavily customise their profiles and their online page which is organised and used like a bedroom. This flexibility has kept MySpace popular with

Generation Y and Z despite the growth of Facebook – which has an interface which is much less customisable.

Last.fm is a music streaming site which recommends music according to your personal tastes. If you flag that you like a particular singer, then other songs from singers of a similar genre will be streamed to you. Any song you don't like will be removed from your individual playlist and there are opportunities to share your favourite music with others in your network by tagging your songs.

Updates

Plurk is a Twitter-like microblogging tool which shows user timelines and conversation history. It allows you to set your mood and track your followers' moods also. It is popular in Asia, but less so in Europe and the US.

There are thousands more of these sites, covering every genre imaginable. With the perpetual beta of Web 2.0, new sites pop up weekly and less popular sites fade from prominence. There are some sites that seem to have withstood the test of time. These sites cater for our primary business needs. Buying and selling things.

CLASSIFIEDS

When it comes to information, education and things to purchase, you can find just about everything on the Internet. There are directory sites pointing to other interesting websites, sites that sell and sites that advertise. But apart from huge, direct selling sites like Amazon, where do you go for classified ads, the sort that you find in the back of your local paper?

Craigslist is an online classified advertisement site that began in 1995 when Craig Newmark started to email his friends in the San Francisco area about local events. People placed paid adverts onto the site covering myriad products and services, including personal ads and adult services. It's now ranked 30th in the world in terms of page views per month, which is surprising for a site with such a simple design (see Figure 5.1). It has no images and allows minimal web page customisation and it now spans over 60 countries and over 700 regions.

Word of mouth about these local events ensured that both Craigslist subscribers and postings grew quickly. Craigslist soon also began to carry postings about job vacancies and small ads, which led to new categories being created. Unfortunately, lack of moderation on the site led to some underhand activities such as robbery, rape and murder.[11]

As Craig Newmark says, Craigslist works because it gives people a voice, a sense of community trust and even intimacy. Consistency of down-to-earth values, customer service and simplicity are also important.[12] But, there are always people who will use these networks for their own, not necessarily honourable means.

In addition to the usual definition of classified advertisements, there is also the concept of bidding for a product on auction sites. The market leader here is eBay,

Figure 5.1 Craigslist classified advertising site

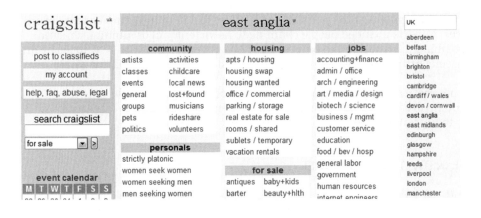

which has listings advertising almost everything you can think of. The success of eBay from a reputational point of view is that you can read feedback about the seller by the buyer of the item. This fosters a sense of community amongst the buyers. If one buyer criticises the seller, the seller's reputation falls below 100% and never recovers. All feedback remains permanently attached to the seller's profile, along with a list of items that the seller has sold or purchased.

Some of the items for sale turn out to be much more successful than originally anticipated, or are sold at inflated prices as a result of viral notoriety.

Viral notoriety

Amusing or strange items for sale are often emailed around the Internet, adding to their notoriety and ultimately their saleability. This phenomenon has produced a new challenge. Some sellers will post a picture of the item for sale, with the naked image of the photographer in the photograph.[13] Reflectoporn, as it has come to be known, is where a person takes a photograph of a reflective object, such as a kettle or cutlery, while they are naked. Their image appears in the reflection of the item. The seller then puts this item up for sale on eBay with the photo to accompany it.[14] The link to the eBay item is then forwarded around the web virally. Other items spread virally due to their comedic nature. I remember a forwarded email with a link to an eBay wedding dress. A man modelled his ex-wife's wedding dress and included several photos of him wearing the dress complete with pony-tail, beard and t-shirt. He explained that he was 'selling it hoping to get enough money for maybe a couple of Mariners tickets and some beer.' The $1200 dress sold for $3850.

Another eBay item which spread virally across the Internet was the Haunted Painting[15] which was viewed over 30,000 times in February 2000. According to the seller, the painting carried a form of curse. The description on eBay claimed that the characters in the painting moved during the night, and that they would

sometimes leave the painting and enter the room in which it was being displayed. News of the listing was spread virally by Internet users who forwarded the link to their friends or wrote their own pages about it. Some people claimed that simply viewing the photos of the painting made them feel ill or have unpleasant experiences. Reports included people claiming to be violently ill or fainting, children screaming upon seeing the painting and observers were said to be gripped by an 'unseen entity'. Bidding began at $199 and the painting was sold for $1025.

So notoriety and visibility do seem to enhance sales. And notoriety, as the wedding dress seller discovered, can inflate the price far beyond anything originally anticipated.

THE INSTANT NEWS CHANNEL

Twitter seems to have evolved to being at the centre of news. It's a real-time hub where there are opportunities for sharing of information, news and media from any other social media source, whether it be a YouTube video, photos from a shared photo site, a link to comments or a new post on a blog. Everyone can propagate information, news and stories within moments and the man on the street can broadcast a story that spreads around the world in a flash. Everyone has a voice on Twitter and, joined together, it's a really powerful voice. The power of the crowd is enormous. People can create their own news.

Take for example, the Trafigura news story. In 2009, the *Guardian* newspaper in the UK claimed to have conclusive proof that toxic waste had been released in Côte d'Ivoire and reported that it had been prevented from covering remarks made in Parliament. Guido Fawkes, a political blogger, speculated that this injunction was linked to the Trafigura case. Although there was a news blackout in the UK, the Twitter community ensured that the story remained current, topical and at the forefront of news. Trafigura became a trending topic on Twitter, with thousands of messages all tagged with the hashtag #Trafigura. The gagging order on the *Guardian* was lifted the next day and the paper confirmed that Trafigura had been the source of the order.

This is really significant. Every member of the community has the ability to become a broadcaster and a commentator on the news.

The broadcaster gains credibility with their audience. Writers build relationships with their readers and the interaction between the newscaster and the readers becomes more personal.

Often people don't initially see the value of Twitter. They don't see the benefit of the real-time interaction with a huge potential audience. One of my friends, James, could not understand why people used Twitter at all. He felt that it was a stream of constant chatter distracting him from his day job. Now Twitter keeps him in touch with some of the key influencers in his industry, and he can have a

useful dialogue with them on a far more regular basis than just at PR and industry events.

Twitter and Facebook can be linked together with status updates from Twitter appearing on Facebook and vice versa. Twitter has also integrated with LinkedIn so that status messages from Twitter appear on the feed at LinkedIn. The bringing together of parts of the Web 2.0 world in this way means that the edges of the worlds of each conversational tool are starting to blur more and more. These applications are no longer used in isolation, and this symbiotic relationship brings benefits on all sides.

But is Twitter leading or trailing edge? Does Twitter make the news, or just amplify some of the messages made by the few leading edge influencers on Twitter? Is **any** news broadcast mechanism leading edge? Or are we all just avid consumers and followers of the news? This news could be any type of information which happens to be reported by a Twitter user and comes to prominence as more and more people refer to the item so that it becomes a trend?

When you need to find out what's happening, where do you go? You probably don't pick up the newspapers, which might have been printed 18 hours earlier. Do you turn on the TV? Or do you listen to the radio? You will find out the news from your trusted advisers and they, very likely, will have got their information from the instant news channel – Twitter. Time and time again Twitter has had information and pictures about world events long before any other news channel has been able to begin broadcasting. When it comes to emergencies, Twitter seems to be quicker at disseminating information than the popular media channels. In the Australian bush fires in February 2009, the Australian fire authority sent out alerts using Twitter. In Mumbai in 2008, Twitter users helped to compile a list of the dead and injured during the attacks and announced locations where volunteers could go to donate blood.

Images uploaded to the web from a mobile device are also used to very powerful effect. In 2009, US Airways flight 1549, which had just taken off from New York's LaGuardia Airport, experienced a bird strike. The plane had to land on the Hudson River, which was a fairly routine simulator exercise for the pilot to do. News propagated around the world fairly quickly. The plane landed at 3.31 p.m.; within 6 minutes it was being reported in blogs and tweets, and images were being uploaded to photo sharing sites on the web (Figure 5.2). The time in the image below, shows the local time on, my computer and not the local time where the plane landed.

Photo sharing sites such as Flickr, YFrog and Twitpic, which permit the uploading of photos from mobile devices, guarantee worldwide transmission of images and on the spot access to eyewitness accounts. In an hour or so, more than one hundred pages of Twitter messages about the crash were generated and accessed by newsfeeds around the world. By the time the TV cameras and crews arrived, the passengers were being rescued and the plane was being moved to the jetty. I was looking at Twitter watching the news unfold in text and images. Where were you?

Figure 5.2 Tweet about the plane landing on the Hudson River

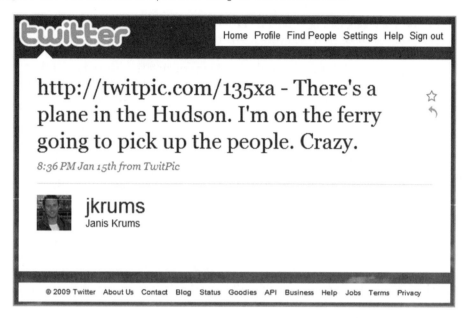

When J.F. Kennedy was shot, the world held its breath watching the grainy footage of the last few moments of his life. This 8mm film was shot by an amateur who was watching the motorcade. This footage was played over and over again as experts tried to analyse where the bullet came from. When Elvis Presley died in 1977, the world was informed by an official press release which hit the newspapers and TV some time later. His LP records immediately rushed to the top of the charts. When Michael Jackson was rushed into hospital at 1.14 p.m. on 25 June 2009 with suspected cardiac arrest, the news didn't trickle out from normal media channels. Community generated news site TMZ, which relies on 'hot tips', news snippets and images uploaded by its readers, was the first to break the news – well ahead of any traditional media outlets with reporters and paparazzi. This information spread around Twitter at an unprecedented rate. Biz Stone, co-founder of Twitter, said: 'We saw an instant doubling of tweets per second the moment the story broke. It is the biggest jump in tweets per second since the U.S. presidential election.'[16] By 10.30 p.m., tweets containing the words 'Michael Jackson' accounted for approximately 12% of all Twitter traffic (Figure 5.3), and there were so many requests for 'Michael Jackson' on Google that it was deemed by Google to be a denial of service attack.

Hundreds of memorial sites soon appeared across the Web and on Facebook. His albums rocketed straight to the top of the charts, and the film of his rehearsals for his concert zoomed into the top 10 movies within days. Michael Jackson's death, occurring in the glare of the beady eye of Twitter and the digital spotlight, has ensured that his star status will not fade for some considerable time yet.

Figure 5.3 Comment on Michael Jackson dominating Twitter traffic[17]

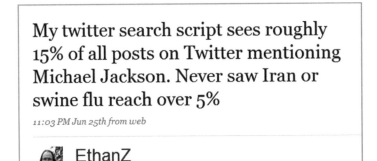

> My twitter search script sees roughly
> 15% of all posts on Twitter mentioning
> Michael Jackson. Never saw Iran or
> swine flu reach over 5%
>
> *11:03 PM Jun 25th from web*
>
> **EthanZ**
> Ethan Zuckerman

SOCIAL NETWORKS AND THE YOUNGER GENERATION

Generation Y is changing the way we work. Their ability to engage with multiple streams of communication, tools and websites and ably deal with the fire hose of information flooding at them will define our future working patterns. Generation Y thinks email is *passé* and tends not to use it. Generation Y graduates are moving into fast track management. They will be the next leaders of business and industry. Their current ways of working will become the new way of working for the baby boomer generation and Generation X – whether they like it or not.

Different online networking sites tend to be populated by different age groups. Teenagers and young adults tend to focus their attention on MySpace, Facebook, Bebo and Piczo. Adults of all ages now use Facebook for social and business purposes. The largest growth sector on Facebook is currently women in the 55–65 age range. Teenagers use these types of sites to network and form social groups with those in their peer group.[18] They join subgroups and share information among their friends.

TEENAGERS' BEHAVIOUR ON SOCIAL NETWORKING SITES

- Teenagers heavily customise their online profile as it is an easy way for them to express themselves.
- They update their profile and modify their status and other information regularly. They do this as an extension of their personality in much the same way as they will customise their bedroom.
- Their profile names are adorned with non-alphanumeric characters.
- They have mashups of media associated with their profile and the text in the 'about me' section changes frequently.
- Teenagers' online profiles are used as an extension of their status updates and their online identities.

This is a completely different form the way Generation X and older people use their profiles on these types of sites.

But why is this important in business? It's important to have a good understanding of how Generation Y and Z behave on social networking sites, and how they use their profiles, mobility and connections to live their digital life. Knowing these behaviour patterns gives you a great opportunity to effectively tune your social media architecture so that you can attract the correct audience to the right place. If your product sells to the young, then marketing your product in a way that is attractive to the young will give you credibility in their world and a positive return on your sales and marketing investment.

Have you considered your community and digital online conversation strategy at your company? Have you thought about how you can use social media to bring marketing by your community of friends into your customer and partner marketing campaigns today? Do you consider this strand of conversational marketing important at all? Are you looking at your competitors and watching how they are using online community tools to gain advantages over you? Do you currently have a two-way, push–pull marketing strategy or do you plan to promote your brand using the voice of the community talking about you and creating user generated content on your behalf?

THE NEW WAY OF MARKETING

By looking at best practices from leading companies and reviewing what others are doing today in their engagement with the community, you can start to create your strategic plan. You can integrate community marketing and your learning from online user behaviours to engage, share and drive conversations with customers and partners online. Using social engagement technologies, you can explore how to create demand and excitement for Web 2.0 interaction. You can create new marketing and selling opportunities and you can gain new insights into your audience.

> You can use conversational marketing to drive your own local marketing efforts to capture mindshare and increase satisfaction amongst your customers.

Perhaps the term 'social media' has skewed your perception about this new form of marketing. Underneath the glitz, the viral propagation and the news, is this really the way that you want to communicate with your customers? Do you already engage in some form of social communication? Are you communicating with your customers, partners, friends and competitors? Are you helping out your community, are you working with your virtual friends? Are your friends amplifying your message or are you collaborating with intent? And if you are collaborating with intent, what is the benefit to you? What is the value to your customers?

Every link we share, every blog we post, every video we upload adds to community collaboration and contributes to the conversation.

Comments, rebroadcasts, interaction and discussion add to brand awareness. The 'word of mouse', as Seth Godin terms this phenomenon, increases potential sales. An increase in sales leads to revenue growth and a better ROI for your digital marketing efforts. But before you launch your brand onto all of the engagement channels, you need to clearly define and develop your strategy and plan. You need a comprehensive plan and you need to define goals for what you want to achieve.

Once you have a strategy and an objective to achieve your goals, you need to think about how your brand will be perceived. In the next chapter we'll start to think about your online brand.

SUMMARY

- Classified social media sites are useful for B2C opportunities.
- Choose your site wisely. There are social networking sites for every purpose.
- Getting your campaign to go viral can be very good for business.
- Twitter can be used to broadcast and receive relevant news in almost real time.
- Generation Y uses social media sites in a different way than older users, and this should be taken into account when planning marketing campaigns.
- Conversational marketing increases mindshare and increases satisfaction.
- Does your strategy take into account push–pull marketing and conversational marketing? It should.

6 THE ONLINE BRAND

The first thing to consider about having a presence online is, quite simply, what you want people to think when they first meet you. By 'you' we might mean your product, your firm, or your cause, rather than you personally. The essence of that first impression is important as it is continued through repeated social online interaction. That essence is something you need to determine before showing your face at the party or getting your foot in the door.

Part of presenting your online brand is considering the medium and the tools you will use.

This is really critical because not all businesses should use all tools.

This chapter will show you what goes into distilling that essence into something that works for you as well as your customers. But how do you get the best out of the web?

Think about how you intend to promote your brand on the web and also how the 'personality of your brand (whether your brand represents a product or your own persona) works well in the social media world. It's no coincidence that the medium most often used to demonstrate the fun or quality of a new video game is video. Only through movement and monitoring actual game play can customers get a sense of what's in it for them when they purchase the new first-person shooter. If you are a better public speaker than writer, you may well consider having audio podcasts or video as your online medium of choice, because it will show your ideas and yourself in the best light. Likewise, if you are more a person of words than pictures, choosing a medium that relies more heavily on deftness with text (Twitter, blogging, Internet Relay Chat, etc.) may be the place to begin. The expense to the business has to be weighed against what the business wants to get done. Small businesses won't necessarily have the money to spare for big fancy video or sound production equipment.

As part of this discussion we will also look into what can go wrong when using the online tools. We will look at issues such as identity theft, reputation damage, profile-jacking, and harassment. While these may not deter you from an online presence, it's best to consider what can go wrong and to try to protect against these scenarios from the beginning. We will also consider what can be done when clones of you start to appear across the web. We will look at how

you can measure your online brand effectiveness or reputation. Just as a partygoer may need a trusted friend to help her realise there is piece of spinach caught in her teeth, so do businesses and business people need measurable and objective targets to gauge how well they are doing online. We will cover some of the ways to determine if things have gone horribly wrong as well, if your brand or personal identity has been hijacked, or if the customers are not reacting as well to your brand as you'd hoped.

Finally, we will look at how brands can change over time. An online brand may be slower to change than its human makers –but brands can and do change, and figuring how to finesse an existing brand morphing into a new one is a good and potentially profitable exercise.

MANAGING YOUR BRAND

Managing your online brand is key to your success. It is important to make sure that the information you want to be released is on message, accurate and positive. And with this type of personal engagement offering the potential for things to go very wrong, it can be rather daunting.

> There is a lot of buzz around social media and social networking sites at the moment, and in order to keep your business at the forefront of your industry you need to be part of the conversation.

The move away from traditional push marketing to pull marketing and the word of mouth network is creating a more dynamic and engaging marketplace for your brand. If you are looking to buy a book on Amazon, you'll often look at the recommendations from others who have bought the book. You may also look at other recommended books to go with your original choice.

> Peer recommendations are powerful and can clinch deals.

Listening to your online and offline friends is much more powerful than buying from a static website. People buy from people, so an effective and positive brand is an important tool to have.

Good PR, bad PR

A great example of a company carefully managing its online brand is Apple. Everything that gets out into the 'open', so to speak, is carefully managed and controlled from a PR, messaging and brand perspective. This approach ensures that Apple's outbound messages are exactly what the company wishes to convey. This generates a huge amount of excitement among Apple fans desperate for news about future products. Forums, blogs and tweets abound speculating about the latest releases. The fans of Apple products create buzz and excitement from tiny snippets of the corporate message and no access at all to early versions of the products.

Compare that style of messaging with the approach taken by Microsoft. When Microsoft prepares to release a new version of its software, it releases very early beta copies of the code out to thousands of software and hardware testers. These testers have signed a Non-Disclosure Agreement, yet copies of this beta code sometimes find their way out onto peer to peer file sharing sites such as Bit Torrent. The early version of the code is discussed and speculated upon at length by the community and by technology journalists. If Microsoft subsequently decides to withdraw a component from the product build for whatever reason, or decides to fork, or create a new direction of the software build, perhaps deciding to drop certain features as they move forward with product development, then their brand and reputation can suffer in the press as a result.

These different approaches to product marketing seem to have very different results. Microsoft's apparent openness, which works really well with the concepts of social media marketing, often disappoints the audience. Apple, on the other hand, with its obsession with secrecy and lack of openness in social media spaces, generates an evangelical following by saying almost nothing.

So how do you manage your brand effectively? Brand management is all about making certain that you have a consistent message. It's about making sure that everyone inside the company follows your messaging guidelines and knows what to say. It's about damage control if there are problems further down the line. It's about consistency and communication. It's actually about empowering your employees and trusting them. And it's very hard to do that well without proper guidelines in place.

Your Twitter messages (tweets) can be seen by more people than you can imagine. James Andrews, who tweets under the name of @KeyInfluencer, was due to do a presentation in Memphis. James worked for Ketchum, a global PR management agency, and his presentation was intended for the Communications group at FedEx whose head office is in Memphis. He arrived at the airport in Memphis in January 2009 and sent a Twitter message (Figure 6.1) to his followers.

Figure 6.1 The tweet that upset a FedEx Employee

True confession but I'm in one of those towns where I scratch my head and say "I would die if I had to live here!

10:58 PM Jan 14th, 2009 from twhirl ⤺ Reply ⇄ Retweet

 keyinfluencer
James Andrews

A FedEx employee saw the tweet and wrote an email. He copied his mail not only to the Ketchum directors and vice-presidents, but also up the management chain at FedEx. FedEx was founded in Memphis and is the city's largest private employer. The Employee Communications team responded to James:[19]

> Many of my peers and I feel this is inappropriate. ... A hazard of social networking is people will read what you write.

Two days later, James posted a response on his website:[20]

> Two days ago I made a comment on Twitter that was the emotional response to a run in I had with an intolerant individual. Everyone knows that at 140 characters Twitter does not allow for context and therefore my comments were misunderstood. If I offended the residents of Memphis, TN I'm sorry. That was not my intention.

Ketchum responded in a statement: *'It was a lapse in judgment and we've apologized to our client. We greatly value the longstanding relationship. It is our privilege to work with them.'*

Now there may be an underlying story other than the one splashed all over the blogosphere, and reading through the many comments after his post, there were speculations about other reasons. But I suppose it comes back to a simple tenet about publishing on the Internet:

> Quite simply, don't publish anything online that you wouldn't want to be written on your headstone, or indeed, quoted back at you by a barrister in a court of law.

STARTING TO CREATE YOUR PERSONAL BRAND

I'm often dismayed at some of the photos I see on Facebook and other sites which have been uploaded by people who aren't in my immediate network of friends. These photos are visible to me through the fact that the photos of my friends have been tagged by **their** friends. Unfortunately some of these photos are inappropriate and not photos I'd want to see on the page of one of my team. I'm a manager and I look on various different networking sites like Facebook and LinkedIn to find out information about people who could be potential employees. I'm saddened to see the lack of thought and discretion by some people in my extended network. These people are not my direct acquaintances. They are the friends of my direct acquaintances, so they are one step out of my immediate network. People are also sometimes indiscreet on Twitter too. James Andrews's tweet could potentially have damaged a good customer relationship, which is certainly not the thing to do in these uncertain times. In the run-up to the 2010 general election in the UK, Stuart Maclennan was removed as a candidate from the Scottish Labour Party after 'totally unacceptable language which he has expressed online'

On Facebook, the profile settings allow you to display various pieces of information on your public profile. You can include your private email address on the public page. This does have its drawbacks, however. Sometimes when I've been researching potential employees, or business partners, I've been hesitant to take the conversation further due to some of the information I've found on the public profile.

If you're considering starting off and creating your own personal online brand or you wish to project a more positive image of yourself than might already be on the web, there are some basic steps you can take to get you started.

- Search for your name on the Internet. If someone has written something bad about you then it's likely that your prospective employer will have seen it. If you are searching for a job a recruitment agency will also find any information about you when they search for your details.

- Try to connect with all of your contacts online. Find the relevant addresses and make the connection with everyone in your network. Be careful, however, that harvesting contacts from your work contacts list might be in breach of your company privacy policy.

- Get a website – or, if you're hesitant about your coding skills, get a blog. You need to have a presence on the web. You may consider your website to be a static business card with your online curriculum vitae and details of your skills. If you have a blog and ensure that it is regularly updated, it will rise higher in search stack rankings and make your investment in time pay off in the long run.

- If you're publicising your email address to one and all, make sure that you have sensible email names. Names like studmuffin@mymail.com and evilbitch@yourmail.com may be funny when you're still at college, but you need to consider whether a prospective employer wants to hire you for that top job you've been looking for.

- Makes sure your LinkedIn, Facebook and Twitter profiles display appropriate information. You may think that the information that you've put into these is pithy, witty and humorous. Consider whether your next employer would think that your brand is appropriate.

- Contribute to the conversation. Don't spend your time lurking on sites that you find. If you have something interesting and relevant to say, add to the conversation and get your voice and ideas heard.

- If you do blog, remember to link, link, and link. Refer on your blog to quality posts you find, and acknowledge people that link to you. Links equate to reputation and credibility. Retweet interesting tweets and thank people who retweet your messages.

- Be careful what you say on your Twitter, Facebook and LinkedIn feeds. Do you really want to share too much information and go into detail about your personal life? Bleeping the swear words out with *** doesn't really help if you're trying to create the correct image online.

- Consider the friends of friends networks. I may not follow you on Twitter directly, but I may follow someone who follows you. How can you guarantee that people who contact you are not saying something in a conversation to you that will upset a prospective employer? Use the blocking feature of Twitter if you're concerned about someone's continued use of inappropriate messages.

- Create a business card with your email address, Skype name, Twitter name, LinkedIn profile, Facebook page and blog URL. Make your online brand addresses visible and make sure that you drive everyone to your online brand.

- If you use Facebook for your private and public personas, then learn to use the privacy settings within the application (Figure 6.2). Make sure that only the information that you want to publicise outside your network of accepted friends is actually the information you wish the world to see.

- Publicise your brand. Everywhere. The most successful online experts are everywhere you happen to look. They contribute and interact with their friends and colleagues on social networks, they comment on blogs and they are very vocal. They are also very well known across the web.

Figure 6.2 Where to apply Facebook privacy settings

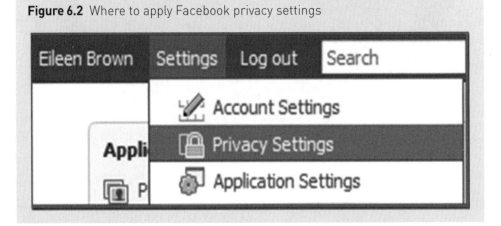

I use the privacy settings on my profiles across the various websites I use regularly and layer different settings like an onion (Figure 6.3). As you get closer and closer to me and get to know me personally, you will find out more and more about me. Visiting my website gives you a limited amount of information about me, viewing my profile on Twitter gives you a little more. Finally I use my Facebook account for the most personal aspects of my personal life and my business life.

Corporate pages on Facebook
Investing in brand management takes time and effort. You will completely underestimate the investment in time required to make your digital brand successful. It's not at all easy to keep up an interesting, regular flow of articles,

Figure 6.3 My 'onion layer' approach to my privacy settings

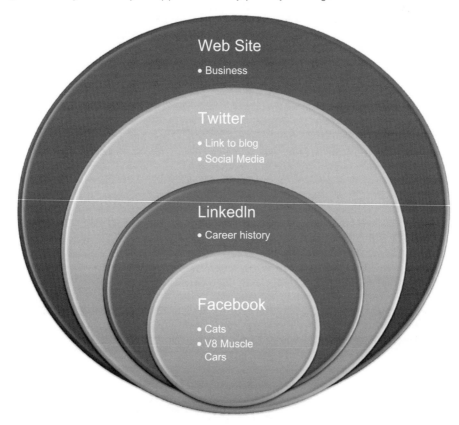

status updates and information for your audience. However, if you keep your messages topical, thought provoking, interesting or even controversial you'll see the conversation intensify and will start to reap the rewards.

Facebook has been used for personal friendships since its inception, but over time, with the increase in the number of users, companies have started to get involved. Companies have pages dedicated to promoting their business, and Facebook allows groups to be created, which fans can join, so that businesses can promote their special offers and encourage people to become fans. Facebook recognised the need to have corporate identities using unique names on the site. In May 2009 Facebook permitted personal user names for profiles and pages. Your Facebook profile or page for your business appears as

http://www.facebook.com/WorkingTheCrowd/

instead of

Entering a Facebook username as a search term on Facebook or searching for that name on the web enables people to find friends and organisations with common names.

Companies, who own the right to their company name, sometimes find that their name has been pre-registered by cyber squatters. Fortunately they can make the business case to Facebook to have their name restored to them. Facebook states that it reserves 'the right to remove and/or reclaim any username at any time for any reason and that if someone's username infringes a company's intellectual property rights then there are ways to reclaim that name by filling in the IP infringement form'.[21] Hopefully you might still be able to claim your rightful company name on Facebook if you haven't done so already.

Pseudonyms and staying anonymous

There's a cartoon that's been doing the rounds on the Internet for years. The image is of a dog at a computer and the caption reads 'On the Internet, no one knows you're a dog'. It was created by Peter Steiner for the *New Yorker* magazine back in 1993. It's a classic cartoon of the Internet age, and it highlights just how easy it is to fool everyone online because it's so easy to send and receive messages in relative anonymity.

Many bloggers enjoy posting without revealing their identity, and indeed some bloggers turn their hobby into a successful and lucrative venture. An example of anonymous blogging hit the news at the end of 2009. 'Belle de Jour' was a pseudonym for a blogger who wrote about her activities in the sex trade. She used her earnings to finance her PhD studies. Her blog was noticed by the *Guardian* newspaper which gave her the 'blog of the year' award in 2003. Her extremely well written blog appeared to be tailored so completely to male sexual fantasies that many journalists speculated that she was actually a man.

Her candid and scurrilous blog was published as a book, *The Intimate Adventures of a London Call Girl.* This book was subsequently turned into a TV series in the UK, starring Billie Piper as Belle. In November 2009 Belle decided to disclose her identity to the broadsheet newspapers in the UK, as she believed that a former boyfriend was about to reveal her identity in the tabloid press. Surprisingly enough, Belle revealed herself as Dr Brooke Magnanti. Brooke is a student of informatics, epidemiology and forensic science who works at Bristol University's Centre for Nanoscience and Quantum Information. Revealing her identity totally smashed the misconception that she was male or that she had been forced into the sex trade for other reasons than she stated in her blog.

There are different schools of thought about whether it matters if your messages online are from you as a representative of the company, or if you are communicating under a pseudonym. There are some bloggers who hide their identity in order to be more candid about the company that they work for. An example of a hidden identity is the Microsoft blogger who uses the name 'Mini MSFT'. Mini has been blogging anonymously about the inner workings of Microsoft since 2004 and has a huge readership. He or she has a policy of total anonymity which encourages employees to have an open discussion about the company and its inner workings on his blog. He is credited with changing some of the company's internal processes around the end of year pay review process which has led to greater transparency throughout the organisation. The blog called Fake Steve Jobs was written by someone who hid his identity for over a year before being revealed as the journalist Daniel Lyons, a writer at *Newsweek*.

Whilst these kinds of anonymous postings on blogs didn't detract from the quality of information, or do much damage to the writers involved, there are much darker sides to consider. There is a fundamental requirement to protect children from the darker parts of the Internet, and the new applications, with sharing, collaboration and interaction, can be a potential minefield for keeping our children safe online. The media portrayals of danger give individuals a grossly inaccurate view of what is actually happening which is influencing companies to create fixes and offer new technologies that are often not fixing the real problem. It is important to understand how to help your children be safe.

We hear stories of Internet grooming, and read about the efforts of CEOP (Child Exploitation and Online Protection) to try and encourage children to report any specific activity. Paedophiles engaging in grooming activities try to trick children into meeting them. They often pose as teenagers and post messages, complete with spelling mistakes, poor grammar and abbreviated words, to impersonate the younger generation. Unfortunately there are often news items reporting about teenage girls who have been lured into meeting older men with whom they have struck up a friendship on Facebook or similar social networking sites.

There are laws and guidelines on marketing to children, with restrictions on junk food marketing and using children's programs for product placement. You need to be aware that your marketing activities across these social media tools may be seen by children and you should take this into account when constructing your messaging activities.

Using authenticity to build trust with your customers

When blogging for an enterprise or corporation it is also important to remember that you are using these sites on behalf of the company so there are rules, adopted by most large companies, which essentially boil down to being authentic and disclosing your true identity. The journalist posing as Fake Steve Jobs never purported to be the real Steve Jobs, but his information appeared to be accurate enough for readers to speculate. Mini MSFT definitely works for Microsoft and is rumoured to be fairly senior, judging from his conversations at executive level. The identity, although fake, gives a valuable look into the inner workings of a large company and the anonymous comments from real Microsoft

employees give the blog authenticity, even though the blogger's true identity is not revealed.

When you blog on behalf of the company, you should fully disclose who you work for from the start. If you are using engagement tools to communicate on behalf of a client or business relationship you should disclose this relationship. It doesn't need to be a paragraph of legal jargon, just a simple like 'I work for xxx and the views on this blog are my own and not those of the company'. You should never use a false identity or pseudonym to hide your true identity. If you blog on behalf of a product, brand or for another business reason, then the identity itself should identify the company it represents.

One of the main issues with concealing your identity and operating under an alias is the brand itself.

> Authenticity is key to building and developing trust with your audience, and operating under a pseudonym – especially if your true identity is exposed at a later stage – can often lead to disappointment and lack of trust. Lack of authenticity online alters perceptions of your brand offline.

There is a much deeper issue around online authenticity and authenticity in general. Without a deep level of integrity and honesty which has got to be ingrained in your corporate culture, achieving authenticity online is difficult. People can easily see through online activities that don't show authenticity or any degree of transparency. This can lead to loss of reputation and poor brand perception.

> Things to consider to improve perception about your brand:
>
> - Engage your audience little and often. Communicate regularly and avoid intense bursts of activity followed by deathly silences.
> - Don't spam your audience with the same message over and over again. They will soon tire of the message.
> - Social media works because it is a dialogue between members of the community. Listen to your audience. Engage them and interact with them.
> - Don't disparage the competition. Your own company has its faults too.
> - Be authentic. Show your audience the human side of your company.

It is so easy to add a new media channel for every campaign you launch and to focus your efforts entirely on achieving your reach metrics, interaction or engagement levels. But social networking is not a panacea for all digital marketing efforts. You will not improve poor brand perception with a short marketing campaign. Online execution is like adopting a healthy eating plan.

Only with diligence, dedication and long term adherence to the plan will you get the results you desire over time.

THE POTENTIAL FOR REPUTATION DAMAGE

Companies that have communities are well aware of the need to monitor and maintain the positive effects of the community, and that means instilling a sense of community health. Moderators use sophisticated tools to search for content that is considered inappropriate, or to watch for patterns of behaviour that could be deemed unsuitable. Bullying, impersonation to groom children for nefarious means, abuse, and child pornography need to be monitored very carefully, and stopping unsuitable behaviour is an urgent imperative. But in these task-rich, time-poor days how often do you look at your network to watch for these effects?

If you're using a system where friends of friends are free to post content you need to be very aware of what is happening outside your immediate network. For example, if someone is posting pornographic images on their own profile, what effect is this having on their friends? What are your friends doing? What are **their** friends doing? Issues like this then become more than an individual problem, they become a network problem. The US Air Force cancelled their online profile on MySpace due to precisely these concerns.[22] Col. Brian Madtes, chief of the Recruiting Service's strategic communication division, said:

The danger with MySpace is we got to the point where we weren't real comfortable with the potential for inappropriate content to be posted [on the page of] a friend of a friend. We didn't want to be associated with that ... and tarnish our reputation.

But everything isn't always as clear cut as it seems. If you chop off whole parts of the established network then the network will fragment and crumble. The health of the community has a great deal to do with the network. Using appropriate monitoring tools and judiciously blocking miscreants might be better in the long term than pruning whole segments of the environment. And it may have a much larger impact than you think. Google, which carries out continuous monitoring, took a bold stand in January 2010 when it stated that it was pulling out of China as it believed that sophisticated cyber attacks were being attempted on human rights activists in the country. However, consider the effect on the majority of the Chinese people who use the service. Prune your network wisely.

Vitriol, harassment and spite
There is also the issue of people with personal brands who are targeted by others, being bullied and terrorised. Kathy Sierra, considered to be one of technology's 'A list' bloggers, experienced this at first hand. Kathy, whose blog is called 'Creating Passionate Users', received death threats and harassment from unnamed persons. These threats and comments terrified her so much she stopped going to public events, stopped blogging and disappeared from the public eye for quite

some time. Fortunately, with her excellent personal and online brand and reputation, she received considerable support from the blogosphere which helped her return to online life.

Some people on the Internet create fake IDs, send out cruel backbiting messages and place comments on sites using these fake IDs. Such behaviour, which can turn vitriolic and nasty, is thinly disguised harassment delivered by cowards.

Preparing for negative PR

There are lessons to be learned here. It is hard to build a great reputation, and it can easily be destroyed. Nestlé, one of the food giants, has long been criticised over its poor environmental practices over deforestation and palm oil and its 'unethical use and promotion of formula feed for babies in third world countries'.[23] Nestlé has a Facebook page which became the target of many unhappy people advocating a boycott of the company over these practices. The administrators of the Facebook page took a hostile approach to the comments made on Twitter and Facebook and responded on Facebook accordingly.

With Facebook numbers currently at almost 600 million users, and the concept of friends telling friends, this PR disaster has amplified very quickly.

It no longer takes years to reach millions of users, it now takes minutes.

Nestlé representatives complained about some of the comments from Facebook users on their page. They initially deleted posts which were critical of the company and complained about use of Nestlé's altered logo. Unfortunately, the situation quickly appeared to get out of hand, with hundreds of negative comments appearing on Nestlé's Facebook page. This is not the first time that Nestlé has been in the news; Wikipedia has examples of previous issues concerning Nestlé. The interesting phenomenon here is that the use of social media has accelerated the runaway propagation of information into almost meltdown proportions. This is something that may do damage to Nestlé's reputation entirely due to their initial attitude towards their Facebook fans.

I heard an interesting story at an event I attended recently about a social media site which has become notorious in a very short time and has got its social media PR entirely wrong. The site is called Fit Finder and it has the tagline 'Witness the Fitness'. This site isn't very politically correct but it has a huge following. Fit Finder has a feed for each college or university where you can post information anonymously on where the good-looking students are. All you do is fill in a form so that anyone subscribing to the feed can see where they are right now.

As I said, the site isn't politically correct, and one of the universities had a couple of complaints about harassment. The college, which has a policy of not blocking sites, then sent out an email telling everyone not to visit the site. Traffic to the site rocketed, which led to more complaints about the content on the site.

JANET (the Joint Academic NETwork in the UK) then blocked access to the site. This meant that all universities, schools and colleges had no access from their PCs. However, anyone with a mobile device or other wireless connection could access the site and log on to see what the fuss was about. Another major spike in traffic happened and awareness of the site grew. The *Guardian* and the London *Metro* covered the story, with *Metro* further reporting about the start of the mobile revolution occurring. The Facebook page grew to over 4,000 fans and the feed at all college locations is updated regularly.

JANET, after multiple complaints from universities around the UK, unblocked access to the site again. There are regular updates – lots of them seem to be by girls commenting on boys, so there do seem to be roughly equal numbers of comments for both males and females on the site.

There are a couple of lessons that can be learned about managing social media PR:

- Don't tell people not to visit a site, as it's the first thing that they will want to do – especially if the site seems scurrilous or controversial.

- A blanket blocking by an organisation such as JANET will drive people to visit the site using other means. Mobile device updates, Facebook updates and Twitter notifications keep awareness right up there.

If no one had said anything, traffic to the site might have fizzled out in a few weeks or months. Instead, its notoriety has ensured its continued success. Fit Finder follows a similar model to Facebook, which is now 7 years old and hugely different now than when it started. I wonder if Fit Finder will have the same sort of success. It seems to have started off rather well.

A simple YouTube video can also trigger a similar propagation explosion. In early 2008 Dave Carroll, a musician in a band, flew with his guitar from Nova Scotia to Nebraska via Chicago on United Airlines. One of his band mates saw the baggage handlers heaving around the guitars with 'wanton disregard'. Dave complained to the flight attendants but his comments were met with indifference. When he arrived at his destination to play at the event he found his guitar was broken. He played at his gig, and complained to the airline upon his return and for several weeks afterwards. He spent $1,200 repairing the guitar and claimed compensation from the airline. Unfortunately this claim was denied by the airline because he didn't complain 'in the right place or at the right time'. Dave told United Airlines that he was going to write a song and post it on YouTube, but the company ignored his threat.

The 'United breaks guitars' video went viral very quickly, and soon had over 8 million views on YouTube.[24] This online video managed to connect with the airline. United Airlines responded to the video and 'put things right' for him. By eventually responding to the issue and fixing their customers' issues, United showed that they could reverse the impressions created by their original poor service.

Tackling customers' problems in a timely and positive manner can bring significant benefits to the company. After investing your efforts to create a positive online brand, this is certainly something worth considering as your brand grows in prominence.

So you now have a brand and a presence on the web. People already have a perception of your brand, so now let's have a look at how to make the brand more successful. With success come challenges, and we'll consider what to do so as to stay within your guidelines. What guidelines? Let's now have a look at how to create a framework for your staff to work with.

SUMMARY

- You need to be part of the conversation.
- Don't underestimate the power of peer recommendations.
- Consider your current approach to marketing. Will it still work in the social media world?
- People will read what you write. There is no delete key.
- Consider your privacy settings in each application and review them regularly.
- Consider creating a page in Facebook for business.
- Manage your reputation carefully and take prompt action to rectify any damage to your brand.
- Be aware of the impact on your brand reputation and image if there are issues.

7 BRAND IMPACT AND BRAND SUCCESS

In this chapter we'll start to look at what makes your brand successful amongst your audience. We'll look at how customers want to feel about your brand and your engagement with them. We'll talk about how companies like Dell have used this to their advantage and obtained measurable financial results. We'll also look at how companies adopt policies and guidelines for their staff. We'll look at good and not so good examples of policies and innovative ways of getting the message out. We'll talk about legal aspects and consider some potential issues around intellectual property and copyright. Finally, we'll look at established brands and how they tackle brand migration. Some have managed this brand shift very successfully, others less so. We'll have a look at some things to consider in the digital world if you feel that you want to do the same.

THE IMPACT OF SOCIAL MEDIA INSIDE YOUR BUSINESS

You know what your business is all about. You have defined objectives and metrics that you measure. You have specific actions that you refine regularly and you're ready to add social media marketing to your digital marketing strategy. Unfortunately, this is often where things start to go wrong.

> This flood of communication and interaction has been building for more than 25 years and it is fundamentally changing the way that businesses and customers interact.

It is as vital to business success as was mass production in the industrial revolution, the impact of the PC and the growth of the web.

> This interaction is very important for you, your business and your customers.

Why are networks so important to you and your business? Social media impacts your sales, gives a great insight into market intelligence, and gathers information directly from your customers. It can refine your logistics, contribute to your research and refine your product development cycle. It is crucial to your success in business. You may pay for market analysis, look at your click-through figures to find out unique visitors to your pages and where they are from, but that's

about it. How can you find out how these users are grouped? Is there a network cluster that you can define? Is there a social graph connecting your users? Is it strong and growing? Or is it fragmented and weak? Where are the strong and weak ties in your network? How do you know who your influencers are?

When you're deciding to introduce these conversational tools into your traditional marketing approach, you know that you want to get your marketing message out to your customers. Unfortunately, some companies tend to use all of the channels that they know. This sometimes comes across like a message distributed by scatter gun to the audience. The 'launch' of a blog, the fanfare over the creation of a Facebook page, a new Twitter name, a Friendfeed list or a YouTube channel are all great ideas which will prove valuable to you if you've identified the appropriate channel for your message.

> Many companies forget what type of messages they are trying to broadcast to their customers and the response they are trying to achieve – the message comes before the medium.

Knowing your customer

When preparing to complement your marketing activities with your social media plan, consider what motivates your customers' behaviour online. This means that you need to think about separating your customers into different groups according to their behaviour. And that means looking at their age.

GROUPING CUSTOMERS

- If you're targeting customers who are aged between the ages of 20 and 30, think about competitions. This age group tends to be competitive. They set themselves ambitious targets and compete with their peers.

- Between the ages of 30 and 40, customers like to have an understanding and awareness of who they are and where they fit into the larger model. Perhaps they have defined themselves as working class or middle class. If they know how important they are to your brand they can understand why you are communicating with them and how they can help.

- Customers aged between 45 and 60 tend to seek affirmation that the decisions that they have made are the correct one, so brand value plays a large role in their decision making process.

Essentially, the consumer wants you to acknowledge that they are valued.

> It's all about me – understand me, acknowledge me, and know who I am and what I represent.

Once a brand has done this, then your business is well on the way to persuading them to become advocates and enthusiasts. You also need to remember that your business mind is quite different from your customer's mind. For you it's about revenue, profit, power, growth, status, work, money and sex, whereas customers will be thinking about family, home, F1, football, celebrities, kittens, money and sex. Since the dotcom boom, consumers have moved towards a more web-centric method of purchasing and interacting. The web is now widely used for shopping, and with social tools displaying birthdays and status updates people are much more willing to share more personal details about themselves online. This new attitude contrasts completely with our face to face lives, when only our closest friends get to share the personal details of our life such as our birth date, relationship details and hobbies.

USING TWITTER TO GROW YOUR BUSINESS – DELL STYLE

Dell is a great example of an organisation that has benefited from using the new communication tools. It had very a specific and targeted business purpose, which was to increase sales revenues and decrease support costs. It decided to spread its methods of communicating with its customers across several channels. Dell has blogs, four Twitter accounts, several Facebook pages and a YouTube channel. Dell features time-limited 'special offers' in its Twitter feeds; its YouTube channel has over 500 videos. These videos showcase new products, feature discussions with product managers showing innovation in products, and display the results of student competitions. In this case, Dell knows how the under 30s feel the need to compete with each other. Dell's blogs are full of useful information from the product team, but there is also a wealth of information from people who have knowledge of the product set.

DELL'S COMMUNITY SUCCESS

Dell's community is contributing to the expansion of knowledge by effective peer to peer support. This support is lowering the cost of each support call to Dell. The answers to customers' questions can often be found on the forums, written by another member of the community.

This approach has brought Dell measurable results. Figure 7.1 shows the number of people following the Dell Outlet Twitter account from March to June 2009. On 7 March it had around 117,000 followers, on 7 June there were almost 609,000; by 1 January 2010 the number exceeded 1.5 million.

These followers are looking for Dell offers that are exclusively announced on Twitter.

These offers are retweeted by many of the Dell Outlet Twitter followers, which creates buzz for Dell and has helped to grow Dell's follower base.

According to Stephanie Nelson, who started tweeting as the @DellOutlet account, deal hunters are especially attracted to Dell's Twitter presence.[25] Dell Outlet sells

Figure 7.1 @Dell Outlet Twitter follower growth March to June 2009

(Source: TwitterCounter.com)

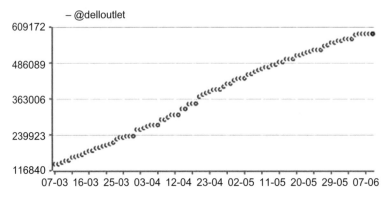

refurbished Dell products at great prices, but inventories fluctuate, making it difficult to know when products are available or on sale. Dell Outlet uses Twitter as a way to message out coupons, clearance events and new arrival information to those looking for Dell technology at a discounted price.

This innovation has generated Dell over $3 million in revenue (to the end of 2009), and as a global brand, Dell has recognised the need to duplicate this success in other countries.[26] Now Dell has other accounts: @DellOutletUK, @DellOutletIE, @DellHomeSalesAU and @Offertas_Dell_MX, to name a few. Dell has even linked its Twitter activity to a web page on its site to round the experience out for the consumer, which seems to have done a great deal for its brand image too.

CORPORATE GUIDELINES AND POLICIES

Companies are starting to regard social networking sites, forums and message boards as significant to the business. These forums contain important content, and companies recognise that they need to apply policies that govern the acceptable use of this content. But is it possible to define an acceptable standard for user generated content? Do you apply something that prohibits the use of social engagement tools in any form whilst inside the corporate firewall? Some companies prohibit blogging, or they block Facebook and Twitter through the corporate firewall. Some companies issue such severely restrictive policies that they are almost impossible to comply with.

ESPN, the sports news channel, has issued very specific and detailed guidelines for social networking for any of their staff engaged with the public discussing sports news:[27]

- Personal websites and blogs that contain sports content are not permitted.
- Prior to engaging in any form of social networking dealing with sports, you must receive permission from the supervisor as appointed by your department head.

- ESPN.COM may choose to post sports related social media content.
- If ESPN.com opts not to post sports related social media content created by ESPN talent, you are not permitted to report, speculate, discuss or give any opinions on sports related topics or personalities on your personal platforms.
- The first and only priority is to serve ESPN sanctioned efforts, including sports news, information and content.
- Assume at all times you are representing ESPN.
- If you wouldn't say it on the air or write it in your column, don't tweet it.
- Exercise discretion, thoughtfulness and respect for your colleagues, business associates and our fans.
- Avoid discussing internal policies or detailing how a story or feature was reported, written, edited or produced and discussing stories or features in progress, those that haven't been posted or produced, interviews you've conducted, or any future coverage plans.
- Steer clear of engaging in dialogue that defends your work against those who challenge it and do not engage in media criticism or disparage colleagues or competitors.
- Be mindful that all posted content is subject to review in accordance with ESPN's employee policies and editorial guidelines.
- Confidential or proprietary company information or similar information of third parties who have shared such information with ESPN, should not be shared.

Any violation of these guidelines could result in a range of consequences, including but not limited to suspension or dismissal.

These steps are logical and considered, but perhaps a little too restrictive for employees. Some of the bullet points seem to oversimplify certain details. A lot of these guidelines could form part of the standard employee guidelines and be set out in an employee handbook, and reference made to this from the company's social media policy.

In the 1920s the United States applied prohibition to alcohol, which immediately led to hundreds of illicit outlets springing up and operating illegally. There are indications that this level of restriction may foster similar behaviour online. Users will start to use their personal mobile devices to engage in digital conversations whilst at work.

Telstra, the Australian telecommunications and media company, had an innovative way to announce its social guidelines for its staff. It published its training guide on the web in an easy to read comic book format. This guide has links to videos, two of which have been published on YouTube. This is a great way to make sure everyone inside and outside the company sees the guidelines that Telstra has published, and knows how they work. They're simple and straight forward too. Publishing in this way, online for everyone to see and search for on the

web, is a great initiative. Telstra certainly appears to be leading the way here, and should be applauded for its efforts. The new form of engagement is all about discoverability, communication and channelling the torrent of information into something manageable, constructive and useful.

So what would a good corporate social media policy contain? Here are some core principles that I believe are a good foundation for policy guidelines:

GENERAL SOCIAL MEDIA POLICY GUIDELINES

- Be respectful of others. Don't insult, disparage, libel, defame, inflame or attack others.

- Be true to yourself. Authenticity and integrity must underpin all of your communications.

- Be accurate. Fake social media campaigns are soon exposed and credibility is soon lost.

- Be respectful of corporate intellectual property. Protect copyright or confidential corporate information.

- Bring value to your readers. They are potential future clients and connections and their satisfaction matters.

- Be humble. You cannot be right all of the time. Acknowledge your errors and apologise with humility.

- Be generous. Acknowledge other authors where you've used their work.

- Be responsible. You are the company spokesperson in your external messaging.

- Be thoughtful. An off the cuff comment can do immense damage to your reputation and corporate brand.

- Be careful. Think before you post.

- Do not speculate on matters that may prejudice your company in any legal case.

Another good tip when you're writing your social media policy is to be concise. A good social media policy needs to be less than one page so that the contents are remembered. Keeping it simple is a great idea. IBM[28] has a simple, easy to read blogging policy and social media policy, as does Intel,[29] including these tips for engaging in global conversations:

- Stick to your area of expertise and provide unique, individual perspectives on what's going on at Intel and in the world.

- Post meaningful, respectful comments—in other words, no spam and no remarks that are off-topic or offensive.

Intel's rules of engagement follow similar themes to other companies which have published their guidelines on the web and can be summarised as follows:

- Respect brands, copyrights and trademarks.
- Add value to your customers and readers. Build a sense of community.
- If it gives you pause, pause. If you're about to publish something that makes you even the slightest bit uncomfortable, don't shrug it off and hit 'send'.

Twitter guidelines

With the rise of Twitter for customer interaction, there are other specific policies that could be applied to microblogging. If you're using Twitter as a way to communicate with your customers and provide great customer service from the brand, you might want to modify your style somewhat.

GUIDELINES FOR USING TWITTER

- If you get customer questions, respond quickly to keep the dialogue flowing.
- Ask questions of your audience – don't just broadcast.
- Do not be derogatory about your competitors.
- Twitter should not be the only tool used for customer maintenance. All requests need to be redirected back to the appropriate support team for action and recording.
- Respect corporate legal guidelines, and confidentiality.
- If you're using a specific Twitter name, like SubaruSupport, make sure that your messages are relevant to your brand.
- If you have a corporate account, keep to corporate messages and don't flood the stream with information about your personal life.
- Tweet about what you know – stick to your area of expertise.
- Make sure your messages are interesting or compelling or newsworthy.
- Make sure that you are committed to maintaining your Twitter presence. Co-opt others into helping you populate the Twitter stream.
- Be careful who you follow, and don't automatically follow everyone who follows you. Watch out for automated bots, and aim for quality not quantity.
- Use hashtags to talk about themes so you can search for tweets using these themes to track your metrics. Try to keep these hashtags short. You only have 140 characters, so #followfriday has, over time, been shortened to #ff to save space.
- Retweet other interesting tweets.
- Use short URLs like http://bit.ly which have metrics showing click-through totals.

If you have a clearly defined social media policy and blogging policy and you have raised awareness amongst your staff and everyone follows the rules, then you don't really need to not worry. Over time, you will find that internal conversations occur within your organisation, the users will self-police their behaviour, and brand advocates will ensure that your brand message stays consistent. However, you need to consider things that may go wrong.

Keeping things legal

Who are you on the web? What do people know about you? If you search for your brand you will find mentions of it, but there may be items on the web that you might never have known were there. On a personal level, these facts may be innocuous, like your daughter talking about you and the job you do on her Facebook page or Twitter feed. It may be others in your network tweeting about your holiday antics in Spain last summer, your rugby skills, or a photograph of you downing that last vodka shot in a club. These exchanges are out there on the web, and you can't do anything about them – because you don't actually own them. They are out of your control and they have the potential to do your reputation great harm. In addition to effective corporate policies and basic common sense over what you broadcast on the Internet, a question arises about where the legal boundaries lie.

During the snowfall in February 2009 a blogger in the UK, Ben Marsh, created a mashup application on the web. He used a Google map and overlaid the map with Twitter hashtags showing where all of the snow was falling in the UK. He also displayed the tweets marked with the hashtag #uksnow as they appeared on Twitter from users around the UK. The hashtag #uksnow was widely adopted and reported in the media. Rory Cellan-Jones from the BBC received a message from a reader, Julian Bray, who said that he had 'invented' the hashtag and claimed it as his intellectual property.[30] This seemed to be the first time anyone had claimed intellectual property rights over a hashtag – after all, it's only a word. The http://hashtags.org website documents millions of hashtags in popular use on Twitter, and it's almost impossible to claim ownership of a word. The ability to do this could raise some interesting battles.

Twitter and copyright

If someone plagiarises content from a book and republishes it elsewhere, then the author has due recourse to the law of the land. If a piece of music is copied, cloned or reproduced, and the owner of the original piece of music can prove that the music has been plagiarised, then they also have a legal advantage in court. Trademarks are enforceable by law and counterfeit art is illegal. But what is the legal case if you repeat information that you found on Twitter or Facebook? Do you actually have any rights at all to the information you broadcast?

According to Twitter, what you write is yours.[31] Twitter copyright policy states:

Twitter respects the intellectual property rights of others and expects users of the Services to do the same. We will respond to notices of alleged copyright infringement that comply with applicable law and are properly provided to us. If you believe that your Content has been copied in a way that constitutes copyright infringement, please provide us with the following information:

(i)   a physical or electronic signature of the copyright owner or a person authorized to act on their behalf;

(ii) identification of the copyrighted work claimed to have been infringed;

(iii) identification of the material that is claimed to be infringing or to be the subject of infringing activity and that is to be removed or access to which is to be disabled, and information reasonably sufficient to permit us to locate the material;

(iv) your contact information, including your address, telephone number, and an email address;

(v)   a statement by you that you have a good faith belief that use of the material in the manner complained of is not authorized by the copyright owner, its agent, or the law; and

(vi) a statement that the information in the notification is accurate, and, under penalty of perjury, that you are authorized to act on behalf of the copyright owner.

Facebook has multiple approaches to copyright information, but their main policy says:[32]

We respect the intellectual property rights of others and we prohibit users from posting content that violates another party's intellectual property rights. When we receive a proper claim of IP infringement, we promptly remove or disable access to the allegedly infringing content. We also terminate the accounts of repeat infringers in appropriate circumstances.

So does this mean that if you retweet or share a comment on Twitter or Facebook, you are breaking copyright law? Theoretically, yes. However, tweets and comments are attributed to the owner of the tweet, typically via a retweet. Comments are attributed to the originator so that credit is given for their original quote. The United States Copyright Office Circular 34 states that copyright law does not protect names, titles, or short phrases or expressions.[33] Twitter is limited to 140 characters and theoretically a 'short phrase' as opposed to a long paragraph of text from a publication or online article.

But who actually owns these tweets? Twitter and Facebook both say that it is the originator of the message who owns them. Of course, if you were so obsessed about copyright, then perhaps you wouldn't broadcast your intellectual property on such a public site in the first place. Unless, of course, you want to have your information broadcast by your friends and your message amplified.

There might be someone on the web who may take issue with something you write.

Who owns your content?

Facebook changed its terms and conditions to reflect their stance about ownership of content:[34]

> You hereby grant Facebook an irrevocable, perpetual, non-exclusive, transferable, fully paid, worldwide license...to (a) use, copy, publish, stream, store, retain, ...reformat, modify, edit,... and distribute..., any User Content you (i) Post ... or (ii) enable a user to Post, ... and (b) to use your name, likeness and image for any purpose, ...

The important bit is this:

> You may remove your User Content from the Site at any time. If you choose to remove your User Content, the license granted above will automatically expire, however you acknowledge that the Company may retain archived copies of your User Content.

Several blogs picked this up from Facebook and an outcry ensued. Facebook reverted to its old terms within a few days. But what does this mean? Well, hopefully those photos of you downing vodka shots at the rugby reunion were taken by friends who have protected their Facebook profiles with appropriate privacy settings. Any photos which were not taken by you but have been tagged with your name and placed on other, unprotected profiles can be seen by anyone who searches for your name. Privacy settings are very important (and Facebook gives you the chance to untag any photos that you don't wish to broadcast further). Once you have set your privacy it is a good idea to regularly check your settings. Make sure that your specific settings are still valid as this will stop any problems if Facebook changes anything in the application which could potentially open up your data and photos to a wider group of connections.

If you have not spent some time setting your privacy settings correctly, think about this. In 20 years' time, when you're in a respectable position at work or you are thinking about becoming a councillor or a politician, remember that those Facebook photos can be accessed by anyone. Without the proper settings in place, they could come back to haunt you and your reputation.

It's certainly worth a thought. Vodka shot, anyone?

MANAGING REBRANDS AND BRAND MIGRATION

Things change at the speed of a mouse click nowadays. Change is inevitable in the Web 2.0 world. So how do you manage your brand status whilst preparing for a rebrand? There are right and wrong ways to go about the migration of your brand which will be largely determined by how much you want your customers to be influenced by your new brand and how much you want to change customer perception.

Have you considered the reasons for your rebrand? Mergers and acquisitions are often a great opportunity for a brand revamp. Symantec acquired Quarterdeck in November 1998 and renamed its product CleanSweep to Norton CleanSweep. Symantec subsequently repositioned the entire product line by bundling a suite of products together and naming it Norton SystemWorks. Other reasons to rebrand could be due to a decline in product perception amongst consumers. The rebranding of the Philip Morris brand to Altria was done to help the company shed its negative image when a court in the US ordered Philip Morris to pay $3 billion in damages to a smoker suffering terminal cancer who claimed he wasn't warned of the dangers of smoking.[35]

Things can go wrong with the product rebrand if it's not carried out to customer satisfaction. The UK Post Office's attempt to rebrand itself as Consignia proved to be such a failure that millions more had to be spent rebranding again to become Royal Mail. The branding of New Coke lasted 77 days before Coca-Cola switched the drink back to its original formula and renamed it Coke Classic.[36] People seemed to be more upset about the withdrawal of the old formula than the taste of the new one. The psychiatrist hired by Coca-Cola to listen in on phone calls to the company hotline told executives that some people sounded as if they were discussing the death of a family member. Pepsi has changed many of their brands. It recently renamed Mountain Dew as Mtn Dew and it has adjusted the Pepsi logo slightly. The red and blue areas within the circle have been modified to represent a series of 'smiles' on each of their product range.[37] Will it be successful? Only time and consumer conversation will tell.

A rebrand can be a great opportunity for you to take a long hard look at how your product is perceived in the digital world. Your traditional approach to your product sales on the Internet may be in the form of bricks and clicks marketing, integrating both an offline (bricks) and an online (clicks) presence. You order the product online, but you go to collect your product in person at the store. Any attempt at rebranding or brand migration needs to be effectively handled. Customers need to be made aware of the new plans through external marketing, and internal staff need training so that they can also talk about the new product or brand. A good design agency needs to be engaged early on in the process so that tight co-ordination can keep everyone on message throughout the process. Successful rebranding projects can yield a brand which is better regarded than it was before. The new company identity and brand could also be launched in a methodical manner to avoid alienating your existing customers, while aiming to attract new business prospects. Microsoft successfully achieved this with its search engine, Bing, which was an evolutionary step forward for their Live Search product and relaunched at the end of May 2009.

Controlling these marketing messages does seem to work. Figure 7.2 shows that when Bing was launched, searches performed on Google dipped for each spike in Bing.[38] Each of these spikes equates to an announcement about Bing – for example, the announcement that Bing was going to add Twitter real-time data to search results as well as indexing static Twitter profiles.[39]

If you're planning a similar brand migration, how do you migrate your brand to take advantage of the digital market?

Figure 7.2 Top search engines in the US from May to December 2009

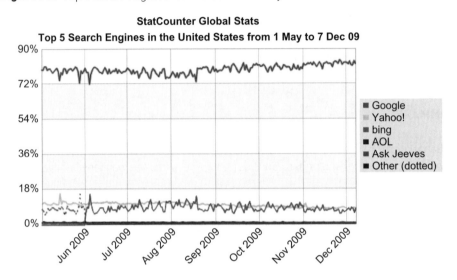

StatCounter Global Stats
Top 5 Search Engines in the United States from 1 May to 7 Dec 09

Legend:
- Google
- Yahoo!
- bing
- AOL
- Ask Jeeves
- Other (dotted)

MIGRATING YOUR BRAND

- This is a business move. Take the emotion out of the decision and try to be objective about it. An external agency can bring a fresh approach – without the emotion that you will have invested. The family firm that has been in business for years probably hasn't moved its brand strategy forward for a while.

- Companies usually start small and expand, sometimes exponentially, without a formal brand strategy in place. Make sure you have a strategy in place before embarking on a rebrand.

- Your brand is already successful. It's time to analyse which parts of it will work in the digital age. Is it the name, the image, the logo, the tag line, or even the colour? Make sure you keep the parts of the brand that are important to you.

- It doesn't have to be a major change. Think of the success that rebranding the term 'gambling' to 'gaming' has brought for the industry.

- Smaller companies find that there is lots of room for a major rebrand, while large companies, such as the Post Office, Hewlett-Packard and Microsoft, have to make sure that they avoid upsetting their existing customers. A rule of thumb is: the smaller the company, the larger the opportunity to rebrand, which is a great opportunity for entrepreneurs.

The mighty Disney Corporation, which has Mickey Mouse as one of its best known assets, is considering rebranding this iconic figure. Disney has created a new Mickey Mouse for a video game. Epic Mickey[40] has new cunning personality

traits which he exhibits as he traverses the game. This brand migration of their most beloved character is risky, to say the least. But if Disney can pull this brand migration off with Mickey Mouse, then anyone can.

You now have a brand, a presence and guidelines to work with. What next? The next chapter gets you connecting and growing your network.

SUMMARY

- Social interaction is fundamentally changing the way we do business.
- Correctly classify and understand your customers and the way they behave online.
- Consider using Dell's approach to get business through Twitter.
- Create effective social media guidelines for your staff and educate them on your digital policy.
- Be aware of copyright and legal issues around repeating content.
- Consider the effects of rebranding and take steps to manage it properly.

8 CONNECTIONS AND REPUTATION

Connecting to others in the social networking space is simple. With social distance decreasing, and the friends of friends networks becoming closer, it seems easy to reach potentially anyone across the connected world. In this chapter we will look at how the web has morphed into a socially connected environment where users' behaviour has evolved over time and has grown to incorporate all ages, tastes and styles.

Discoverability is key to your success with social networking.

We'll consider ways to manage your reputation and how recommendations are vital to build a community and discover your influencers. We'll talk about the apparent differences in the way news propagates and how different types of networking applications cater to these styles. We'll also see how easy it is to monitor sentiment for your brand and to gauge your reputation. We'll work out some ways to mitigate brand-jacking and think about how to build your reputation if the worst does happen. Finally, we'll discuss the dangers that can occur if your identity is cloned and we'll look at some best practice ideas around managing passwords across different websites that you visit on the web.

MAKING SENSE OF SOCIAL NETWORKING

Do you have friends on Facebook, or do you prefer to connect on LinkedIn? Are you a tweeter, a lurker or a Plurker? Do you live in the world of instant news, video uploads, or do you constantly watch your status updates? Is your avatar a taller, thinner, better-looking and more exciting version of you? Do you live in your Second Life because it's more exciting than your first life? Do you aggregate your RSS feeds for viewing online in Google Reader, or offline with Sharpreader or Outlook? What is your favourite news feed service? How compact is your social graph? Where are you on Technorati? Meebo? IceRocket? What's your favourite wiki?

The web has morphed into something that lends itself perfectly to interaction, both synchronous and asynchronous.

The term 'Web 2.0' was first coined by Darcy DiNucci in 1999.[41] She predicted that the browser experience which delivered web content in 'static screenfuls' was 'only an embryo of the Web to come'. She said that the web would be used as the 'transport mechanism, the ether through which interactivity happens'. Her comments, now more than 11 years old, were far ahead of their time and are so true today.

The term 'Web 2.0' disappeared from general use but reappeared in 2003. Web 2.0 is now generally associated with Tim O'Reilly, who discussed the term at the Web 2.0 Conference in San Francisco. Even in 2003, Tim recognised that interaction between users was a significant business benefit. He brought industry leaders from companies like Amazon and Yahoo! to the conference to deliver their predictions. They talked about the emergence of the web as a platform which would deliver the applications, and the browser to deliver the application experience for the users.

Now the phrase of the moment seems to be 'social media'. Social media is actually an evolution of the term 'social software'. It's usually used in technical circles and is also known in academia as 'groupwork'. Social media is the latest in a long line of buzzwords. It is used to describe the collection of software, tools and services that brings users together into a massively collaborative environment. Here they can share, inform, gather, play, co-ordinate and communicate. These collaborators create user generated content which is used for the greater good of others. Wikipedia is a great example of the community freely giving their time and expertise to contribute to a document entirely to benefit others.

To delve into this evolutionary shift, we need to consider three factors:

SOCIAL NETWORKING EVOLUTION

- Social networking originally appeared to be attractive to the younger age groups and niche technologists. This has now changed, with all age groups from all walks of life engaging in social connection activities.

- Social networking sites have achieved a tremendous groundswell of followers. This network effect has rippled around the world gaining significant traction in many social circles, demographics and societies.

- With all groundswell effects we need to consider where they are going and what will be next in this behavioural interaction.

To understand how social networking works, we need to try to work out which aspects of social networking activities actually glue these communities together. There are certain behaviours that are important to the structure of engagement and interaction.

SOCIAL NETWORKING BEHAVIOURS

- Discoverability. With the sophistication of search, it's now fairly easy to find someone who has been posting content online. Historical content is saved and stored somewhere on cache servers. Search exposes us to a far wider spread of information due to these mechanisms. Unfortunately, this information can be used for bad activities as well as good.

- Location. With the rise in location based applications, you can add location and presence to your digital communications. Think about geocaching applications for example. With geocaching, objects and clues are hidden at specified places and discovered using geographic coordinates. With location aware services on mobile devices, we now have the opportunity to take a photograph, or a video, upload and share it immediately on social networking sites. If you add tagging to this functionality or recommendations from others, you can discover who else has been in the same location, when they were there, and what they thought of it. This functionality helps you to connect virtually with the community from your current physical location. This virtual location can now take you to any location across the world.

- Propagation. People forward on emails, cut and paste text from useful snippets and forward them on. Whether this is in the form of a status update, a retweet or a re-shared link, the value to others is the propagation of this information. Unfortunately, the ability to modify the original text to suit your opinions has the potential to replicate false information across the Internet.

- Recommendation. This is a double edged sword in social applications. Receiving recommendations can improve your profile, lead to referrals from your extended network and be of mutual benefit to both parties. However there are times when this interaction can also cause problems. Malicious rumours, negative comments, and ill chosen words can propagate around the Internet, doing significant damage to a reputation in a matter of hours. This propagation of information, once it is out there, is permanent.

- Connection. If I know someone whom I think you would benefit from meeting then I can connect you both together. This connection extends your network and can amplify any message you want to broadcast. You can decide whether you want to make the connection, for mutual benefit or business reasons. You can also decide not to proceed.

- Reputation. This is of enormous value to the user. If someone recommends you, a link you've shared, or likes your online status, your reputation increases in the eyes of your peers. MMORPGs have recognised this status and award badges, medals and tier points for obtaining arbitrary goals in the game. Reputation in gaming is similar to the value to the seller having an unblemished 100% feedback score on eBay, and it is visible across most online games.

Having the correct mechanisms in place to make effective connections is important. However, you also need knowledge about how communities interact, participate and lead the conversation. With this as a foundation, you can start to think about your social media architecture. You will then be able to formulate what your approach might be and how to create your strategic plan.

The digitally connected world

Much has been made of the term 'six degrees of separation'[42] to explain how connected the world is. The term actually originated in a book of short stories written by the Hungarian author Frigyes Karinthy.[43] The book talked about 'friendship networks' which could traverse great distances. Despite being physically separated by distance, the shrinking world and the increase in human population density make this 'social distance' appear much smaller than it has been in the past. The hypothesis about the six degrees of separation came about as a result of an experiment which speculated that any two people could be connected to each other by at most five connections. This concept actually influenced the early thinking about social networks.

Further experiments were conducted later by Stanley Millgram. Millgram tried to calculate the average path or hop length of a social network. He wanted to count the number of ties between any two people who passed a packet of information from Omaha and Wichita to Boston in the United States. People in these regions were randomly selected and sent packages explaining the purpose of the study. They were asked to send the package on to their known connections. There was a list on the package for the recipients to record their name and which part of the link they participated in.

Recipients of the package were asked to forward it on to someone they knew who might know the end recipient in the chain at Boston. If the end recipient was known, then the package went straight to them. Often the letters would arrive at the intended target in one or two hops; others would arrive at their target after more than nine links. The average number of hops to the destination seemed to be about 5.5.

An interesting facet of human behaviour appeared during this study which explains some people's behaviour on social networking sites. In some of these studies, the packages never arrived at their intended destination at all. Some of the recipients refused to forward the packages, bringing the chain to an end. In some tests, around 80% of packages were not forwarded on to their intended destination. In other cases, 66% of the letters were handed to the destination recipient by the same person. This person, a 'Mr Jacobs', whose occupation had something to do with clothing, must have had significant connections or ties to several of the other networks in the chain, making him a great connector. Malcolm Gladwell, the author of *The Tipping Point*, speculated that connectors are 'people specialists'. They know and like a lot of people, they collect acquaintances and they remember people in their network. Mr Jacobs must have been a great connector in his own network to receive so many packages to deliver on to his other networks.

COMMUNITY CONNECTIONS AND RECOMMENDATIONS

Starting your implementation for digital engagement requires careful planning, a lot of thought, dedication and, most of all, a significant investment of time. So it's important to understand the different strands you need to think about when you create your plan. There are several things that you need to consider when you build your community or ecosystem and make it self-sustaining and thriving. Imagine a citizenship project at your company. The project moves along defined tasks and timelines to a defined set of milestones. It is driven by one person, the project manager, who co-ordinates the rest of the team when required. But what if this project is driven by social networking? This project would engage volunteers for the project who felt that they had something to contribute. The volunteers would use their shared knowledge to come to a consensus about where the project was heading. Friends of the contributors, who also wanted to contribute, could also potentially work on the project, sharing their knowledge. The combined skills of the community of project workers would drive the outcome of the project.

Successful companies let customer feedback, based on experience and knowledge, drive their future direction.

> The three most important things that you need to make your project successful are community, content and connections.

You also need to listen to the community. Your customers are out there talking about you and your brand. It's very worthwhile listening to what they are saying. Listen to what they say about your brand, your products, and listen to their experience with you from a consumer point of view. Are they positive, neutral or negative towards you? Are they vocal in their praise about you? Are they detractors or, even worse, critics who influence others to become critics too? Without this level of market intelligence, you can run the risk of setting off in the wrong direction with your product and alienating your customers. Gaining product feedback from your customers in the form of online conversations is really important. You can elicit votes and comments on your website and you can ask questions.

> The answers that the community will give offer you a huge amount of information that rounds out your standard web metric results and will give you a different perspective for analysis and response.

Demonstrating to the customer that you are listening to them is important for your long term business goals and will allow you to create initiatives that will enable your business to grow and help to connect effectively with your customers.

Listen before you leap

This programme is a long term investment for your company and it will take some time before success and a positive ROI can be measured.

Starbucks listens to its customers and has produced some great results. Starbucks has a site called My Starbucks Idea (http://mystarbucksidea.com) where customers can suggest ideas to improve Starbucks. The site has polls where you can vote for your favourite kind of coffee or decide on a new initiative. Customers have persuaded Starbucks to sell Jamaican Blue Mountain coffee, sell decaffeinated iced coffee and bring back oatmeal and chocolate chip cookies. Since My Starbucks Idea launched in early 2008 Starbucks has had over 79,000 ideas submitted by the community, and the company has over 13 million friends on its Facebook page.

STARTING TO LISTEN

- Spending time collecting information about the audience before you embark on your customer engagement strategy is vital.

- The approach has to be communicated to your staff so that they can also become online advocates.

- Ultimately, your communications strategy will be embedded in your staff approach to customer engagement and it will become part of the values of your organisation.

Until that happens, the goals you set need to be realistic, flexible and focused on what your customers want. If the needs of the customer change, then the goals also need to change and it is important to bear this in mind when you create your plan.

Your trusted advisers

Referrals are really important when you are building your network of influencers and advocates. Just as a doctor may be asked whom he trusts when it comes to patient referrals, so **key people in your network will also be used by the community as super-referrers**. These super-referrers have a key set of good connections across several different networks, and information given to them has the potential to be spread broadly across a wide set of interconnected areas. These community members are very well connected, they are often first to try out a new product and they are considered to be influential amongst their groups. They are often not self-proclaimed experts, but they are genuine enthusiasts about their technology, and other members of the community go to them for thought leadership and trends. These leaders often have more reach and influence than traditional self-proclaimed experts. Experts already assume themselves to be thought leaders and often are not as interested in what others in the marketplace are actually doing. This makes them slower to adopt new practices, gadgets or technologies and slower to talk about them to others.

Beware the self-proclaimed experts.

You don't necessarily need to engage with the people who have the largest number of apparent connections. These people might not necessarily have the greatest number of strong relationships amongst their connections. Monitoring their blogs, status updates and forum entries will give you a good idea of how they interact within their social circle. Watching in this way will give you an indication of the strength of their networking ties and how many good strong and weak connections they have. These strong relationships will be more valuable to you as they indicate a trusted adviser status amongst their followers and friends.

Networks such as Twitter are useful for broadcasting ideas and discovering trends, but the word of mouth network is often hidden and poorly explored here.

Marketers have their work cut out to discover who maintains strong ties across their network and who propagates valuable and relevant information. Often marketing teams have relied purely on the number of connections that someone has and have not exploited the hidden links within a network. It's often the interaction between the 30 or so 'real' friends within a network that will bring the most value to the conversation.

You also need to consider the people who work inside your organisation.

Identify your existing evangelists, enthusiasts, pragmatists and any detractors you might have.

These are the people who might already be speaking publicly about your brand. Make sure you've prepared them to communicate externally with an effective, practical and workable social media policy. Give them training on the different types of tools that they will be using, remembering that tools that are in vogue today may be out of favour next year. Allow for change in your plans and make sure these are effectively communicated internally to the digital natives who will be contributors to your stream.

One of the most important benefits of effective engagement is the development of your 'voice'.

Whether this voice is the voice of yourself, the team, the organisation or the company, make sure that the voice is human. Leave the corporate style messaging to your PR team. The audience want to develop a relationship with you, your brand or your company in a way that isn't possible with structured PR messaging.

Try not to use any form of automated response. Just as auto-responders in email often irritate and turn customers away, so automated broadcasts will drive your followers away from your transmissions. To ensure that you create and maintain a strong relationship with your customers it is important to engage directly with your audience to give them that personal connection that they value. Investing in the personal touch will in time develop your relationship with them and will prove rewarding in diverse ways. Your connections will become your advocates, benefiting from being your first tier 1 influencers in your social graph, and having an indirect and positive influence on your sales.

If you want to improve your customer satisfaction ratings, reach out and engage with your customers. Regularly engaging with customers, quickly responding to their issues and engaging in open and honest dialogue will demonstrate a high level of customer care. This regular and personal interaction will start to alter customers' perceptions of you and your company.

CONSOLIDATING YOUR APPROACH

I was talking to a client about various different Web 2.0 options and I was going through various tools that she could use to complement her traditional marketing approach with an effective digital marketing strategy, and I was reviewing the different types of networks and tools that she could use to get started on her strategy. I mentioned Facebook and Twitter and ways to use each of these. 'Do I need to do both?' she asked. 'They seem very different.'

Facebook appeals to people looking to reconnect with old friends and keep up with the activities of family members or find new friends online. It also appeals to companies who wish to interact with their fans, offering them the chance to discover new products and services and engage in discussion with each other in a forum style environment. Twitter, on the other hand, encourages you to grab ideas in bite-size chunks and use your updates as pointers to other places on the web, or you can just let others know what you're up to at any given moment without any pointers or links. Dialogue is generally between the Twitter account holder and the person responding and there is less opportunity (and fewer characters) for a forum style discussion to take place.

On the surface, these seem to be completely different styles of applications. Facebook appears to nurture relationships and Twitter appears to broadcast news. But is this the case? Twitter certainly appeals to anyone who seeks the instant update or the news of the moment. Facebook, on the other hand, seems to group like-minded people together along common interests.

Twitter has the ability to move from simple real-time status updates broadcast to all, on to replies, retweets, direct (private) messages and finally on to face to face relationships. It's easy enough to initiate a conversation with people you follow on Twitter, who may then decide to follow you. This mutual following gives both of you the ability to send each other direct messages. Over time, as your relationship develops, your conversation can then progress to email,

Facebook, LinkedIn and ultimately face to face. The ability to add your Twitter feeds to Facebook means that you can connect different platforms together and streamline your updates.

Getting the cluster effect you need in your networks to grow your digital engagement efforts is fairly easy if all of your users have access to the same platform. Unfortunately the sheer variety of networking platforms can cause problems when trying to connect different networks together. Currently it doesn't matter which browser you happen to use on a day to day basis, you can still access your usual networking sites like Facebook, MySpace, LinkedIn and Twitter. This allows your network to grow and clusters of connections to be formed, regardless of operating system, regardless of browser. You need these clusters to grow your network and you need network effects for your news to spread effectively across these different types of networks.

Syndication
If you feel overwhelmed by the amount of potential updates that you have to do for each of the Web 2.0 sites that you contribute to, then there are syndication tools that can help you broadcast across several networking platforms at once:

SAVING TIME THROUGH SYNDICATING

- The Twitter Notifier is an add-on for Live Writer, an offline blog authoring tool. It can be configured to update Twitter every time you publish a blog post. It also provides a shortened URL so that Twitter followers can click the link to reach your blog.

- There is a Facebook application for Twitter which can update your Facebook status with each Twitter update you make. This can be found by searching Facebook for 'Twitter' and installing the application.

- You can update Twitter from Facebook. Search for 'Twitter updater' from within Facebook and install the Facebook application.

- LinkedIn has the ability to pull Twitter updates to display in your LinkedIn feed and can be configured from within the profiles setting area.

- http://ping.fm can update multiple networking sites at once from one status update. The application just needs to know the login credentials for each site you wish it to update.

Facebook Connect was introduced by the developers at Facebook and it pioneered the ability for website developers to access Facebook visitors' social graph information. Social graph information includes information about the users themselves, the users' friends, their status updates and other personal information stored on Facebook. This information is initially accessed by the application when the user explicitly authorises the application to use personal data.

> Applications can access all of your information to display actions and other details on the Facebook news feed.

For example, the Farmville application on Facebook publishes data about the farmer's progression through Farmville by publishing updates on the user's main status feed. Incentives, such as the offer of a free gift or bonus, can be used to entice friends of the farmer to also play Farmville. Incentives like this appearing on your profile page can encourage your friends to join in the game and lead to the acquisition of a greater number of players in the game for the application. Facebook Connect can be used in other ways too. Profile information, photos and other data such as birthday information can be used to deliver a more personalised experience to the user's status feed. Other applications can use the presence information provided by Facebook to take advantage of instant interaction and engagement between Facebook users.

Twitter has an authentication mechanism, Oauth, which allows single login across applications. You can create synergy with your updates across different types of applications and you can get interaction from people across networking platforms.

> Applications communicate with Twitter using a secure application channel to validate credentials.

Your login credentials are cached if you allow the application access so you don't need to maintain separate login details for both applications. This approach can be valuable to the community who can keep interacting with the tool of their choice whilst maintaining the connection across different applications.

YOUR EXISTING BRAND

It's fairly easy to find out what people are saying about you online. All you need to do is type your name into Google and have a look at the results. If you sign up for an alerts service like Google Alerts, Windows Live Alerts, Yahoo! Alerts or Bing News Alerts, you can get a daily digest about what is being said about you or your brand. If you have a blog there are search engines like Technorati or BlogPulse which specifically search through 200 million or so blogs and give you references to your name or other search terms that have been used on other blogs. Again, this is a useful way to find out who is talking about you – especially if there are no physical links or trackbacks to your blog from the originator's blog.

Most of the new interactive applications have search facilities for you to gauge the mood and sentiment of the social media landscape. Facebook, LinkedIn and Twitter all have search tools so you can find out what is being said about you or your brand. Twitter and most of the third party clients that connect to its

application programming interface have search facilities. Twitter allows you to search for and retrieve a list of historical tweets for your hashtag, phrase or user name (Figure 8.1).

Figure 8.1 Twitter search

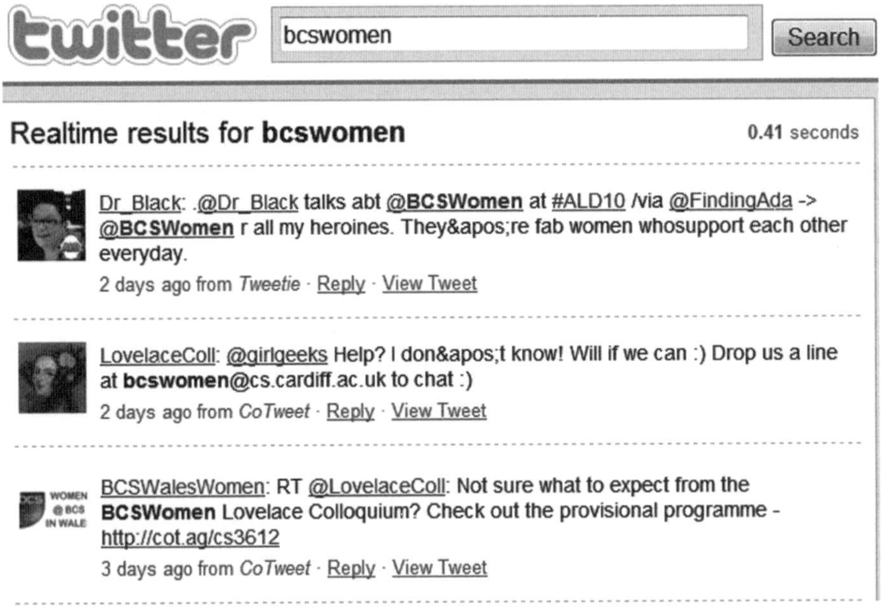

Searching for your brand in this way can give you an immediate sense about how your customers feel about you and lets you listen to their feedback, good or bad, about your company. It's a good idea to regularly search for your product name, brand or company so that you can see what people are saying about you, identify changes in almost real time and, more importantly, have the opportunity to change customer perceptions based on your early actions and response.

Preserving your online reputation

As you already have an online presence on the web, with an established personal or corporate brand you will already have some sort of online reputation. You may think that it's not relevant to you at all, but in the Web 2.0 world everyone has an online reputation, whether they realise it or not. Hopefully your online reputation is good at the very least. It would be nice to know if it's neutral, upsetting if you find that it's negative and absolutely devastating if it's vilified or targeted by cyber bullies. So it's important to consider how you can preserve your online reputation, especially as perception about you can change almost instantly.

The first thing that you could consider is to preserve your brand name. Take a popular enough name like that of my husband, Steve Brown. Typing his full

name into the address bar returns a URL which redirects me to another site selling various things. Someone else has thought of registering his name like this before we have. They have registered the domain name http://SteveBrown.com and they are trying to make some revenue from someone who would like to purchase it – like him, or other Steve Browns across the world.

These names need to be registered on a long term basis with a domain hosting company. If you can manage to, try to purchase domain registrations for periods of longer than 2 years. After all, you're not intending to change your name (unless you're female and intending to change your maiden name when you marry). Securing your domain on a long term basis will ensure that no one else will be able to 'brand-jack' your domain name if you forget to update the registration. If you have several corporate products which have brand identities in their own right, then it's a good idea to register these too. There may also be trademarks which need to be considered in a corporate environment and registered with the appropriate trademark authority.

This all seems very innocuous so far, and only applies to someone who wants their own personally named domain. Imagine the problems that might arise if you were famous, in the media, or politics and someone was cyber squatting on your name. What if your name URL redirected to a very 'unsuitable' site, and even worse, the fake 'you' sites were turning up top of all of the search engines? What can you do to try and rectify things?

One of the best ways to be proactive about this is to buy all of the combinations of your name as domain names – including the unsavoury versions. So for our Steve Brown site example you could also buy:

> http://SteveBrown.net
>
> http://SteveBrown.org
>
> http://SteveBrown.co.xx

You could also consider purchasing other combinations of the name that you can think of – even the domains that are 'seedy', abusive, or unsavoury. So you might buy:

> http://SteveBrownS***s.com
>
> http://F***SteveBrown.com

and similar names.

Once you've secured the domain names use one of your registered names to start to build your positive online reputation. You could start to publish a blog on the domain. Wordpress and similar blogging platforms offer a simple way for you to redirect your own domain name to their website. If you want a website that is

optimised for search engines (SEO) you need to make sure that you update the site often so that the web crawlers find fresh and updated content on a regular basis. Try to blog regularly in small manageable chunks so that the site is fresh and updated with frequent posts.

The search engine spiders will begin to crawl your website or blog, they will find updated content on it, and the spiders will start to visit it more regularly. Slowly, with diligence, your site domain name will rise up the page ranks and the site that you don't actually own will slowly move down onto the second page of search results where people hardly ever look.

> Pointers to your blog or website with fresh content will take precedence due to your regularly updated fresh content.

It will take some time to achieve this, but eventually you'll be able to recover your position in the search engine rankings with positive messages about your site which will improve perception about your reputation. Remember: prevention is always better, and cheaper, than cure.

Damaging your reputation

On Facebook, or MySpace, if you have created pages for your brand, you might want to consider the security settings on the application. You may not wish to have inappropriate content posted on the page of a friend of a friend and find that the content is linked to your page and tarnishing your reputation. It only takes a few moments for your reputation to change. Humorous behaviour can also do reputational harm. Early in 2010 the UK suffered from an extended and unprecedented fall of snow which paralysed the country for several days. Police officers in Oxfordshire,[44] wearing their high visibility jackets, were filmed using their riot shields to sledge down a snowy hill. It all seemed like fun, but these officers they were on duty. These videos were filmed using a mobile device which had the ability to immediately upload to YouTube. The viral nature of YouTube ensured the propagation of the links until it reached the eyes of the media, which took a dim view of their antics. Were their actions fun or irresponsible? Had the snow 'brought out the child' in them, or did the policemen overstep the mark? The decision is yours.

> The community decides and the power of the people has the ability to quickly change perception one way or the other.

When Steve Jobs was allegedly rushed into hospital with a heart attack, Apple's stock plummeted. In October 2008, bloggers reported that Steve 'claimed to be suffering from chest pains'. The story had started on a site which was linked to the CNN network. Apple PR categorically denied[45] the unfounded rumours. With citizen journalism, unsubstantiated rumours, **and no validation from the company itself**, there were a few upsets. Apple's stock took a tumble, CNN's credibility was in question in the media, and a Silicon Valley insider was heavily criticised for reporting on the story in the first place.

Sharing too much on Facebook

I've always smiled at the phrase 'What goes on tour, stays on tour', and I'm sure that lots of us could share some stories if that sentence had never been uttered. However, in this world of digital connections, mobile phones with cameras and immediacy, I think we need an updated version:

> What goes on tour stays on Facebook.

Facebook, with almost 600 million users, is growing at a fantastic rate. It took less than 9 months to add more than 100 million users to Facebook and there are over 1.5 million pieces of content shared daily. Some of this content isn't suitable for viewing outside your immediate network, but it all too often slips through.

> With Facebook's friendly interface and connections to your friends and family it is often easy to forget that it is a public website with extensions to your connections.

Unfortunately, Facebook can be much more public than you realise. Some Facebook users publish information that should often be kept private. Your own Facebook privacy settings may ensure that no one outside your immediate family can see your photos or your status updates, but there is nothing to stop any one of your friends taking a screenshot and broadcasting your message more broadly. There are hundreds of examples of foolish status comments that have been propagated by email, blogged about and propagated as a .jpg screen clipping throughout the web.

Sixteen-year-old Kimberley Swann, who worked at Ivell Marketing and Logistics at Clacton on Sea, Essex, posted comments on Facebook complaining about her job from the first day she started work.

> first day at work. omg (oh my God)!! So dull!!
>
> all i do is shred holepunch n scan paper!!! omg!
>
> 'im so totally bord!!!

Unfortunately her boss found her comments on Facebook, called her in to his office and terminated her employment. He said: 'Following your comments made on Facebook about your job and the company we feel it is better that, as you are not happy and do not enjoy your work, we end your employment with Ivell Marketing & Logistics with immediate effect.'

Crystal Bell was fired via Facebook, according to the *Kelowna Daily Courier*. She had been working for Faces Cosmetics & European Day Spa in Kelowna, she had missed a meeting on her day off and didn't call her boss to tell her.

> It's a good thing I checked my Facebook (site). I had one new message, so I went in and found that I had been fired by my boss.
>
> Her message to me said she found it very unprofessional that I didn't call and say I wouldn't be at the meeting, and that I should find another job.
>
> Firing someone on Facebook is not a professional way to do it.

Large companies also take a firm stand when finding out about indiscretions by their staff. Virgin Atlantic sacked 13 members of staff after they referred to their passengers as 'chavs', a term referring to their perceived social standing and intelligence.

> Following a thorough investigation, it was found that all 13 staff participated in a discussion on the networking site Facebook, which brought the company into disrepute and insulted some of our passengers. ... It is impossible for these cabin crew members to uphold the high standards of customer service that Virgin Atlantic is renowned for if they hold these views.

Direct complaints on Facebook aren't the only way to lose credibility. Status updates showing passive-aggressive behaviour can also be detrimental. Passive aggressive messages can include comments such as:

> I love it when the client cancels our meetings.
>
> It's fantastic when one of my customers think that they have exclusive rights on my time.
>
> Why can't the support team be more helpful?

If you have a public persona for your team or company, people will know if you're talking about them, even obliquely. They could imagine that you're talking about them and become concerned about your hidden meaning. Facebook status updates are not the best place to vent your frustration. Your reputation and credibility will suffer and you may turn clients away. Being negative online has far reaching effects and as your customer engagement goal is to try and grow your business, and improve perception, refraining from being rude or belligerent is a

very good idea. It's easy to destroy your reputation with a few ill chosen words. It's also very difficult to discover the source of some reputation attacks as some choose to hide their true identities when launching an attack.

Cloning and faking your identity

Identity fraud is distressing enough for the individual, but what would you do if your brand was being cloned and used to execute business on your behalf? Your website could be copied and used for illegal purposes, or used as a phishing site specifically designed to extract confidential, personal or financial details from the unwary user. Banks often have to deal with these issues as copied sites are hard to distinguish from the genuine article and unwary users can be tricked into sharing personal details. You might have a significant customer satisfaction issue and poor perception about your brand or the security of the website through no fault of your own. People may also impersonate you when playing MMORPGs such as World of Warcraft, perhaps to gain status, award points or to damage your own standing in the game.

Designer labels have long been victims of piracy, with fake versions of designer items, usually produced in the Far East, appearing across Europe at cut down prices, but fake websites also abound to trick the unwary. Ugg boots are favoured by celebrities and mere mortals alike. They are sold in physical shops and also increasingly found online on websites and on eBay. Unfortunately there are also a lot of websites that offer fake Ugg boots. These are of inferior quality, and customers have complained about them. This poor quality fake merchandise has done damage to Ugg's reputation. Ugg has been proactive in stamping out fake websites that pretend to be genuine Ugg websites selling genuine boots. Ugg Australia has a page on its website advising what you can do in order to purchase genuine Ugg boots and works with customs agencies and Internet service providers to stamp out instances of fake shipments and cloned websites.

Corporations such as banks now have stringent processes in place to search out fake copies of their websites which are used to phish information about bank accounts for fraudulent use. Generally these fake websites appear as hyperlinks on a phishing email, which, when clicked, direct the unwary to a copy of the original banking website, ready to receive your data. Once a fraudulent site is uncovered, there are several procedures in place to remove the DNS record for the site so the DNS name no longer resolves to an IP address at the website. There is also a process for longer term disputes over websites names. The Uniform Domain-Name Dispute-Resolution Policy (UDRP) can resolve disputes over Internet domain name registration. The policy applies to .biz, .com, .info, .name, .net, and .org top-level domains. It can also include some country code top-level domains and the UDRP can be engaged to act on your behalf if the domain name in question is identical or similar enough to be confused with a trademark or service mark owned by another company and the registered domain name is being used it 'bad faith'.

Preventing online identity theft

There are some precautions you can take, however, to try to prevent identity theft. To completely avoid identity cloning on a personal level, you need to be

extremely cautious when you are on the web. Make sure you remain aware of your transactions and activities, and you need to always protect your personal information. Here are a few ideas you could consider:

Use different passwords for each online site you use, and don't use sequential passwords to avoid phishing attempts on one site using the same or sequential logon details across other social networking sites that you use (LemonApple42, LemonApple43, LemonApple44 for example).

Use complex passwords with mixed case letters, numbers and a non-alphanumeric character. A good example is to use passwords that are not related or are not proper names. For example, you could use the first character of each word in a sentence to create your own acronym. Take the poem: 'Mary had a little lamb; its fleece was white as snow'. This would produce the following set of letters for your password:

Mhall,ifwwas

Use numbers to replace certain letters. You might use 1 instead of the letter I, 3 instead of E and 4 instead of H. Your original acronym becomes following complex password:

M4all,1fwwas

This makes your memorable sentence and the process to create your password process logical. It makes complex passwords easy to create and easy to change especially if you have a long piece of text to draw inspiration from. Adding non-alphanumeric characters like %, & * ! ; ^ makes the password even more difficult to guess.

You can change your birth date. When you register on a website consider adjusting your birth date so that it is one or two days different from your actual birthday. You could adjust the year of your birth by a year or so. If your actual birth date is needed, the website will probably have a mechanism where a manual check, performed by a human, will highlight the difference and contact you to confirm the real date. The only slight irritation of changing the date of your birthday may be that your friends will send you birthday wishes on a different day than your real birthday. This is a small price to pay for knowing that your true date of birth does not appear on any website and your real identity cannot be used for other purposes.

You can never be totally safe from identity theft or cloning, but if you put as many challenges as possible in the way, you can help to mitigate this risk.

Now we're online and active. We're going to find our audience and search for the job or that candidate that we really want to find. Let's now start to really publicise our online presence!

SUMMARY

- Discoverability is key to online success.
- Learn the behaviours that are important to user interaction and engagement.
- Listen to the community.
- Set goals based on what your customers want.
- Find your experts who have a true passion about what you do.
- Beware the self proclaimed experts.
- Use syndication to cross walled garden sites.
- Develop your voice.
- Use search facilities to check for information about your brand.
- Take steps to preserve your online reputation.
- Try to mitigate the risk of online identity theft.

9 DISCOVERY

'Create a community and it will come'. This is a great idea, and your community will come – however, they will only come if they know where they can find you. Your brand, both personal and corporate, needs to be discovered and needs to be advertised. In this chapter, we will look at ways to improve your search engine rankings through the intelligent use of social tools, and the need for you to keep active in online circles. We'll talk about how recruitment has been turned on its head, both from the ease of finding a role online, and the visibility that you have to potentially millions of recruiters. We'll find out how innovative use of social media has managed to put a whole musical orchestra together and we'll see how important the extended social network now is to recruiters and companies alike. We'll give some tips to think about if you're looking for a new role and want to try a different channel to publicise your skills, and we'll learn from recruiters and what they look for when they search for candidates.

We'll talk about how to grow your online audience and how you can find friends to connect with across different social networks. Finally, we'll look at how you can increase the number of connections you have and some techniques you could try for extra reach to your connections in your next digital marketing campaign.

CREATING AND PUBLICISING YOUR BRAND

What makes software popular? For many it's the feature set of the product. But now perceptions have changed, and this is entirely due to the new way we interact with each other online. Different types of websites attract different types of visitors. Features, interactive widgets and animations are designed to attract and entice. Early adopters, techies and enthusiasts will go to a site for different reasons than mainstream followers. One of the main reasons why you will visit social networking sites is that your friends, colleagues and people in your immediate network are engaging with their friends and interacting there.

> Having your contacts grouped together amplifies the network effect and significantly extends your potential reach.

The ability to connect outside your immediate network to include people further out in your social graph is important. These second degree connections can

significantly add to the spread of networking and adoption of the site or application. You have your connections to your friends and you wish to extend your network outside your immediate circle of friends. You want to find those useful connections and work them into your network. LinkedIn, Facebook and Twitter all have search facilities where you can find others who are interested in the same things as you, whether in business, personal, political or scientific. You can connect directly or get connected through one of your first degree networks.

If you want to use the community approach to gather new connections, then you can use broadcasts to find your audience. Your audience are people who are interested in the same things as you are. If you blog, tweet, or update your networking sites regularly then others who are searching for similar topics will find your postings. With regular broadcasts and responses to your audience you will start to generate a relationship with your audience that will bring you more followers, extend your network and create potential new advocates for your brand.

As soon as you publish online, you'll get some kind of audience. But who are they? A lot of them are silent lurkers, they are visitors to your site who may have stumbled across your information accidentally and then move away. These visitors may be invisible to your eyes, they spend their time watching and waiting for you to connect with them. These lurkers are waiting for some information that resonates with them. It's hard to connect with these people if you don't know who or where they are.

You do know that these people are out there watching and listening, so there are things you can do.

> Consider adjusting your 'voice' to a different style to try to reach the people you don't currently know about.

If your style consists of opinions and commentary, you might want to try a different tone, such as information sharing, or questioning your readers. Your message has the potential to become diluted or taken out of context. It may be replicated elsewhere through different channels or it may not be replicated at all. There's always a chance that you won't connect with your original intended audience. Persistence always pays off, and it's worth bearing in mind that some people will never connect with you no matter how hard you try. Don't be disheartened. If you make sure that your site can be discovered easily by your audience, eventually the interaction will come.

Getting your website discovered requires some tweaking so that search engines like Google can find and index the site. Search engine optimisation, the art of improving the ranking of a website in search results, has been around for some time. Using keywords or meta-tags on your web pages can get your page higher up the search engine rankings, or get you some 'Google juice'. It's simple enough to use intelligent keywords, image keywords and keyword hotlinks on your web page. SEO specialists can register your site on search engines so that the spiders and search bots come to visit your page, but these are manual processes.

Fortunately, with the advent of status updates and online profiles, Web 2.0 techniques can improve your rankings with very little effort. User generated updates by their nature are dynamic, and having dynamic, frequently changing information on your site is a good thing. Dynamic updates ensure that web bots will visit your site more frequently and improve your rankings across the search engines. Google Bing and Yahoo! now index social media updates such as those from Friendfeed, Twitter and YouTube, so your recent communications on these sites can appear in the results fairly quickly. There are other considerations for SEO and practices you could put into place to publicise your brand or profile.

PUBLICISING YOUR BRAND

- Try to have a consistent naming strategy. If your company is called Best New Media Marketing Ltd, try to find a name that matches across all of your profiles. If you're going to use this name as your alias on Twitter, with its 140-character limit, you'll need to use short status messages as you won't have many characters left in the message.

- Try to reserve your brand identities by registering them. Use http://namechk.com to check whether the username you wish has already been registered on other networking sites.

- Think about your brand attributes. Are you reliable, efficient, dynamic, energetic, innovative, strategic, structured or creative? Make sure you include these attributes whenever you post online updates.

- Make sure your visual image portrays the brand you want, both in your corporate identity and your personal brand online. Consider whether using a headshot in your profile is the best for your brand, or whether your logo is the image you want your customers to see.

- Decide on your personal and professional brand limits. Decide where to draw the line. With suitable privacy settings, lock down any settings that you don't want broadcasted.

- Focus on quality and consistency in your message. Remember content is king and freshness is queen.

- Post information regularly. Find a schedule which works for you and stick to it. Whether you have the time to update once a day, or once a week, the key message is consistency. Avoid bursts of activity which will confuse the web crawl spiders and turn your readers away.

- Create channels for your brand. YouTube and Slideshare are just two examples of channels that you can customise with your logo and configure a background to the page in your company style. Facebook pages and LinkedIn groups, when well configured and maintained, promote your brand and encourage dialogue with your customers and partners.

- Cross-link. Refer to your Twitter feed, your Facebook page, your blog or your LinkedIn Profile on each of your sites so that each of them can be accessed

from the other. If you want a single destination point, make sure that all of your profiles point to that site.

- Vary the content. Talking about the same thing using the same URL time after time will make your updates appear to be spam and your followers will go elsewhere.

- Keep the content on message. If your business is about ballet shoes, then make sure that the term 'ballet shoes' appears regularly in your blog posts, or on Twitter. You'll eventually turn up in search results for 'ballet shoes' if you regularly post ballet related updates on each of these sites.

- Comment on other blogs. Your comment profile will appear as a URL on the other blog site which links back to your site. Web crawl spiders will notice the links and give your site more relevance and ranking amongst other similar sites.

- Be generous with your links to other blogs which will draw traffic back to your site.

- Use several platforms and remember that you can link each of these. Content goes across most of these platforms.

The key thing is to make sure that the content is fresh and updated regularly. Appearing at the top of search engine results is not something that happens overnight. If you are diligent and organised about creating fresh content, then you'll be surprised at how quickly this can happen, and you can measure your success in weeks instead of months.

USING SOCIAL MEDIA FOR RECRUITMENT

Finding a job and recruiting for a role can be daunting and a huge time sink. You need a plan to market yourself and a plan for your approach.

Consider marketing yourself in the same way that you would market the feature set for a new product.

This approach can bring benefits. You can become innovative and creative in your search for a job. Adding digital media activities to your job finding pipeline can extend your reach and improve your chances. It certainly worked for one job hunter. Alec Brownstein is a copywriter who was looking for a new role with a creative agency. He went about it in an unusual way by purchasing Ad Words on Google for the creative directors' names he wished to target.[46] When they Googled their names, his ad appeared at the top of the list. He was offered two jobs.

Having an online presence which states your capabilities in a positive way can expose you to a potentially unlimited number of potential employers. Streamline your profile so it is seen by your target audience, and focus their attention on your key skills.

Social networking sites allow you to segment your interests. You can join specialised groups focusing on your specific interest, skills and aspirations. These specialised groups are followed by your intended audience and thus anyone searching for skills in a particular area is more likely to find you there. LinkedIn is an excellent example of this, with almost half a million groups to choose from on politics, technology, recruitment, networks – anything, really, as you can easily create your own group which is searchable from within the groups directory. You can easily find specialised groups on Facebook too, and YouTube categorises its videos for easier searching.

A new way to find a job

YouTube has been used to successfully recruit a specialist band of people. In February 2009 musicians from around the world were invited to audition exclusively using YouTube as the medium.[47] They were asked to upload a video of themselves playing a segment from a piece of music. These videos were voted on by YouTube viewers around the world. The winners were selected to play at Carnegie Hall in New York in April 2009 under the direction of Michael Tilson Thomas. A mashup video was created of the event which is also on YouTube. Jim Moffat, who played French horn in New York, said about his experience:[48]

And so to my own romantic foolishness, an attempt, courtesy of the YouTube Symphony Orchestra virtual auditions, to create a decent rendition of one movement of Mozart's earliest horn concerto – commonly known as the second. It was maddening. I discovered how to create semi-watchable video and passable audio, in my dining room. And how to concentrate for five minutes, never an easy task. There I stand, naked but for my underwear. You may see with your eyes a man relaxing in a comfy cricket jumper, but hear with your ears a man starkers.

Finding a job using social tools is not as easy as joining a new networking site and announcing 'Give me work'. You need to build up your reputation and your online profile so that your connections can get to know and trust you. Your profile needs to be comprehensive, clear and concise. Start connecting, link to others who have the same interests as you. Respond to queries, make recommendations to people you've connected with, make new connections and keep existing connections alive with communication and interaction.

Once you've created your profile, you need to keep it fresh so that your changes continue to appear on the pages of your connections. You might like to change something on your profile every few days to alert your followers to new content. If you're using a tool like LinkedIn to manage your profile and connections, every modification you make to your profile shows up in others' timelines and draws their attention towards you if you have allowed this on your privacy settings. Update your status regularly so that recruitment agents know that you're looking for new opportunities.

Your second level connections are also important to you. These are the people who have a greater social distance from you. Your immediate network may not be able to help you but **their** networks might have the answer you need.

The 'friend of a friend' network can prove to be an extremely powerful asset to you.

The connectors and key networkers in your immediate networking circle may be very useful to you in recommending you to one of the connections in their network. If you start to build up your own valuable connections and develop a good relationship with them, you'll find that your extended network grows significantly and can have great potential.

Searching for jobs

If you're searching for a new job, you need to have a good online presence and brand. Your online brand is the first thing that recruiters will search for when they want to check out your credentials. Publicising your profile online is a great and free way to advertise your ability and build your brand. You can use some of the techniques I've mentioned to find your perfect role. Now that you know that recruiters are looking out for you, it's really important to tidy up all of your online profiles to make sure you give the right impression to your potential new employer.

FINDING A JOB

- Most recruiters turn to LinkedIn first to check out details of your CV, so make sure that your LinkedIn details match the CV that you submitted to the agency.

- Ensure your LinkedIn profile is 100% completed. If your LinkedIn profile is sitting at 75% and you're sure that you have completed all of the fields, you need to get recommendations about your recent work from your connections. Recruiters want recent testimonials about your work, so make sure these referrals are up to date.

- Make your LinkedIn public profile name easy to remember. For example, http://LinkedIn.com/in/eileenbrown is much easier to remember than http://uk.linkedin.com/pub/eileen-brown/2/5b7/978. It's easy to change the URL in your profile settings.

- Link your online accounts to each other and link them to LinkedIn. If you link your Facebook account to LinkedIn, make sure that you have your appropriate privacy settings in place to avoid any personal data migrating onto your professional page. If you use Facebook for entirely personal reasons, then protect your Facebook profile and don't link it to LinkedIn.

- Search for job-specific keywords on Twitter, Google and Facebook. Recruiters may be advertising for roles on these sites using the same phrases. Use the RSS feed functionality of Twitter to save any tweets that appear to your RSS reader for action at a later stage. Set up Google Alerts for job-specific words.

- Post your CV online if you're openly looking for a role. You could create a link to your curriculum vitae on your blog or you could create a visual CV on Slideshare if your speciality is in design. Syndicate it across your other network sites so that everyone is aware of it.

- Search for your target keywords on LinkedIn. Someone may be advertising your dream role.

Be active, consistent and current in these areas. You and your online profile will bubble up to the top of the search results and your second degree network might turn up the role designed specifically with you in mind.

Recruiting from social networking sites

As a recruiter, if you don't use sites with a high degree of audience engagement and conversation to find candidates you may be missing out on some top notch candidates who do use these types of sites to find their next role. Advertising on job boards gives you access to half of your potential candidates, telling your story on as many sites as possible, and actively searching out candidates will significantly broaden your horizons.

> The purpose of social networking in a business context is to engage with others. If you are not using social media, you will never know who else is out there.

Regularly advertising your presence on Twitter using keywords can bring benefits, and if requests are phrased appropriately, you can avoid the flood of inappropriate CVs. Anyone doing keyword searching will find you and your job. Many human resources professionals who aim to recruit use sites like LinkedIn and Facebook, not only to check out your employment history but also to look for your recommendations from your previous employers. According to a survey of human resources professionals, over 48% spend more than 3–5 hours per week searching for suitable candidates whom they otherwise wouldn't know or couldn't contact.

Cisco uses this form of communication very effectively as a recruitment tool and to communicate with and engage Generation Y. Cisco EMEA (Europe, Middle East and Africa) conducts graduate recruitment through Facebook groups and has a very successful master page with over 4,000 fans. There are three pages pertaining to EMEA: a high level graduate recruitment page, 'Cisco Graduate Recruitment', with other groups such as 'Emerging Markets East' – Middle East region, and the CIS region. Cisco provides information on upcoming campus events, and offers programmes and opportunities for graduates across various disciplines. The team respond to questions related to the overall graduate recruitment process and discuss graduate roles on the pages. Fresh content and activity on the page keep the page activity growing. One of the benefits of having a Facebook page with so many fans is that Cisco then has the opportunity to check out potential candidates if it chooses to.

Executive search agencies and consultants use tools like LinkedIn to trawl through profiles, searching on phrases like 'looking for new opportunities'. You won't be able to guarantee a good hire, but if you're smart about your use of searches, and make good use of the resources out there, then you'll get a very good idea of the available talent. A key benefit of using sites such as LinkedIn is that you can ask those in your LinkedIn network if they know of anyone in **their** network who might fit your criteria. This allows you to take advantage of your extended network, the second degree connection. The candidate may not be suitable for a role offered by your colleague, but they may dovetail perfectly into the role you're trying to fill. Take advantage of your second degree network, it could bring you unexpected benefits.

It's a good idea also to check whether anyone already on your shortlist has a presence on sites that you may not be aware of. Technorati will find blog entries, Google or Bing will find tweets, email addresses and entries posted on other social networking sites that you may not be aware of. You may find evidence of skills that didn't make it onto the candidate's CV. This may be due to space constraints on the original document, but it can give you a different insight into the candidate. Perhaps your candidate does charity or pro bono work, perhaps he leads communities or interacts with a wide circle of influencers, and perhaps he has published papers online.

When you are considering a candidate you can check sites for the candidate's writing style, patterns of behaviour, grammar, spelling and general attitude. You also have the opportunity to see what other people are saying about your candidate online, and have a look at their interaction on Twitter. Lots of the under 30 age group tend to favour Facebook over LinkedIn, using Facebook for their social and business interaction, so be sure to look there. If you happen to find an unsuitable photo of your candidate, don't necessarily rule her out completely. Her transgression may have been simply a one-off which her other entries on different sites show to be out of character. You can, however, get a feel for her other activities from online profiles that may not be obvious at first look. There may be drug and alcohol use or abuse, a poor attitude to work in general, negative feelings about a former employer or humorous stories about missing work. These clues can add to the general impression, good or bad, of a candidate and help you effectively refine your choice.

Social networking sites will never replace the recruitment screening process entirely, but they will help you to reduce some of the legwork required, circumvent some of the questions, and gain a great understanding about your potential new hire.

DISCOVERING THE INFLUENCERS IN YOUR AUDIENCE

If you're intending to market your product or services using conversational media, then you need to identify the correct part of your audience, and find who your influencers are. Depending on the type of business you're in, your audience and potential customers are active in their own specific spheres. They may be decision makers inside the firewall, they may not hold budget themselves, but they may have significant influence over the decision makers at your customer. Your influencers may be key technologists in the community, considered trusted advisers in their field. They might be geeks who are visionaries in your industry, they may be early adopters or trend setters. These people will help you advance your business, they will help in achieving a measurable ROI, and you would benefit from making them your friends.

Seeding these influential members of the audience with information is your challenge.

How can you ensure that these people are the hubs in their network and will extend your buzz across their own networks?

Traditionally marketers have looked for influencers who are active in a structured network, but research has shown that networks are often split into zones or smaller hubs within the network. The key to finding your influencer is not to search for the hub of the whole network.

> It's about finding the right individual who will spread the message across all of the different subgroups within a network.

These individuals, with their links to many subgroups, are known as **super-connectors**. These subgroups may be classified by technology, geography, interests or social activity, but careful examination will find those users who transcend these networks and, more importantly, link different networks together. To effectively market to these people, take a closer look at who these super-connectors are and who they communicate with regularly. Then you can start the discussion with the right connector.

Online 'friends' are very important. They will help you to expand your network beyond the initial circle of networking contacts you have. Like the six degrees of separation experiment where each person is one step away from each of their direct contacts and two steps away from their contacts' contacts, everyone on earth is theoretically connected by at most six steps.

> The important thing to remember is that these steps are not equal in strength. Some of your close friends are bound by extremely strong ties, and other casual acquaintances are connected to you by much weaker ties.

Social structures are modelled using both weak and strong ties, and it is often the case that weaker ties become stronger for a time, in order to perform some transient social function. This function might be something as simple as connecting you to one of their strong ties to form a bond. This system of social hubs and routing hubs, strong ties and weak ties, forms the basis of all connections. It is dynamic and fluid, and it changes all the time.

Finding your audience and friends

Hubs, people who have a collection of friends who feed them information, routers who pass information onto other hubs, and endpoints who receive output from hubs and routers are very useful in your network. However, you may want to discover easy ways to increase your audience. For example, you may be launching a new campaign and one of your metrics is to get 'net new' visitors to your site and increase your audience by driving page views to your target campaign site.

There are hundreds of social networks, some are specialised and designed for specific interests, and perhaps hobbyist or music sites, and some are more generic.

You may know and use LinkedIn for your business contacts and Plaxo to connect your email contact list to others. You might use Last.fm, MySpace, Pandora and Spotify for music, and Facebook, Hi5, Orkut and Twitter for your social connections.

These websites are 'sticky', they are simple and popular, they encourage connections and they drive huge amounts of user engagement.

Users tend to spend a lot of time on their sites, they store a lot of their data on them, and there are tools such as Facebook that allow friends using different social networks to connect with each other. This amount of engagement means that there's a great opportunity here for advertisers to take advantage of these websites and connections. A simple example would be the opportunity for job search and recruitment companies to have a tight tie-in with LinkedIn. LinkedIn could display job advertisements targeted according to the user's online profile. There is also an opportunity for consumer brands to advertise across Facebook and YouTube, and opportunities to drive traffic to the website using Twitter updates – providing, of course that they have compelling and eye catching status messages.

There are many ways to automatically find new people to follow on Twitter via an array of tools which offer free and paid-for services.

These services offer automated ways to gather new followers and ways to follow those who tweet about keywords you choose.

Several Twitter clients – including Tweetdeck, Seesmic and TweetGrid – allow search strings to be placed into a separate feed column to discover who is talking about your product, service or brand. Whilst this is a great opportunity to gather feedback, it still requires manual intervention to follow these people if you so choose.

Searching for the right information is easy. There are tools to help connect you to anything you want on the web, whether it's stored in a web page, a YouTube video or a blog. Tools like Technorati and IceRocket search blogs, while Yahoo! Search, Google and Bing search content on web pages and across social networking sites. MetaTube and Redlasso search for videos, and CrowdEye is used for social searches. Most of these tools offer targeted online advertisements, so there's a potential business opportunity to increase revenue on these sites.

If you have a presence across several networks and you have fresh and interesting content, you'll be seen by your target audience. Some of your followers will link to you and their friends will notice this presence and amplify your message on your behalf.

Increasing your following

If part of your customer engagement strategy is to increase the number of your followers then you need to think ways to engage your new audience. The mechanisms for increasing followers are pretty much the same whatever tool you use, and whether you want to spread your message across the Twitterverse or score large numbers of hits for your YouTube video.

> Your strategy needs to consider the fact that once you've identified your audience, you need to get them to follow you or subscribe to you, so the most important thing here is to provide interesting content.

Your broadcasts need to have useful, relevant and informative information to capture their attention and keep them engaged. This information could be in the form of news about an upcoming event, a product or beta launch or a new piece of business news. It could be a simple 'how-to' article. I love the 'how to fold a t-shirt' videos on YouTube. These 'how-to' articles appear at the top of the search engines. Try it!

Whatever your information is, it needs to be useful enough for people to recommend it to their connections, who recommend it to their connections and amplify the message.

STARTING YOUR SOCIAL MEDIA PLAN

Unfortunately there are lots of poor quality campaigns and things can go wrong. Some marketers continually spam their followers with the same message over and over again. Adverts like 'Don't pay for tooth whitening. This Mom discovered the secret to white teeth for under $5' repeated across each of your sites will not give you the profile you desire. If the tooth whitening solution is one of the few products that you market, then you need to be creative about the different ways you can broadcast your message.

BROADCASTING YOUR MESSAGE

- Find the active conversationalists, influencers and leaders in your industry and follow them. Subscribe to their blogs, follow them on Twitter, and connect with the people they connect with. You'll then get great insights into the way they use online marketing to get their message across effectively.

- Search for the types of people you want to notice you and follow them. Use keywords to narrow your search to the target market. Comment on their blogs, photos and video uploads, link to them and follow them on Twitter. This will increase their reputation in the community and bring you to their attention.

If you follow people in your industry and post interesting things, it's likely that they will follow you back.

- Decide on a sensible name for your channels. People are much more likely to follow realistic companies like 'WhiteTeeth' than they are to follow channels such as 'Awesome Tooth Whitening Products'.

- Make sure your channels are populated. People won't subscribe to a blog that isn't updated regularly, nor will they follow a blank Twitter feed or an uninteresting YouTube channel.

- Try to broadcast realistically. If you insist on talking about your amazing tooth whitening products all the time, you will appear to be spamming your audience. Try instead to ask poll questions like 'Which tooth whitening product is your favourite?' or 'Which tooth whitening product would you try?' Your consumers are intelligent and will move away in droves from a poorly executed strategy.

- If your social media strategy centres around Twitter, make sure that you don't follow everyone. You will be overwhelmed with information and will miss out useful snippets in the fire hose of communication. Make sure that if you choose to follow lots of people on Twitter, then your Twitter client software allows you to create groups of key influencers, friends, and business associates, so you can filter out the noise.

- Post interesting news and information about your product, and advertise your message regularly. Also make sure that you also talk about other products to give yourself credibility across the market. Highlight news across your industry sector to show balance. If others post relevant and interesting news on Twitter, use the retweet function to broadcast this to your own followers. Re-share Facebook pages with your friends with interesting links and broadcast interesting video uploads. Use trackbacks to link to blogs with relevant content.

- Use URL shorteners so that your links can be forwarded easily. You might want to publicise a link on your blog, or on Facebook. Use one of the many URL shorteners to create a smaller link that people can easily share within Twitter's 140-character limit. If you use a shortener with metrics tracking facilities, then you can track the click-through numbers from the link.

- Search for your brand name on blogs, videos, and Twitter. Respond to any comments or questions. If there are any issues, then make sure that you try to get a solution for the customer. The customer will know you are listening, and their perception of your brand will improve.

Once you have been discovered, then you need to take advantage of your network of friends and your friends' friends. If you have a small team, or are attempting this yourself, then your next challenge is to think about scaling your network activities and working the crowd.

SUMMARY

- Group your contacts together to amplify the network effect.
- Have a consistent identity and broadcast pattern.
- Use LinkedIn for recruitment and to find a new job.
- Provide interesting and fresh content for your followers to find you.
- Plan the way you broadcast your message.

10   SCALING NETWORKS

Taking advantage of the opportunity to join in the great conversation isn't without its problems. If there are restrictions on your budget, headcount and time then it may be difficult for you to find the relevant people to help you extend your network. In this chapter we'll talk about engaging the right types of people to help you propagate your message, the sorts of rewards that motivate these people and how you can get them to become your advocates. We'll have a look at the different behaviours of different age groups on social networking sites and how they engage with their peers. We'll see how different ways of sharing data have evolved and the potential for community and enterprise mashups to be put to good use for both community and businesses. We'll also have a look at the differences of behaviour inside the firewalls.

> Inside companies, reticence in adopting the new way of communicating has resulted in huge amounts of data storage and ineffective collaboration, information islands and siloed data repositories.

We'll also look at opportunities to change this approach from the ground up and we will look at ways to change the way of working from the traditional 'top down' hierarchical approach. Finally, we'll look at how these tools have encouraged companies to use social media as a customer connections tool to gather market intelligence about their products. We'll explore how they can quickly respond to customers with problems and build effective relationships that validate the investment in their digital engagement activities. These activities will enable them to scale to a much greater level than their traditional customer service approaches currently do.

SCALING NETWORKS

It's all very well having a social media strategy, a plan to reach millions of potential new customers that will charm your army of advocates into buying your products, but there may be something niggling at the back of your mind. Scale. How on earth will you single-handedly reach such a large number of people? With IT departments stretched to breaking point with no staff to spare, this is going to be a challenge. You have limited budget, minimal time to invest in your carefully crafted 'execution policy' and no other resources at your disposal. You probably

feel that this new edict from above is impossible to achieve. You can't implement your digital marketing strategy alone. Of course, if you consider yourself to be a sole trader or you are running a small business and have no other resources at your disposal then you might think that you have no other option.

However, there are potentially millions of helpers at your disposal. You could use this super-connected network of extended friends to build up a set of connections for you.

> These connections are not just a band of happy followers who love your product and buy every new version or revision that they can get their hands on.

These are your loyal football fans. They have the season ticket, they attend every match that they can – even the away games – and they buy all of your merchandise whenever a new club design comes out. But most of these 'football fans' stay silent – apart from when they're actually at a game of course. These followers do not actually help you get your word out to your new potential customers. They are the silent majority. These types of people will always buy the same brand of baked beans, toothpaste or tampons. They have done so for years and they don't intend to change on a whim.

> The problem with the silent majority is that they won't evangelise your product for you. For this you need to reach out and find your 'noisy few'.

The noisy few exist in your immediate network, your tier 1 network, and they are vocal. They may be positive, they may be negative, but they are communicating with you. They **want** to talk to you. All you need to do is connect with them and start a conversation. The noisy few will relish the opportunity to communicate with you. They will form a relationship and engage in regular discussions with you about your brand, product or feature set.

> Over time these noisy few will become your advocates, and your friends. Your noisy few will tell your story on your behalf.

OUR BEHAVIOUR IS INFLUENCED BY OUR AGE

The way that grownups have approached social media is totally different from the way their children use the tools. Adults don't tend to have free flow conversations with each other on your Facebook wall and they don't tend to send many virtual hugs. They don't tend to use quizzes to the same extent as the younger generation, nor do they join hundreds of groups and subgroups. They do tend to contact their friends with birthday wishes, they will comment on their friends' status

messages, and they will click on the 'like' tag on Facebook. They will even 'favourite' a particular tweet on Twitter when something captures their interest. Their behaviours tend to be very different from their teenage children, and this behaviour even filters through to the way they use their profile information on their network.

Adult behaviour

Adults tend to complete their initial profile when they set up an account on a site. They use their profile primarily to promote their business; they add links to their website or blog. As far as the social aspect is concerned, they will display their hobbies and interests and they will complete most of the personal sections of their profile. Adults only tend to complete their profiles to a minimum level, presenting a minimal framework of their activities which becomes a permanent record of their account.

This is totally different from the way that young people treat their profiles. Teenagers' and young adults' online profiles are a living, breathing, organic record of their personality, mood and situation at that moment in time. Their status updates and their moods are frequently changed, often several times a day. They join numerous groups and interact and modify their home pages on the site.

Adults' use of social networking sites reflects exactly what these sites were originally intended for, which is primarily to connect and communicate with their friends from now, and from their past. The networking site, Friends Reunited, is a prime example of this online 'school reunion' where everyone can find out what happened to their classmates and work colleagues. They can communicate with old friends, comment on old enemies and rejoin the dots of their history.

Teenagers and social networking

For young people in the US, online services have become the place to go to socialise.

It's a little like the online version of the youth club, it is the place for people to congregate, gossip, agonise over teenage relationships, socialise and exchange information. The term networking, which tends to be used by adults in business environments, is not an alien term to young people.

They congregate in groups of friends they know and they tend not to reach out to new groups. However, they don't really need to socialise outside their immediate school or social group. If they use sites like Friendster, MySpace, Bebo and Facebook, they can exchange information, chat with their online friends, enhance their profile and customise their page to suit their personality. They can advertise the things they like, the books they read, and films they watch, and create lists of their favourite foods. They can take quizzes, adopt virtual names and personalities which they change on a regular basis and they can express themselves to the world. This social behaviour seems to help them prepare for the transition into

adulthood; it's a type of social grooming amongst their peers that helps them to operate in the adult world whilst in the safety of their own social circle, with their own language, habits and social rules.

Teenagers use sites that allow them to interact within their social circle. They can update their status, they can join groups, and they can change their mood or their relationship status to alert their friends to what is going on right here, right now. They use emoticons to share the mood of the moment with their friends, not their parents. They are horrified that their parents are also on Facebook, though they might also connect with them or follow them on Twitter. This group of teenagers wants to hide certain things from their parents, whilst still telling all to their immediate social circle. They need to have a balance in information that is propagated.

I've seen blog posts that speculate that there aren't too many teenagers who use Twitter. Perhaps this could be due to the very public nature of Twitter, where your every status message can be seen, unless your profile is locked. The nature of Twitter encourages sharing information in a wide public forum. Perhaps teenagers prefer to grade their broadcasts to different groups, and the only way to hide your updates in Twitter is to secure the stream. This doesn't seem to be of benefit to the broadcaster who secures their status updates. Twitter is all about the broader conversation, and perhaps it appeals to an older age group. A Twitter update can potentially become a news item – as celebrities and politicians are increasingly finding out.

OTHER WAYS OF BROADCASTING YOUR MESSAGE

Video sharing

There are many ways to extend your brand using mechanisms other than the written word. YouTube, the second largest search engine after Google in terms of items searched, has over 100 million videos that you can search. Videos are created by corporate teams, film and video companies, end users, and now it is really simple to quickly upload a video captured on a mobile device. And there are many other video hosting and sharing sites too – Viddler, Vimeo, Hulu, Brightcove, MetaCafe, to name just a few. You can broadcast your video stream in real time too. Services like Ustream, BlogTalk radio and Justin.tv use livecasting, streamed video and tools for broadcasting in real time to your audience.

There are services that enable you to add telephone dial-in facilities to host a multi-party video conference. You can save the audio files or the video stream so that users can download the session as a compressed MP3 file at a later stage – ideal for any users that didn't get to hear the original broadcast. You also have the opportunity to upload documents to accompany the session. There are options in some of these tools for a Twitter stream to be embedded alongside the broadcast so that questions can be tweeted in for the presenters to answer. This instant delivery allows a host of opportunities for companies who can use video for educational services, training, product launches and PR campaigns. You can secure the

channel to host your own private business meetings if you don't have a comparable conferencing solution in house.

Asics, the shoe company, created a video for YouTube about the origin of the company – all done using origami. The video quickly went viral with comments about the beauty of the video and the story of how the company was created. This viral video had a secondary effect. Within a few days of the video being posted, the company saw a huge upturn in traffic on the main Asics site and a much greater awareness of the brand.

Audio broadcasting

Podcasting (personal on demand broadcasting) has been around for a few years now and is very popular. It is really easy to download audio files from the web to listen to selected snippets of a radio show at your convenience. You can also create podcasts for use in learning and training, for capturing vox pops at events, and to record facts and narratives. These audio files are a good way for technical people to showcase their expertise in a specific area. This might be a series of podcasts documenting the Second World War in manageable session 'chunks' or it might be advice for people who need personal coaching to appear more confident. There seems to be podcasts for every conceivable subject. Podcasts can be placed on the web for anyone to download to their PCs or devices, or delivered via a specific service like podcast.com to specific users.

Currently one of the most popular mechanisms for listening to podcasts is Apple's iTunes, but there are other services such as Podbean and Rhapsody that you can use. One of the key advantages of podcasts is that they can be any length you want. This means that you can deliver short targeted broadcasts of a few minutes, with snippets of useful information, or record a series of lectures of an hour or more.

Let the community categorise the content

With the move away from structured taxonomies on the web and the wide adoption of folksonomies, much richer data can be tagged and found on the web. You can tag photos that you upload to photo sharing sites, in addition to naming them. This extra information gives applications a wealth of resources to take advantage of. Imagine a mashup, with a mapping service like Google Maps or Bing Maps. Users can visit a location and see photos of the area that have been taken by the community and uploaded to a photo sharing site like Flickr or Yfrog. Now imagine a 360-degree panorama of the area consisting of photographs that have been taken by different people and merged using photo stitching software. This technology already exists and has been demonstrated to great acclaim at the TED conference.[49] Imagine user-created videos attached to the location map so that upon looking at your destination you can take a virtual tour of the location and see it from the community point of view. It's a really powerful concept that brings social photo sharing into enterprise applications – and provides a great opportunity for website owners and advertisers to take advantage of.

The Landmark Trust, which lets out unusual buildings for people to stay in, doesn't have many pictures of its fascinating-looking properties. There are

castles, lighthouses, gatehouses, forts and towers. However, visitors to the Landmark Trust have taken photographs of these amazing places and uploaded them to Flickr where they are tagged with the name of the property and also the tag 'Landmark Trust'. This is a great example of the community getting together, following no hard and fast rules for categorising these photographs, but using their own way of tagging to provide order and structure for the greater good.

INSIDE THE FIREWALL

Businesses may not yet be using social media in a structured way, but with the groundswell of adoption, especially amongst the Generation Y and Z crowd, the use of social tools in a business setting will become more and more widespread.

HOW GENERATION Y WORK

Generation Y are your future managers, executives and engineers, and their adoption of social networking methods for communication and collaboration will shape the next generation of communications platforms products and services. These people are 'prosumers'; they use social media, networks and any tool at their disposal to effectively and efficiently do their job.

This has a huge and far reaching impact on business. Industries that embrace this new world of work are enjoying success – look at how Dell have benefited by being agile in this area. Ultimately, for your business success, you need to be there too. There are huge opportunities created by word of mouth networks, and smart businesses see the need to collaborate in these areas where there are opportunities for marketing your products and brands. Collaboration inside the firewall is just one part of social networking.

Collaboration enables companies to exchange intellectual capital with colleagues inside of their company.

Corporations invest huge amounts of money in storage systems to store corporate data – but as soon as a file is stored on the corporate network, the data effectively dies. With poor enterprise search tools, this dead data is no longer a corporate asset; users spend more and more time trying to find the documents they need amongst the ever growing mass of data.

If you implement a system that enables effective and contextual search to discover the data, use meta-information to tag the content appropriately and add multi-user editing and version control, things change. This data becomes discoverable, updatable and, more importantly, alive. And it's the living data that becomes a strategic asset to a company and enables corporate agility.

Having live up-to-date documents instead of terabytes of archives can reduce the need for storing duplicate data. Your new, modified versions of the original documents are used from the document store, and document versioning keep the original version intact.

The term 'social media' conjures up images of tools like Twitter and Facebook and brings to mind their use and misuse on the Internet. Often companies are wary of opening ports to allow the use of social software inside the firewall because of the potential risks that it may bring. Companies either ban sites through use of firewall block lists, or they monitor usage through audit trails and policies. Restricting your staff from using these sites will drive them to communicate with their friends from their mobile devices, or use other WiFi networks to access the sites in their lunch breaks. But social networking applications can also be used to enhance efficiency and productivity inside companies. In this context it tends to be known by a different name: social computing.

Social computing: the new productivity

With the growing use of social computing within companies, users are starting to reap the benefits of enhanced productivity. If a company has implemented a productivity suite with a unified mechanism for collaboration then it can start to communicate in real time. If it has installed an application that can display a list of colleagues and show whether they are online, away from their desk or on the phone, then this information can also be embedded into other applications to provide dynamic information around the company. Staff can easily communicate with their colleagues using instant messaging without the need for email and the associated disk space. If they use and manage dynamic websites instead of static pages, they can take advantage of the knowledge capital that the business already has and keep their data alive. Collaboration offers significant value to companies, but without the dynamism offered by socially connecting, exchanging information and chatting with your friends, collaboration can only give value in one aspect of business life.

Social computing doesn't necessarily mean embracing Facebook, Twitter and MySpace inside the firewall. It's about using the collaboration tools you have in a new way. Using wikis for group work, or changing your intranet pages to wikis instead of static web pages, means that as data changes at the company, updating the system involves only a small amount of work. Adding document versioning and meta-information to your documents means that information can be discovered in a new way. Instead of searching for 'consultancy proposal for NHS', for example, you can search for 'NHS Surrey project management 2010' or 'server refresh Surrey hospitals'. This richer meta-information allows for more targeted searches and more relevant results which ultimately improve productivity.

Searching for information

The average user in a large company can spend up to 10% of their time searching for documents on the intranet, so implementing social computing can soon improve productivity. Adding presence information to the document repository and landing pages means that document authors can be contacted immediately to clarify any queries. Status updates and out of office messages can bring richness to intranet sites and encourage greater interaction.

In the short term, this new way of working does require a shift in behaviour. Think about how your team interacts at the moment. You might email documents around for review by the team, which can often cause bandwidth and mailbox issues if you send large files. You might call your team on the phone, leaving voice-mails, and then email them to follow up on your voicemail. You might have a set of file shares on the server where all of your project documentation is stored. Think about how much more productive you could be if you could only change the way the team works.

This shift in behaviour could lead to everyone in the team storing their documents in a dynamic way on the document management system. You could use instant messaging with presence information to see whether the person you want to talk to is at their desk. You could then start a conversation by instant message, switching to voice and adding video. You could work on the same document and save a copy of the amended document. You could collaborate with wikis and you could have information updated quickly by members of the team. In the long term, this behaviour will reap benefits to both the information workers and the company through increased productivity and efficiency. Businesses sometimes flinch when they contemplate allowing the use of these tools behind the corporate firewall, but a quick analysis of access logs shows that over 80% of web visits are to social sites such as LinkedIn, Facebook and Twitter.

Collaborating with your colleagues

The desire to communicate with colleagues and friends both inside and outside the firewall will set the direction for the organisation's social strategy. Tools can be incorporated as part of a bottom-up approach to implementing new working practices instead of the current top-down approach to information dissemination. You might consider having an email group that is used for social activities. These social activities could be notices about items to sell, company events, 'how do I?' type emails, and the group could soon grow to become a central repository of information. Microsoft in the UK has an email group for its campus staff. Over half the staff in the UK subscribe to the mailing list, it is policed by its members and it covers topics as diverse as warning drivers about traffic hold-ups on the M4, and advice to people not to go too close to the pond as the resident geese have hatched their new brood of chicks. It also acts as the pulse of the company staff to gauge mood and sentiment about any new initiative or idea that is introduced onto campus.

Companies that decentralise the passing of information like this become a community of individuals sharing and contributing to corporate knowledge. This leads to an enhancement of corporate intellectual property and an increase in connectedness of the silos of information stored across the company. Companies that adopt this approach are inherently more agile than companies that rigidly maintain the top-down approach.

The groundswell of the bottom-up way of adopting social tools inside the agile business keeps companies at the forefront of competitive information and gives them the ability to move quickly if the business needs to.

There are various catch-all names for social applications inside the firewall, from collaboration tools to contact managers, portals to productivity applications. Having information about your users embedded within these applications enhances the user experience and makes the collaboration site more engaging. Document versioning keeps track of multi-user edits, wikis provide up-to-date web pages and data points, and a good enterprise search solution keeps data alive. There are inbox rules to control the messages that flow into your mailbox, alerts to control changes to your documents, and status changes to control who can view your online presence; there are also ways to harness social computing tools. Using collaborative software will make your work inside the firewall more productive and effective, and users will not feel restricted. Capturing those chats around the coffee machine and harnessing them appropriately can spark the next business advantage you otherwise may have missed. You can transform your dated intranet to something that teams actually want to use.

Using the internal web

Intranets have been around for a while. They are generally searchable. They are repositories of data that contain historical documentation, facts and perhaps an organisation-wide telephone directory. Occasionally there may be a web page that contains news articles, social events and items to sell.

But there's so much more you can do with an intranet. Think of how you could improve it if you had a social computing platform for collaboration and customised it well. NASA is developing an intranet site called Spacebook.[50] The site will be useful for staff wanting to find out what's going on and engage with their colleagues, with real-time status updates, announcements and people search.

Sites like these appear to have all of the prerequisites for an engaging site. Staff need the ability to search for people and groups with similar skills, interests and job functions; the ability to capture status updates from colleagues on your friend list; the ability to add meta-information to documents so that popular documents about the topics you care about bubble up to the top of the intranet page. Furthermore, information about where your colleagues are right now means you can directly connect and interact with others in the team, group or organisation.

Keeping your data alive

Having a clear, simple to use site that is engaging and updated regularly is key to successful engagement inside the firewall. Collaboration suites such as Lotus Notes and Microsoft SharePoint are frameworks that can be installed out of the box to give a simple collaboration site, or they can be extensively customised with add-ons and scripting. This customisation provides the collaborative and engaging environment that your business requires and can, with the appropriate add-on software packages, turn an out of the box product into something that even NASA could be proud of. That can be the key to successful collaboration. If you build an effective interactive engagement network you will ensure that your staff will visit the site. The intranet site contains fresh and updated data and employees will regularly want to return to the site for their information. This keeps your data alive and turns the information into a strategic asset for the business, not terabytes of dead data taking up storage space in your data centre.

CUSTOMER SERVICE

Twitter helps turn around negative attitudes to products in almost real time – as the attitudes are actually forming amongst your audience. There are some superb examples of this effect. I've been really impressed with the way that companies use Twitter to connect with their customers. A friend of mine, Andrew, told me about his own personal experience of excellent and speedy service results through an initial conversation over Twitter.

Andrew and I both have a really slow broadband connection. We each get about 0.5 Mbps. So any calls that we make using Voice over IP (VOIP) can sometimes be a bit tortuous with the latency that we have to endure. The quality reminds me of my days in the Merchant Navy, using the VHF radio and speaking simplex commands like 'roger', 'over' and 'over and out'. The latency, especially using shared bandwidth after school hours, is sometimes very bad. Andrew complained about the speed of his broadband service to one of his contacts on Twitter:

> @raybooysen BT broadband running at 0.5 mbps (paying for 8) , no BT Vision or XBVox live for me sob!
>
> *9:11 AM May 29th from TweetDeck in reply to raybooysen*

BT obviously monitors mentions of its name on Twitter using the search feature in its Twitter client and it responded within an hour of Andrew's original tweet.

> @raybooysen super impressed with BT they have already been onto me after the tweet
>
> *10:01 AM May 29th from TweetDeck in reply to raybooysen*

BT and Andrew had a few private conversations which were not visible on the main Twitter feed, so after a few tweets on Friday morning and a BT visit on Tuesday evening, Andrew was happy to report:

> BT improved my,broadband to 2.4 Mbps from 0.5 with a simple bit of rewiring and a dedicated faceplate, thanks guys
>
> *7:24 AM Jun 3rd from TweetDeck*

Which brought a response from BT:

BTCare: @DeepFat That's great news. Glad to hear it!

6 days ago from *web* · <u>Reply</u> · <u>View Tweet</u>

Andrew told me that BT even came down to his house a few days after this tweet to check the connections in the road in his village. BT demonstrated an excellent response to its customer issues, and all of this was initiated over Twitter.

Companies could certainly learn from this type of positive customer service and response using Twitter. This is just one example of how Twitter can be put to good use to change perception and improve satisfaction of a service, product or company amongst its customers. Credit should go to BT for being so responsive and getting great customer satisfaction from just one Tweet. Just think what this could do for your customers' perception of you.

Other companies use Twitter as a way of effectively engaging with their audience to track sentiment after an event. Selfridges in the UK is an example of this, responding to one of my own Twitter comments within 2 hours of my initial broadcast about an event I'd attended, see Figure 10.1.

Figure 10.1 Example of a brand monitoring customer comments

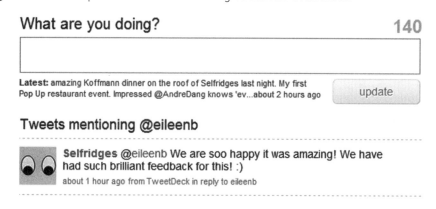

Customer service isn't all about customer complaints and giving the customer actual service. It's the customer connection, customer communication and customer engagement that make for good customer experience and ultimately a good perception of customer service.

The phenomenal popularity of a service like Twitter does bring its own challenges. People with a cause or a grievance will want to air it on the widest possible platform, and with sites like Twitter being watched and searched by millions, naturally these sites are a prime target.

Creating a plan if things go wrong

In the early days of Twitter, users used to complain about the 'fail whale'. This is the image that appears on Twitter's website whenever Twitter is over capacity and struggling to keep up with demand. In August 2009 there were several incidents where both Facebook and Twitter seemed to suffer from denial of service attacks which slowed the site down considerably and prevented users logging in. This caused an outcry as users struggled to access their favourite sites. Similar attacks occurred on LiveJournal, Blogger and YouTube which appeared to be co-ordinated attacks to prevent a prominent blogger from the Republic of Georgia from having any of his messages read by the media. Complaints from outraged users about Twitter and Facebook access became news. In December of the same year, a denial of service attack redirected the Twitter home page to a new screen alleging that the site had been 'hacked by Iranian Cyber Army' [*sic*]. Unfortunately these attacks pose a challenge for business. With increasing corporate and private user dependence on these types of sites, the potential for business disruption also increases if the sites are unavailable. These sites, which are out of your control, could be down for planned maintenance or they could become unavailable due to network issues or even subject to cyber attack from hackers.

When you are planning your influencer strategy using freely available tools, you need to consider the impact if an attack like this happened. What would it mean for your business and for your customer satisfaction? You will need to devise an alternative plan to allow for situations of this kind.

With our plans in place we'll now start to really work the crowd. Let's use the platforms to market our products and generate some fans and let the information flow on in. (Oh, we'd better learn how to manage it too!)

SUMMARY

- Plan your collaboration strategy to avoid information islands and data silos.
- Find your noisy few to tell the story on your behalf.
- Teenage interaction on social networking sites is completely different than that of adults.
- Consider video sharing, podcasting and photo sharing in your channel planning.
- Use collaboration software for the exchange of intellectual capital inside the company.
- Enterprise search keeps data alive.
- Use tools like Twitter to enhance your customer service experience.
- Create a contingency plan in case the tools fail.

11 RELATIONSHIPS AND ENGAGEMENT

No, this is not the start of a soppy story about me. This chapter focuses on how to turn your casual friends into long lasting enthusiasts and advocates for your brand. We start off with a closer look at one of the most popular social networking tools for news propagation and general interaction – Twitter. We look at how Twitter has evolved and been changed by the actions of the its users, and how Twitter itself is changing how the media operates. We'll talk about how to recognise your advocates and consider the advantages of creating brand personalities who can carry the conversation on your behalf if you give them the correct information.

Next we'll have a look at how this new way of connecting to your customers has changed the way companies market their products by introducing a dynamic engagement model to their traditional marketing approach. Getting the correct strategy in place is very important as the two mechanisms complement each other and both need to work together in order to ensure success. We'll have a look at the sort of metrics you can consider when trying to measure your ROI and consider how to effectively capture the new two-way conversation with customers. Finally, we'll look at how to cope with the huge amounts of information coming at you, and consider ways of managing the information and using it to your advantage.

TWITTER FOR YOUR BUSINESS

Twitter has exploded in popularity since it was launched in 2006, and many businesses are capitalising on the real-time news feed by using it as a news broadcasting, customer service and information tool. Twitter is a microblogging service, where users post short 140 character status messages which are read by their followers. It has over 105 million registered users, and 300,000 new accounts are being created every day. Tweets can be responded to in several ways. You can send a reply that can be seen publicly, you can reply privately with a direct message, or you can forward a message to others using the retweet feature so that others can view your posts. You can use Twitter to talk about anything – from what you had for lunch to the government's latest budget cuts.

> On Twitter you can have an audience for whatever you wish to talk about.

It doesn't matter whether what you talk about is life changing or trivial – there is an audience for everything. Businesses are already capitalising on this viral effect.

There are hundreds of Twitter tips and tricks, Twitter do's Twitter don'ts and Twitter get rich quick schemes, but which one actually works? To fully understand the Twitter phenomenon and how to capitalise on it effectively, it's important to understand the fundamentals of how it works and why it's so successful. Is Twitter a broadcast medium, or something used for social conversations? Is it a feedback loop for customers or is it an advertising channel for marketers? Or is it actually all of these? The social media revolution isn't changing the way we use media, Twitter is changing the way we use media, and social networking has to move to accommodate these changes. Twitter has evolved since its inception because of the behaviour of its users. There is no definitive statement on the Twitter website about what it was supposed to be used for.

> Twitter is a mechanism to communicate, connect and stay connected with online friends and co-workers through quick status updates.

Initially there was no standard way on Twitter to reply or to track interesting conversations on a given topic. The @ reply and the # hashtag were created by the Twitter community itself, which meant that conversation threads developed and communities evolved along similar interests. We wouldn't have become aware of the amount of news about the #iranelection, #swine_flu or #followfriday if these hashtags hadn't evolved and been used by the community. Of course, other hashtags had to evolve such as #fail and #misinformation to counter claims and criticisms on Twitter that turned out to be disappointing or untrue.

Making money from Twitter

There are over 15,000 registered Twitter applications, which represent a huge growth in popularity for Twitter.

> Some of these applications aim to monetise Twitter by offering services so you can grow your Twitter followers, make money from click-throughs or analyse the friends and habits of the people who follow you.

If you have a good idea of your customers' desires and wants then you can target your marketing to more effectively connect with them. The majority of Twitter traffic (over 75% of traffic occurs outside Twitter.com) comes from third party Twitter clients and applications, with new clients appearing regularly. Regular Twitter users talk about the availability of the new Twitter client and their friends quickly adopt it if it suits them. Application designers are aware of this and adapt their software to suit this ever changing mode of interaction.

Twitter itself hasn't yet announced a formal advertising model to bring revenue to the start-up business, but it has announced a new advertising platform called 'Promoted Tweets' in April 2010. Promoted Tweets give companies the opportunity to pay for keywords and initialise a tweet in response. Future opportunities might include the opportunity to take advantage of geolocation so that companies with local branches can take advantage of the location to initialise local offers.

With over 19 billion search queries per month, the opportunity for Twitter to make money is huge. However, the value of Twitter as a social engagement tool seems to have reached the mature stage of the application life cycle model. The challenge for Twitter is that, with maturity, innovation has to occur to keep the service valuable and relevant and prevent users from abandoning the service for the next new thing.

Other businesses seem to be slower to take advantage of the marketing opportunity and people power of the word of mouth network. Some corporate teams already use Twitter to effectively gauge the pulse of their audience by evaluating comments and reactions. They support their audience, engage in dialogue, and they benefit from this new engagement with their customers. This online conversation seems to encourage better interaction and dialogue than blogs or forums. Whilst over 40% of Internet users have read a blog at some time or another, only about 5% of users blog on a daily basis. The simplicity of posting a Twitter update means that active Twitter contributors post frequently about things that might not make it into a blog post.

Hype or reality?

Let's be realistic about this, though. Most of us have never tweeted, nor have we ever read a tweet using a Twitter client. We might have heard about Twitter from the newspapers or the radio, but we are certainly not 'active' Twitter users

Almost 90% of the content is produced by only 10% of Twitter users.

This is quite a lot different from numbers reported on other social networking sites, where 10% of users produce about 30% of the content. On Twitter, the average number of tweets produced per user is 1! Most of us will visit Twitter, we might create a profile and we might even broadcast a tweet. But that's all we will do, we won't tend to interact further and discover the value of Twitter. There are followers in Twitter who are consumers of information, they don't post content or updates, but they use Twitter as their source of information. They gather information without needing to post anything.

Marketing companies offer to get your message out to a much wider audience and in some cases can prove that your chosen Twitter phrase or word is becoming a trending topic for your campaign. However, these updates often seem to come from a set of 'fake accounts' with no information about the user, there is no interaction or dialogue with any of their followers. These 'buzz generation' accounts are published from a Twitter client like Seesmic or Hootsuite that has the ability to post from multiple different Twitter accounts at the same time. In reality, these fake accounts hold little value for either the feed consumer or the company commissioning the campaign and have no longevity in an ongoing marketing strategy.

So Twitter propagates information from a relatively small number of key influencers to the rest of us. These news instigators collate information and

disseminate it to their loyal followers who then repost and retweet it to the rest of the Twitterari. This lack of structure and control is changing the way we look at digital media. Traditional marketing and digital media ran campaigns to drive our actions, whether that was clicking on a link, entering a competition or responding to a query. What we do now is changing the way we interact, and traditional media also needs to evolve from its traditional push marketing to conversational marketing. This approach, which has been driven by the interactivity of networking sites, is changing the nature of media messaging. Content is now free to be distributed in any way possible – by anyone with an online account and a device – and this has completely shifted power to the consumer. Everyone now has an opportunity to communicate across many channels. This gives everyone the opportunity to communicate, not necessarily to broadcast, with a select group of friends who can connect with **their** friends and pass the message on.

CULTIVATING YOUR ADVOCATES

When you have an online presence, it stands to reason that people are going to talk about your product, and it makes sense to connect with your customers by joining in the conversation. If you're a part of the conversation, then you have a great opportunity to influence that conversation, change perceptions and to create new advocates for your brand. But how can you scale your activities so that you connect with your audience and encourage **them** to connect with their networks? You need a plan. Your plan and activities must be structured to include everyone in the company who plans to connect with their audience. You need some guidelines.

CONNECTING WITH THE AUDIENCE

- You've recognised that your digital marketing and engagement approaches complement but do not replace your traditional methods of marketing. Traditional marketing is a timed, well controlled message delivered in a push campaign via various mechanisms and tracked via click-throughs, offer uptake and positive press reports.

- Your plan is to adopt some form of digital conversation and to bring a two-way dialogue into your marketing efforts and involve the voice of the customer. The new marketing is not about direct push any more, it's not about a two-way conversation.

- Take advice from others who have succeeded in this space. Successful companies who use these social tools listen first and sell second. In general, they act like aggregators and content providers rather than traditional advertisers, breaking the traditional marketing model.

- New media marketing provides valuable feedback about the brand whilst raising awareness about the brand offering. If the product is in beta, then this feedback loop can often drive the design of finished product which is more attractive to the consumer when the product launches.

Another advantage of using this type of customer engagement to market your brand is authenticity. Consumers value the interaction with the company, whether it's with you as a person, your team, or the organisation more broadly. The value is gained by having the direct connections with the consumer. In traditional marketing, this role is generally fulfilled by the PR spokesperson, someone who has been briefed in corporate messaging and ensures that the correct brand image is communicated. With these types of tools, everyone becomes a spokesperson. Anything you say on networking platforms can be perceived as being the 'official company line' so everyone with a public persona or online brand must be cognisant of corporate guidelines for social media and follow the corporate code of conduct.

Dealing with your company celebrities

Another thing to be aware of is that, by the very nature of this type of communicating, some of the personalities in your company may bubble up to the top of the pile and become individual celebrities due to their activities using social media tools and the perception of their influence by the community. These 'celebrities' can be used to your benefit. They can become your unofficial spokespeople for the company. This can lead to a positive impression for your brand as interest in the personality increases awareness of new features and news.

> Customers can then connect their perception of your brand to a real human being and not a logo.

Think about brands that with personalities at the helm: Victor Kiam and Remington, Steve Jobs and Apple, James Dyson and Dyson vacuum cleaners, Donatella Versace and the Versace fashion house. These leaders are all great personalities; they are spokespeople and living embodiments of the brand. Glossy magazines, offering a glimpse into celebrities' lives, bring awareness of the celebrity, and, by extension, their product, book or film, by this human connection.

The same is true for celebrities who use social media. Sarah Brown, the wife of the former UK prime minister, and Barack Obama use Twitter as a way as connecting to their audience. Ashton Kutcher has almost 6 million Twitter followers, Oprah Winfrey has over 4 million and Stephen Fry almost 2 million. Each of these personalities has brought this connection off the pages of the glossy magazines and into the online world of interactivity.

> The empathy that your social media spokespeople develop with your customers brings a much closer connection to the customer. The bond created with the brand evangelist becomes close and personal, and, by extension, the bond to the brand which can lead to loyalty and advocacy in future.

If you are trying to increase your social media advocates, perhaps consider the following activities to help drive engagement:

DRIVING CUSTOMER ENGAGEMENT

- Build demand. Information fuels itself. Drive the thirst for knowledge amongst your audience and keep them engaged with information that they would find difficult to find externally.

- Drive awareness. Make sure that the consumers are kept up to date about your products. In their day job, they may not have time to discover everything about your product set. Tell them about it, and reinforce the message regularly. Ask the audience questions, interact and inform.

- Show the new. In technology, consumers want to see your product vision and direction. When a product is ready to talk about, encourage your teams to talk about it, show video clips, images and demos. Get the word out and spread the buzz.

- Show value. If used correctly, social media can demonstrate the value to customers after they have purchased your product. Whether this is ongoing support, customer care, interaction, help and dialogue, the connection is there and should be encouraged to develop.

To preserve your brand and maintain its visibility in the markets, it is important to maintain a good ongoing connection with your customers. There are several ways to do this, but Dell certainly shows leadership with several innovative ideas. In addition to their financially successful Twitter aliases, Dell has other community innovations.

Dell have created a micro-site called IdeaStorm which encourages comments, good and bad, about Dell's products.

This enables users to be in direct touch with Dell about the issues that are important, such as customer service, pre and post sales processes and product quality. The rationale behind this idea is that it is better to allow customers to complain and rant about problems directly to Dell, than have detractors complain on other sites where the comments are harder to find and subsequently fix. Sites like these don't stop customers complaining on other sites, but do allow the complaints to be heard by Dell itself; and by listening to their customers, they also gather ideas for future products.

SOCIAL MARKETING

There are myriad social media, social networking, social computing and social business sites on the web, all of them encouraging conversations with millions of people who use various mechanisms to connect, communicate and collaborate through a variety of channels. Traditional marketing campaigns now have to have a digital component to ensure that they are reaching the correct segment of

the audience, and there are lots of case studies about success and positive ROI from web campaigns.

But can social marketing be measured at all? How do you measure your ROI? It's very simple to measure ROI through traditional channels such as printed media, radio or TV advertising. There are methods of measuring ROI from search marketing also – via click-throughs from a web page. Social marketing often isn't measured directly, although there are several tools that you can use to measure how many customers have clicked on your links. Interesting and useful content is transmitted virally, through recommendations, word of mouth, email and link forwarding.

> If you try to sell directly to the customer using social marketing, you might be disappointed.

Tweeting about the same links over and over again or pushing the same message on your Facebook page will drive customers away. You need to think of your online strategy in a different way. Different rules apply to social marketing than in other, more traditional forms of marketing.

But ROI is a very difficult thing to measure through something as intangible as a social media campaign, a blogging strategy or web competition. Case studies are examples of success in the corporate world, and they are also a key indicator of sentiment and success in the social media space.

Old Spice had an innovative way to persuade women to buy Old Spice in the US. They launched an online video campaign called 'the man your man can smell like'. The campaign was launched during Superbowl week and targeted TV programmes where viewers would likely watch together. In the first three months of 2010, mentions of the Old Spice brand captured 75% of all conversations, with half of the conversations initiated by women. Other videos started to appear parodying the Old Spice advert and style of conversation, and TV presenters like Oprah mentioned the brand on her show.

The agency then hit upon a great way to capture the real-time messages on Facebook, Twitter and YouTube.

> The Old Spice response campaign became the fastest growing campaign ever, reaching 5.9 million views on YouTube on day 1.

On day 2, Old Spice was mentioned in 8 out of the top 11 most popular videos on the web. On day 3 of the campaign there were more than 20 million views, and on day 7 over 40 million. This had a huge knock-on effect on the Old Spice Twitter and Facebook pages. The Old Spice website had a 300% increase in site visits and became the most popular channel on YouTube. Financially this campaign has

made a difference too, with sales of Old Spice body wash up by 27% in 6 months since campaign launch. A great return on investment from a TV and YouTube video campaign.

Businesses need to take advantage of the engagement with the consumer, capturing stories and success measures from their online population, and they need to engage with their key customers and encourage their online influencers to become champions for the brand. Some companies toy with the idea of social media, and consider using it to further their market in order to gain a deeper understanding of their audience and improve perceptions, interaction and feedback. However, there are lots of differing opinions on what constitutes an effective social media strategy, without any clear consensus on which is the best way forward. One size does not fit all. Your strategy should suit your company and it should work for your business. There are, as yet, no clearly defined standards for social marketing.

Objective based social marketing campaigns

There are lots of email campaign software packages which will help you track email click-throughs to help you become more effective in determining which parts of your content are successful. It is important to understand what is relevant and important to your audience so you can track key market trends – what is hot at the moment and what is not in your market. Analysing your metrics and performance helps you to get as much data as possible from any analysis tools that you use. It is much more difficult to measure the ROI from social marketing than from traditional marketing, and that's why measuring the effectiveness of any online marketing activities you do is vital to your go-to-market strategy.

There are three basic rules for social media if you think of it in terms of marketing:

- Influence is everything. Strive to influence positive responses from your audience.
- Engage the audience and engender open discussions.
- Use these positive responses and open discussions to develop your online relationship with your consumer.

Your objectives need to be clearly defined from the outset. This approach is often not about the direct sale to the customer, although Dell has managed to use offers delivered through Twitter to achieve direct sales with its DellOutlet Twitter account. Are your current online efforts making the impact you want them to in the market? Are they having any impact at all? If you haven't defined your objectives and end goals clearly enough then your business leaders will be quickly disappointed by the end result, and your investment in time and money will be wasted if your senior leaders come to the conclusion that your approach has no value or is of no help to the company's bottom line.

Bacardi in Ireland has had success in engaging its audience through Facebook. Its distributors switched from micro-sites to a Facebook page in 2008 and created an

application within Facebook for any competitions it would run. Its campaigns focus on user interaction and it encourages comments on each of its Facebook entries. It also engages the users, responds to comments quickly and grows its fan base by asking people to 'like' its Facebook page in order to enter the competition. This is a successful strategy which gives Bacardi great engagement and interaction.

Before you embark on the measurement of metrics it's important to consider the costs of this strategy, which is not only a financial cost to the business, but is also the time that you and your staff have invested in using the tools to promote your brand or product. If you're hosting your own company blogs, then you need to consider the cost of bandwidth, blogging software and server power to cope with the increased traffic your success will bring. When Twitter started out, every tweet sent by every user was in the software, housed on a couple of servers under a desk in the office in California. As more and more people used the network in the early days, it was plagued by downtime and an over capacity message accompanying an image of birds trying to hold a whale aloft – an image that early Twitter users quickly termed the 'fail whale'.

> You need to consider how you would deal with runaway success in carrying out your social media strategy.

You may have created the next darling of the social media world – the next Twitter for example so you need to account for the possibility that this could happen when you create social media strategy and plan. You also need to consider whether the ROI actually is more than the amount you've invested to implement your strategy.

When considering your strategy, you will be faced with a huge number of options and tools that you can use. Try not to use the scatter gun approach and 'launch' in every area you can. Filter out the tools that will not be valuable to you. Should you consider Bebo, which is primarily used by younger users, for example, if you work for a heavy engineering company and want to market tooling?

Use a rating scale for these tools and decide which of your chosen channels will be valuable to you. Grade them on, say, a nine-point scale to make sure you choose the most appropriate for your business. Have a look at your own business and decide whether a social media strategy would be appropriate, or which parts of your business would benefit from using social media to broadcast your message. There are some factors which may negatively impact perception of your brand online and other opportunities to enhance your brand. Try using a SWOT (strengths, weaknesses, opportunities and threats) analysis – just as you would when pursuing a large business deal, to see whether you actually want to go forward with the plan at all.

DEALING WITH THE FLOOD OF INFORMATION

You can easily become overwhelmed when you try to stem the flow of information from the 'fire hose', and might consider having only one 'corporate' presence on the web. There are great advantages to having corporate level social destinations, such as DellOutlet, MarksandSpencer and Google, who are a credible voice for interacting with the consumer, and a great push news channel for the company. But this often detracts from the benefits gained from the interaction with the 'human voice' of the company. These social destinations can play a key proactive role in producing major announcements and could be considered as part of an overall social media marketing plan. Having a centralised blog or Twitter feed makes it easy for consumers to check news when information gets out to the web, but this does have the potential to become just another sanitised news feed for the PR team – which detracts from the concept of direct engagement with the customer.

The chief marketing officer of Novell, John Dragoon, has his own blog and is also a key contributor to the Novell News blog. With eight other contributors, this blog is a single place to go to for news and opinions across the company from senior leaders. This doesn't seem to be a new PR initiative as John has been blogging for 4 years now and also occasionally updates his Twitter stream. Carefully managed, this approach can work well.

Blogs from company bloggers could be aggregated into one centralised RSS feed so that journalists can follow the corporate master feed. Mary Jo Foley, who has followed Microsoft for over 20 years, follows the main feed from every blogger in the company. She uses Google Reader to categorise the news makers, the key influencers and the interesting people, and scans through the rest of the feed when she has the time.

There is also the option to use an RSS feed to populate a master corporate Twitter feed which customers can follow too. My gut feeling is that this feed would need to be filtered so that duplicate information was removed, and irrelevant posts excluded. This would take a large investment of time for larger companies which would need to fully understand every product, brand and marketing strategy across the whole company, and it would be a huge undertaking for the team involved. I feel this would take away the personality from the interaction with the customer – moving this closer to a PR message than the voice of the individual influencer.

> With the huge variety of channels to communicate through, and the vast amount of information flowing through each channel, the potential to become overwhelmed can be huge.

It's therefore a good idea to get teams working together and contributing to the channel, which can give a balanced perspective to the feed and introduce

individual personalities to communications. To track who is communicating on a channel such as Twitter, tools like Co-Tweet, TweetFunnel and HootSuite have the facility to have multiple authors contributing to the feed and allow the user name to be appended to the outbound message.

Applying filters is another good idea to manage the flow. Grouping search results enables you to track campaigns and customer queries. Analytics tools can track sentiment and guide you towards areas that you need to focus on first. If you are aware of the amount of information you need to work through then you can manage the flow appropriately with the correct tools and measurements.

Our social media strategy is going well. We're on track to be successful, but we're struggling with how we can scale. Now let's let the crowd work for **us** and get them to amplify our message.

- Use Twitter to connect with your customers and engage them in dialogue.
- Listen first and sell second.
- Case studies are a key indicator of success and sentiment.
- Encourage your online influencers to become your brand champions.
- Use filters to reduce the amount of information you receive and make sure you only see the kinds of information that are relevant to your business.

12 AMPLIFYING YOUR MESSAGE

Communities aren't a new concept. Communities have existed in face to face interactions since humans lived in groups. It is still possible to create a brand new community from scratch if you need to. If you want to create a community specifically to enthuse about your new product, we'll see how to build a successful community by following a couple of rules. First, we will look at why influencers in the community are so important in sustaining the community and propagating messages. We will look at trust and how to harness the knowledge through the initiators and trusted advisers in the community. Secondly, we'll look at the different ways that buzz is created, starting with an initiator with an innovative idea that goes viral, and then we'll look at the way that large companies create communities. We'll see how the word of mouth network and the power of the people work together to amplify the message, and we'll look at how tools like Facebook have become the mechanism to amplify this message in minutes instead of days. We'll talk about network effects and how social causes take advantage of these effects to raise vast sums of money through the use of online games. We'll see whether placing news sites behind pay walls will reduce these network effects or sustain them, and we'll look at whether licensing deals are the preferred option for companies to access and expose data through search engines. Finally, we'll look at different ways of measuring reach for your social media activities. We'll see how different tools manage and assess social graph data, sentiment and metrics, and consider how lead generation can be measured using social media alongside your normal sales process in the company.

COMMUNITIES AND INFLUENCERS

Communities exist wherever you look, both inside and outside business. There are groups of like-minded people who come together for a short time to support a good cause. There are groups of people who spend time helping others in user forums. There are communities that share news articles of interest and links to interesting topics. There are also people who are dedicated to helping to increase the store of knowledge on the Internet by creating articles on Wikipedia. These people don't expect rewards for their actions.

Their desire to help others is driven by nothing more than just that – a desire to help.

There are a large number of people out there who want to help you achieve your goals, and if you want to build a community you can turn this desire to your advantage. All you need to do is find **the correct people in the community** and channelling it correctly.

Communities are formed when people come together to share knowledge, ideas and support each other in a self sustaining group. Communities tend to have three basic behaviour characteristics:

- **Advocacy.** Members of the community are evangelists for their group and recommend products and services to other members and groups.
- **Connectedness.** Community members have connections to other experts in the industry – or they know who to contact when additional help is needed.
- **Reputation.** Members of the community are recognised experts in their area, they have been discovered for their skills and ability, and they have a good reputation and often a great reach across their sphere of influence.

Without these characteristics, communities often fragment and fade. The simplicity of successful communities often comes down a matter of basic trust. Community members trust other members within the group itself, and they trust other community members for their skills and knowledge within the group. The community, although often appearing to be disorganised and chaotic, actually works in an organic and simplistic way. The weak ties within the community connect with the stronger ties and glue the group together. Unfortunately, as communities grow in size, usually organically, people tend to try to impose some type of order and rules on the group.

> Placing mandates, edicts or over-stringent regulations onto communities can create factions and discord within the community itself.

Sometimes the community may fragment and create spinoff groups who may work against the main community itself. These 'special interest groups' are useful in some ways. For example, you might have a suite of products with a strong following (like Apple has). Apple might wish to encourage the special interest groups that form for the iPad to become completely different groups than those formed for the iPhone.

> Segmenting groups into special interest groups can vastly increase the size of each community, whilst maintaining a consistent messaging framework across the product suite.

There's a great deal of knowledge within a community that can be harnessed if you wish. Knowledge can be spread really effectively if you can find your community initiators and use their knowledge and desire to help you.

An initiator is someone – perhaps a group – with a real passion for their subject.

Furthermore, your initiators will have a desire to broadcast interesting material. These initiators may have created their own area on the web, often a website or blog, which is filled with information and often stored purely for their own interest. They will have collected as much information as they can, store it on the web and add to the store whenever they get new snippets of information. With search technologies and web crawlers the site will become visible to others and more and more people will become aware of the knowledge repository on the site.

If the site has Web 2.0 features embedded which allow comments then users will start to contribute and interact, and the community will start to grow.

Some hobby sites have come to the attention of corporations which acquire them in order to add to their advertising revenue stream. The Pistonheads forum in the UK, which is a place for car enthusiasts, is a good example of a hobby site which has come to the attention of the media.

Creating a community

If you want to create a community from scratch and don't currently know who your community initiator could be, then you might like to think about a new and oblique approach to community-generating activities.

GENERATING COMMUNITY

- For example, you might have a website with a new community upload photo stream that you'd like to draw users' attention to. You could approach various photographic hobbyist sites or clubs, perhaps to encourage a photography competition. You could then have the results shown on your website. This would bring new visitors to your website from the hobby site who may not have been aware of it before.

- You might have a new product that you'd like to test on a different set of users who are not participating in formal beta downloads of technical support forums. One of your approaches could be to target other communities. You could include communities who are advocates for similar or competing products to yours and you could start to engage with them on a regular basis. You may not be able to convert them to become product evangelists for your new product, but you will be able to tap into a community with an existing voice.

- You can try to use a new stream of advertising to find your new community volunteers. You could ask questions in existing communities like 'Would you like to become part of a customer panel or an opinion panel?' or 'Would you like to road-test some new products?' You could watch the responses, both positive and negative, and see who appears to be the influencer in the community. Your initiators will often respond to your initial query in order to further their search for more knowledge.

You may not find your ideal initiator right at the start as the embryonic community emerges. If you give the community time, it will evolve organically and your new community initiators will drive the community forward for you.

Community buzz

There are many different ways to create buzz about your product or brand. The challenge for a lot of businesses is that they may not have the benefit of a large corporation like Google or Kraft Foods behind them. However, with the word of mouth network, individuals can sometimes create enough buzz on their own to sway a whole industry. It's quite interesting to realise that the major industries and corporations don't always have the largest voice when buzz is created through use of the network and tools.

> The voice of the community can often drown out the official message from the company.

Sometimes one person alone can have enough influence amongst his peers and connections to create significant buzz through his social network and his friends of friends network.

An example occurred on Facebook over a period of 2 weeks in December 2009. In the run-up to Christmas every year there is a battle for supremacy in the music industry. Each music company wants its Christmas song to make it to the top of the music charts. For several years now, the reality TV show, X Factor, has achieved this in the UK. The winner of the TV talent competition is more or less guaranteed chart success. Simon Cowell, who has great influence in the music industry, is one of the judges and also owns the rights to the TV show.

When it became apparent that again, for the fifth year running, the Christmas number one record was going to be the winner of X factor, Jon and Tracy Morter, from Essex in the UK, decided to protest. The Morters used Facebook to create a group dedicated to trying to stop the winner of the X Factor competition from reaching in the top of the charts. They wanted a music group called Rage against the Machine to get to number one instead. This seemed an impossible task. The X Factor winner in 2009, Joe McElderry, looked certain to rise to the top of the charts. What the Morters tried to do was to encourage users through Facebook to buy a different record.

Rage against the Machine is a punk band from the US who had released a single which was not expected to do very well in the UK charts. However, Rage against the Machine did have an advantage over Joe McElderry. Their single was only available to purchase as a download from the web. Unfortunately Joe McElderry's marketing team either didn't want or had forgotten to make this purchasing method available from the start. This omission gave Rage against the Machine a huge advantage.

The Facebook group grew to over 700,000 fans in a very short time. There were 200,000 fans on a backup Facebook page and over 500,000 fans on the main

Facebook page. Both pages had the same message and the instructions were really simple. The tactic was to simply buy a copy of the Rage against the Machine single online within a limited time window. So from 13 to 20 December 2009, every member of each dedicated Facebook group was encouraged to purchase one copy of the single from the web. The simplicity of Facebook and the friends of friends system meant that all members of the Facebook page were encouraged to pass on the message and to persuade others in their networks to buy the downloaded single too. This simple method worked very well indeed.

Rage against the Machine reached number one in the UK charts on 20 December. The band were completely unprepared for their massive and unexpected success in the UK and have promised to do a free gig in the UK in 2010 as a thank-you for all the support from Facebook fans. Simon Cowell was gracious in defeat. He called Jon Morter to congratulate him on his Facebook campaign. This upset made the news everywhere. Jon found himself thrust into the limelight both in the UK and in the US, giving interviews in both countries explaining why he did this. This simple effect proves that people power effectively transcends geographical boundaries when a campaign is done well.

This demonstrates just how significant the word of mouth network is. It demonstrates the power of connections. Friends who connect with each other can share information and create enough buzz to have a greater network effect than traditional push. This particular collaborative effort has been achieved without the huge amounts of work that would have been needed in the past in order to rally a huge group like this.

Facebook has become the mobilisation tool of the 21st century.

When groundswell happens like this, it proves that the ordinary person, the man on the street, does have an influence and does have a voice after all.

Together with the power of connections and crowd sourcing, it's a rather powerful voice – as Facebook has proved over and over again...

VIRAL AWARENESS

If you want success, it's a good idea to think about network effects. People tend to congregate where their friends are, they buy what their friends recommend and they use the products that their friends use. This effect is known as the **cluster effect**, and social network applications need to be designed with these clusters in mind.

In early January 2010, when most of the news channels were reporting how the UK was paralysed under a blanket of snow, a ripple effect started to occur on Facebook. Facebook started to display status updates containing only one word (or occasionally two): 'lemon', 'nude', 'black', 'tartan', 'dirty grey'. These updates

caused speculation amongst male users before word got out that this was all about underwear and the colour we were wearing that day. These status updates had a knock-on effect in raising awareness about breast cancer. Facebook groups dedicated to breast cancer awareness gathered over 40,000 fans supporting the cause, with some fans posting images of them wearing bras on the group pages. The Susan G. Komen for the Cure breast cancer foundation reported that, due to the Facebook status updates, their Facebook fans jumped in number from 134,000 to 154,000.[51] 'We're so delighted,' said spokeswoman Andrea Rader. 'We think this is just a phenomenal example of how powerful the Internet can be in getting this message out.'

Another example of a Facebook group being used to raise awareness and get help quickly was for Philip Pain, a student.[52] Philip fell from a seventh-floor balcony in Mazatlán, Mexico, crushing his internal organs and breaking his legs and back. The local hospital didn't have enough supplies of his rare blood type, O-negative, to operate and save his life. Less than 6% of the population have O-negative blood, so shortages can be expected. His parents set up a Facebook group asking for blood, and within hours 12 pints of blood were flown in from Florida. A further 8 pints were donated at the hospital in Mazatlán and other O-negative donors signed up to an emergency blood list ready to donate if needed. Facebook notified enough people so that there were sufficient supplies of blood available quickly, which meant that doctors were able to start the operation to save his life.

These are amazing examples of how individual voices can be magnified and used with the network effect in order to create a viral effect for good causes.

> Awareness grows about the cause, people become mobilised into action and you can reach millions of people by using a site like Facebook.

ONLINE GAMING FOR SOCIAL CAUSES

There are many opportunities for networking tools to be put to good use for social causes. These networks have become powerful in helping to raise money and awareness about social issues around the world. Zynga, one of the leading MMORPG developers has several social games on Facebook with a huge number of players. Their top games are Mafia Wars, Farmville, FishVille, CafeWorld and Zynga Poker. When the Haiti earthquake struck, Zynga responded very quickly to the need for international aid. It offered 'limited edition social goods' including 'non withering white corn within Farmville'. Farmville has over 75 million online users who can use real money to purchase Farmville vouchers and exchange them for high value items. Zynga also offered a 'Haitian drum on Mafia Wars' to its 23 million users and 'a special chip package' in Zynga Poker. They announced that they would donate 100% of the proceeds to support emergency aid in Haiti through its relief fund.[53] Previous efforts from Zynga in selling seeds for Haiti had earned over $1 million and the opportunity to buy virtual pets in YoVille raised $90,000 for the San Francisco Society for the Prevention of Cruelty to Animals.

Other initiatives allowed players to purchase virtual goods to aid the World Food Program.

Social media has benefited good causes many times. In addition to the great work done by Zynga, other social media channels have been used. Twit Cause asks for causes to be nominated and companies offer donations to the cause for each tweet recorded. Häagen-Dazs donated $1 for any tweet which referenced the hashtag #HelpHoneyBees. Other initiatives have included offering $24,000 for cancer research and donating money to keep teenagers off the streets.

> There are opportunities here to monetise your social media efforts in the third sector (Charities and not for profit organisations) and generate significant revenue if you can take advantage of network effects.

Facebook, MySpace and Bebo make money through targeted advertising on their home pages. Twitter, on the other hand, currently loses money as it doesn't yet have a strategy to earn revenue through click-through Twitter messages. However, several of Twitter's third party applications, analytics and sentiment trackers do have paid-for sustainable subscription models. Twitter itself has recently announced a revenue model for sponsored accounts and links which will advertise services and goods.

In order to create a popular site that will draw your users in for the first time and keep them coming back you need to be creative. Think about how you can turn your site into a business which keeps on generating revenue and increasing its online activities in the long term. This can be achieved through advertisements, membership fees, subscriptions or eBook downloads. The *Times* newspaper in the UK has now changed to a subscription model for its web content, which is now hidden behind a pay wall. This move is being closely monitored by other online newspapers to gauge its success and to determine whether other news sites will follow this model. Will every item of news ultimately be situated behind a pay wall? Where will this news be collected from? Will any of the news then get disseminated through social channels? It's difficult to predict at the moment. Wikipedia is determined to provide content for free for its readers. The site's founder, Jimmy Wales, asks for donations for the upkeep of the site through its Wikimedia Foundation and so far has managed to achieve his goals without resorting to paid for advertising.

> Monetisation and passive income generation need to be part of your strategy to make your sites financially sustainable in the long run.

It seems like licensing deals may be an answer to sites that need to think about continued revenue. Microsoft adopted the policy of licensing its software right from the start of its business, and this policy has continued to give it ongoing

revenue year on year as new products are released. Perhaps your business also lends itself well to licensing of your content. There could then be opportunities to offer licensed access to the Twitter stream, your Twitter results will appear on search engine lists and you then have a viable option that will provide ongoing revenue for Twitter itself.

RECORDING AND TRACKING

In the normal course of business, sales leads are tracked for each customer pre-sales engagement and each deal closed is a success. This is also true of any leads that are generated from your digital marketing initiatives. You can track who follows you, or who clicks on your link and visits your website. You can see which site has generated the click-through. You can also see who has continued their journey through the site and which of these visitors actually turns into a valid business opportunity. If you know which social site has generated the most click-through opportunities then there is a great opportunity for you to increase engagement with your audience by increasing your communication on that particular site. Recording and tracking these metrics can give you enough information to create an easy to digest summary of your progress. The decision makers can see that your efforts have been fruitful with month on month growth, brand awareness and presence. This report then can be used to validate your investment in your social initiative.

The use of search facilities on blogs and on Twitter can highlight mentions of your brand name which can then be used to track the increase or decrease in the number of people talking about your brand or product. These statistics can be used to calculate month on month growth (or decline) in brand mentions. This can be automated by the use of alerts or by using a sentiment measuring tool to watch change in satisfaction with your brand.

So you now have all of the pieces in place for a successful strategy. You know how social engagement works and the tools you need to use. You know why you need a great presence and effective ways to create, manage and maintain a good online brand. You are happy with the perception of your brand and how to effectively manage your reputation. You've implemented policies to manage staff use of social tools guided by thought leaders in digital engagement. You know how to find your audience, listen to them and engage with the right influencers. You've taken advantage of the strong and weak ties in your network and explored ways to leverage your influencer network. You've reached out beyond your immediate network and gathered new connections. You have a great understanding about behaviour and scale and you have generated advocates for your brand. You've generated buzz, have a viral effect going from time to time so you can sit back and relax, right?

Wrong. With the speed of change in our always on, always connected, digital world, nothing is fixed in stone. Everything is fluid and changes with the speed of a mouse click.

You need to be ahead of the game for your business to be agile.

Your existing investment in time and money needs to produce results for the next few years, which is difficult in this rapidly changing environment. So how can you stay ahead of the curve and continue to be a thought leader in your business? Predicting the digital engagement trends of the future will help you be one step ahead of the competition.

So let's gaze into my crystal ball and have a go at predicting what sort of evolution we're going to see next and whether we'll need a brand new crowd to work with.

- Find the recognised experts in your area.
- Don't place mandates and rules on the community. It will fragment and separate.
- One well connected individual has the ability to create significant buzz in the community.
- Think about Facebook and its ability to share links for your business channel.
- Try to create something that will go viral.
- Social causes can benefit from online gaming. Think about opportunities to earn revenue for the third sector.
- Keep alert for the pace of change and watch for leading indicators.

13 WHERE IS IT ALL GOING?

In this, the final chapter, we take a look forward. We look at what will happen next in the new world of communication. Just as the dotcom boom changed the way we used the web in the late 1990s, so the influx of social media platforms will fundamentally change the way we communicate and do business in the 2010s. First, we'll have a look at the new way of marketing and how push marketing will have to evolve to suit the new dialogue. Secondly, we'll speculate on the new platform and how search will play an important part in raising awareness of social engagement tools and encourage more people to take part in the conversation. We'll have a look at how hardware will evolve to take the users to the next level of engagement and how the infrastructure will change to support our changing requirements on the web. We'll talk about the blurring of our work and social lives and the privacy and personas that we'll need to adopt online to keep our public and private lives separate. Finally, I'll share a few tips to help you become successful at engaging with the online audience without becoming overwhelmed in the crowd.

Forrester's Technographic ladder (http://bit.ly/bn6fDc) shows that consumers are collectors, critics, conversationalists and creators and that their engagement increases year on year.[54] There is a great opportunity to engage with the audience, have a two-way conversation and complement the traditional push marketing approach.

> This engagement, carried out where the audience spend their online social hours, gives companies a great opportunity to generate brand advocacy and change perceptions and impact.

In order to achieve marketing success with engagement marketing using online social media, a long term strategy needs to be created. This new way of working is a long term commitment and a valuable business proposition, but it cannot happen on its own.

> This approach takes time and effort to reap the appropriate rewards as each member of the team needs to contribute to and invest in the conversation.

Social media activities are not another push medium for marketers but used in a push–pull way to orchestrate engagement and dialogue with their tier 1 influencers. Regular engagement is necessary for sustained channel growth and there should be activity in each social media channel which can be measured as the conversational responses increase throughout the year.

I do have a word of warning, however, in this new world of marketing. Be cautious of relying on recording the volume of users, followers, fans and friends across each channel. This type of metrics monitoring will not bring any great insight to the business.

Take time to develop your own insight into your audience. Work out an appropriate baseline to build upon, and think carefully about the use of any tools which automate responses as these will quickly damage perceptions of your brand.

Longevity is also important. Any commitment to these types of activities should be for a period one of at least a year to allow you to set a baseline and introduce effective monitoring and tracking. This allows appropriate themes to be created and dialogue with influencers to be developed throughout your audience.

THE NEW WAY OF USING THE PLATFORM

There has been a lot of speculation and head scratching about the next version of Facebook, the new Twitter or the next generation of social media platforms. Analysts, businesses and the community are all trying to predict what will dominate the market, and which product will be one step ahead when the new generation of tools appear. There are several conflicting schools of thought here. My own theory about what's going to happen is totally different from those of some of my technical colleagues in the industry, but it resonates well with what others say. The future depends on your point of view of course – on whether you view social media as an enterprise discussion or a consumer discussion. Both are valid points. However, the main methods that tie both of these enterprise and consumer markets together are mobility and search.

One of the biggest step changes we will see in social media is through the advancement of search. Search will play a powerful role in making new social media items discoverable. Currently search engines often display blog posts and forum comments, videos and podcasts. Google has already launched itself into the social space with its Google Buzz service. Real-time items in Buzz already display in Google search results. Facebook, traditionally a walled garden, now has items appearing on search pages and Google Alerts will show the latest tweets for your user name and where they have been syndicated.

As search engines strike further deals with social media application providers, information or status updates will be returned in search results outside the social

media application itself. This is available at the moment, albeit in a limited functionality, but trending news items on Digg, trending topics on Twitter and widely shared items on Facebook could soon appear in search results for your query along with ordinary search results. The exposure of real-time results will have quite far reaching effects on the way we interact. This advancement will bring more people into engaging with social media sites.

People who don't traditionally class themselves as social media consumers or users will be exposed to new forms of media information through searches. This will enable new consumers to interact with each other and engage with your brand. Over time, this new way of interaction will permeate more into the way we use search with search engine enhancements. Perhaps there will be the ability to refine search results by your social group, which may encourage more social types of searches.

As bandwidth available to homes and mobile devices increases, the way we use video will change. Real-time video chat channels will empower the information worker to work more dynamically. This increase means that more and more of us can work from home and have a good video connection for face to face meetings with our colleagues in the office. Free or low cost WiFi will become more widespread and accessible, enabling mobile workers to remain connected wherever they are. TV and video on demand will provide access across many channels to deliver a consistent experience across PCs and mobile devices. Streaming video will be delivered directly to movie theatres so that within 10 years we will be able to see a high quality streamed movie on the day that it is released worldwide.

Applications like Facebook, which provide users with the ability to chat over instant messaging in real time, will dominate more traditional static applications. Switching from instant messages to video within the application will become simple. Social media applications will strive to become your universal inbox. Filtering systems will become more commonplace in applications as users seek to categorise their many different networks of friends and connections.

THE MOBILE OPPORTUNITY

Mobile devices will become the hub of social media communications, and operate at all levels of our connected lives. There will be an abundance of location aware applications providing useful information to connect users face to face who happen to be in the same location.

Consumers will drive the next evolution of social media applications for mobile devices and many applications will disappear as new technologies (such as GPS location aware applications) evolve.

Mobile phone manufacturers are creating applications for the phone, but there's a problem. There are currently no set standards for application development across

mobile device platforms. If one user is using an iPhone and the other is using a Nokia, there are limited chances for interaction between the two devices. Applications which have been developed for different models of the Windows phone need to be modified to suit each different model. Users want technologies and applications for their mobile device but with the lack of cross-platform support in mobiles, it is difficult to get any cluster effects.

Without these cluster effects, the technology will not be widely adopted. Without wide adoption, there will be no impetus to develop new technologies. And with the huge amount of different devices that are available across different platforms, there are limited opportunities to move forward. So how do you get access to the same platform from all these different devices? The obvious solution is to develop your application to work on the browser. You would also need to make sure that all applications that have been written for the browser comply with international standards. This ensures that your application will work across all of the mobile device platforms and all of the different operating systems and hardware. Or you could buy an iPad...

In hardware terms, the Apple iPad will completely redefine the way we think about consumer devices and interaction on the web. Those that struggle with the form factor of the small smartphones or have chunky fingers will welcome this new device. Anyone who has problems interacting effectively with the tiny keypads will embrace this new form of communication. The iPad will drive greater consumer engagement, and social media will be the vehicle of communication. Augmented reality applications on the iPad will bring a new dimension to e-commerce.

Privacy will become more granular, as social media items become more discoverable. Profiles will be customisable for your different online personas. For example, you may want to customise different settings for your work persona compared with the settings for your home persona. Then there are the other roles you might have. You may be a school governor; you may sit on a committee or a council. You may perform charity work anonymously, or you may be a silent and invisible spectator. There will be new mechanisms in place on social platforms which will ensure that the setting you adopt to communicate with your friends will not cross boundaries into your corporate life.

Conversely, collaboration applications inside the firewall will evolve to incorporate social media connectors and features within the enterprise application.

The email client will become much more than just a place to receive email and view your calendar. Email will include threaded conversations, status updates from presence aware applications, video and instant messaging. Some of these features are already present in clients such as Outlook and Notes. You will be able to seamlessly switch between Facebook type applications and your inbox. Your Twitter stream and your RSS feeds will be accessed from one place. Your work life and your social life will blur. The application shift from your work life to your personal life will become more streamlined and transparent. Companies will adopt social software more readily as they realise that effective employee collaboration

in whatever format makes for more productive working environments. There will be a grass roots adoption of social media platforms inside the firewall as an aid to communication and effective interaction.

But most of all, social media, in whatever form, is here to stay. Do you want to join in the great conversation or do you want to watch it happening? Whatever your choice is, I hope you will benefit from the newsmakers, the influencers and the huge amount of knowledge from the rest of the crowd.

SUMMARY

- Search and mobility will drive the future of social media.
- Location aware applications will present a great business opportunity for the developer.
- Collaboration inside the company will be connected to social software applications to pool knowledge and extend connections.
- Social media is not going to go away. Companies must change their plans to incorporate the new way of communicating to avoid being left behind in the marketplace.

NOTES

1. http://en.wikipedia.org/wiki/The_Tipping_Point_(book)

2. http://en.wikipedia.org/wiki/IPhone

3. http://news.cnet.com/8301-1023_3-10312804-93.html?tag=nl.e703

4. www.well.com/

5. www.loundy.com/CASES/Playboy_v_Hardenburgh.html

6. www.ibiblio.org/pub/academic/communications/logs/

7. http://en.wikipedia.org/wiki/Wikipedia:Vandalism

8. www.timesonline.co.uk/tol/news/uk/article1401041.ece

9. www.wifeinthenorth.com/2007/02/blog-to-book-in-60-seconds.html

10. http://wikimediafoundation.org/wiki/AppealCH/uk?utm_source=
2009_Jimmy_Appeal1&utm_medium=sitenotice&utm_campaign=fundraiser
2009&target=Appeal2

11. http://en.wikipedia.org/wiki/Craigslist_controversies_and_illegal_activities_
by_users

12. http://en.wikipedia.org/wiki/Craigslist

13. http://snopes.com/photos/risque/kettle.asp

14. www.jennyhow.com/16-more-ebay-reflectoporn-pictures/

15. http://en.wikipedia.org/wiki/EBay_Haunted_Painting

16. www.dailymail.co.uk/sciencetech/article-1195651/How-Michael-Jacksons-
death-shut-Twitter-overwhelmed-Google-killed-Jeff-Goldblum.html

17. http://twitter.com/EthanZ/status/2333139296

18. www.danah.org/papers/TakenOutOfContext.pdf

19. http://shankman.com/be-careful-what-you-post/

20. www.thekeyinfluencer.com/channel/2009/01/16/twittersituation/

21. www.facebook.com/legal/copyright.php?noncopyright_notice=1

22. http://social-media-optimization.com/2006/09/air-force-says-no-to-myspace/

23. http://blogs.guardian.co.uk/businessinsight/archives/2005/09/01/branded.html
    and http://www.lawyersandsettlements.com/articles/00008/
    baby_formula.html

24. www.davecarrollmusic.com/ubg/song1/

25. http://en.community.dell.com/dell-blogs/b/direct2dell/archive/2009/06/11/
    delloutlet-surpasses-2-million-on-twitter.aspx

26. www.informationweek.com/news/hardware/desktop/showArticle.jhtml?
    articleID=217801030&subSection=E-Business

27. http://mashable.com/2009/08/04/espn-social-media/

28. www.ibm.com/blogs/zz/en/guidelines.html

29. www.intel.com/sites/sitewide/en_US/social-media.htm

30. www.bbc.co.uk/blogs/technology/2009/12/twitter_iran_and_uksnow.html

31. http://twitter.com/terms

32. www.facebook-log.com/intellectual-property.htm

33. www.copyright.gov/circs/circ34.pdf

34. http://consumerist.com/5150175/facebooks-new-terms-of-service-we-can-do-
    anything-we-want-with-your-content-forever

35. http://news.bbc.co.uk/2/hi/talking_point/1375175.stm

36. http://en.wikipedia.org/wiki/New_Coke

37. www.bevnet.com/news/2008/10-13-2008-pepsi_redesign.asp

38. http://gs.statcounter.com/#search_engine-US-daily-20090501-20091207

39. www.bing.com/community/blogs/search/archive/2009/07/01/bringing-a-bit-
    of-twitter-to-bing.aspx

1

40. http://disney.go.com/disneyinteractivestudios/product.html?platform=
wii&game=disneyepicmickey

41. http://en.wikipedia.org/wiki/Web_2.0

42. http://en.wikipedia.org/wiki/Six_degrees_of_separation

43. http://en.wikipedia.org/wiki/Small_world_experiment

44. http://news.bbc.co.uk/1/hi/england/oxfordshire/8458822.stm

45. www.businessinsider.com/2008/10/apple-s-steve-jobs-rushed-to-er-after-heart-
attack-says-cnn-citizen-journalist

46. www.youtube.com/watch?v=7FRwCs99DWg

47. www.youtube.com/symphony

48. http://elastictime.wordpress.com/2009/01/20/i-found-my-horn-on-youtube,
http://smithivanson.wordpress.com/2009/04/02/a-huge-virtual-team

49. www.youtube.com/watch?v=9QFvfHXkd2o

50. http://blogs.nasa.gov/cm/blog/NASA-CIO-Blog/posts/post_1244861198431.html

51. www.telegraph.co.uk/technology/facebook/6954696/Facebook-bra-colour-
status-update-craze-raising-breast-cancer-awareness.html

52. www.telegraph.co.uk/technology/facebook/6953689/Urgent-Facebook-blood-
appeal-saves-British-students-life-after-Mexico-fall.html

53. www.insidesocialgames.com/2009/12/22/zynga-world-food-programme-team-
up-to-fight-hunger/

54. http://forrester.typepad.com/groundswell/2010/01/conversationalists-get-onto-
the-ladder.html

INDEX